HUMAN ONCOGENIC VIRUSES

HUMAN ONCOGENIC VIRUSES

Editors

Jing-Hsiung James Ou
University of Southern California, USA

T. S. Benedict Yen
University of California, San Francisco, USA

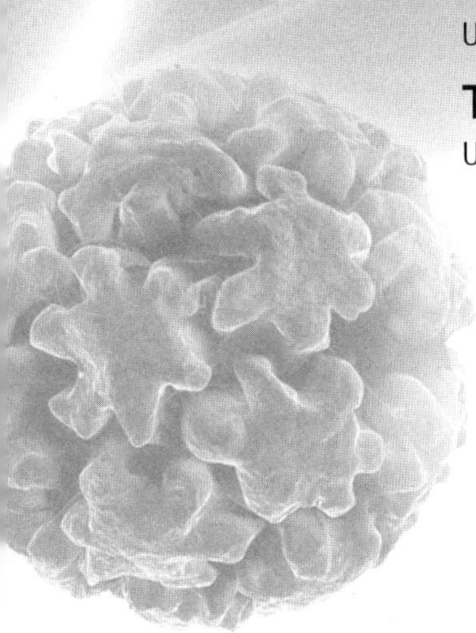

World Scientific

NEW JERSEY • LONDON • SINGAPORE • BEIJING • SHANGHAI • HONG KONG • TAIPEI • CHENNAI

Published by

World Scientific Publishing Co. Pte. Ltd.
5 Toh Tuck Link, Singapore 596224
USA office: 27 Warren Street, Suite 401-402, Hackensack, NJ 07601
UK office: 57 Shelton Street, Covent Garden, London WC2H 9HE

British Library Cataloguing-in-Publication Data
A catalogue record for this book is available from the British Library.

HUMAN ONCOGENIC VIRUSES

ISBN-13 978-981-283-346-4
ISBN-10 981-283-346-3

Typeset by Stallion Press
Email: enquiries@stallionpress.com

Printed by FuIsland Offset Printing (S) Pte Ltd, Singapore

Foreword

Viruses cause more than a fourth of all human cancers. Virus-induced cancers, like all viral diseases, present special challenges and raise specific hopes. The challenges are in understanding the molecular mechanism of the disease, knowing the mode of virus transmission, and obtaining global epidemiological data. The hope is for the development of effective vaccines, antiviral therapies and, ultimately, for the control and eradication of the pathogenic virus.

This book presents a comprehensive survey of human cancer viruses. They include five viral families, the papillomaviruses, herpesviruses, hepadnaviruses, flaviviruses and retroviruses. For most of these cancer viruses, there is a good understanding of transmission, and epidemiological data are extensive. Indeed, epidemiological data have traditionally been essential for establishing the oncogenicity of a virus in humans. The viruses considered here have widely differing impacts on public health. The hepatitis viruses cause acute and chronic infections with significant morbidity and affect millions of people. Infection with oncogenic papillomaviruses is similarly widespread. Papilloma and hepatitis viruses have therefore been the focus of vaccine efforts. These efforts have succeeded for hepatitis B virus and for papillomaviruses; they are still in progress for hepatitis C virus. Kaposi sarcoma herpes virus and human T cell leukemia virus affect much smaller groups of people that are well defined by risk factors and geography.

Our understanding of the molecular mechanisms of viral carcinogenesis in humans shows notable gaps. For some viruses, like the oncogenic papilloma and herpesviruses and for human T cell leukemia virus, specific proteins have been identified that interact with the growth-regulatory machinery of the cell and that play key roles in the oncogenic transformation process. For other viruses, like hepatitis B and hepatitis C viruses, such relationships between viral gene products and cellular regulation are less definitive. The molecular as well as epidemiological insights into human cancer viruses can be summarized in a single conclusion: These viruses are essential, causative components of the oncogenic process, yet they do not act alone. They are necessary, but not sufficient. Other factors play important roles, and many remain to be defined.

Human cancer virology is now a mature field of science, and most of the groundbreaking discoveries have been made. This state of cancer virology invites historical reflection. The initial events that linked viruses to cancer were the discoveries of Ellermann and Bang and of Rous. It took several decades before this basic link was extended to human medicine. The association of the Epstein Barr herpes virus with Burkitt lymphoma and with nasopharyngeal carcinoma was an early signal. Shortly thereafter, hepatitis B virus, human T cell leukemia virus and carcinogenic human papillomaviruses all appeared on the scene. Kaposi sarcoma herpes virus and hepatitis C virus joined the ranks of human tumor viruses later. True discoveries are always unexpected and surprising; each of the critical events that shaped human tumor virology has these attributes. Ingenuity, hard work, instinct, perseverance and serendipity all played a role. The list of groundbreaking discoveries, all under the intellectual ancestry of Ellermann and Bang and of Rous, is short: Epstein and Barr and the Epstein-Barr herpes virus; Beasley and the connection between hepatocellular carcinoma and hepatitis B virus; zur Hausen and the causation of cervical cancer by papillomaviruses; Yoshida and Gallo and human T cell leukemia virus; and Chang and Moore and Kaposi sarcoma herpes virus. The connection between hepatitis C virus and hepatocellular carcinoma emerged more gradually from clinical and epidemiological observations, and credit for this insight is more widely distributed. Most of these openings were achieved by young scientists. Chang and Moore discovered Kaposi sarcoma herpes virus when they were in their middle thirties. Zur Hausen, Beasley,

Epstein and Barr, Yoshida and Gallo were still in their forties when they achieved their breakthroughs. And not all of these discoveries came from established virology labs. Chang and Moore worked outside the virology mainstream and did not even have grant support when they made their spectacular discovery. Beasley's perspective appropriately focused on public health and epidemiology; a molecular approach toward hepatitis B virus and cancer would not have been successful at the time. The igniting spark for the discovery of human T cell leukemia virus came from epidemiological studies that had revealed a unique, geographically confined T cell leukemia in southern Japan.

Government support for medical research has sharply tightened over the past few years. In the US, the structure of funding and the allocation of resources have changed significantly. There has been a shift away from investigator-initiated projects that have been the source of most innovations and breakthroughs. The emphasis is now on larger conglomerate structures. With this collectivization of research funds has come extreme risk avoidance and support of the predictable and the mundane. Few of the research projects that have led to paradigm shifts in cancer virology would be fundable today. The consequences of these developments have been especially severe for young investigators. There is deep concern in the scientific community that much young talent is turned away and lost to science. However, there are now also some encouraging signs that the mechanism for public support of research has become flexible again. Scientists have a great stake in the restoration of individual initiative, prudent risk taking and the spirit of discovery in science funding, and there is hope that this will be possible.

Reading this book and reflecting on the history and the challenges of the cancer virus field will inspire the insight, wisdom and excitement that are needed to advance science.

Peter V. Vogt, PhD
The Scripps Research Institute
La Jolla, California
March 24, 2009

Preface

A relationship between viruses and neoplasia has been suspected ever since the turn of the 20th century, when Ellerman and Bang, followed by Rous, showed that cell-free extracts of a chicken leukemia and sarcoma, respectively, induced the same disease upon inoculation into healthy chickens (Chapter 1). These observations eventually led to the unequivocal demonstration that several viruses of different families can cause malignancies in animals. The hunt was thus on, to search for similar viruses that may cause human cancers. Initially, the biomedical community was disappointed by the lack of positive results, until Epstein, Achong, and Barr demonstrated that Burkitt's lymphoma cells cultured *in vitro* contained a herpesvirus, subsequently named the Epstein-Barr virus. However, the ubiquity of this virus meant that the possibility of its merely being a "passenger" in the lymphoma cells could not be ruled out. The situation changed dramatically with the seminal epidemiological work of Beasley and colleagues, showing that hepatitis B virus infection in men was associated with a dramatic increase in risk of primary liver cancer in Taiwan; this association has since been proven to be causal (Chapter 2). More recently, hepatitis C virus, an entirely unrelated virus, has also been shown to cause liver cancer (Chapter 3). Similarly, the Nobel Prize-winning work of zur Hausen and colleagues revealed that certain types of human papillomaviruses cause cancers of the uterine cervix and other epithelial tissues, such as the oropharynx (Chapter 4). Indeed, the National Institute of Environmental Health and Safety (http://ntp.niehs.nih.gov/ntp/roc/toc11.html) lists these viruses as known human carcinogens. Human oncogenic viruses

Contents

Chapter 1

Oncogenic Viruses, Cellular Transformation and Human Cancers

Yanyan Zheng* and Jing-hsiung James Ou*

Abstract: It has been a century since the initial discovery of the possible link between viruses and tumors. During the past century, extensive studies have been conducted to understand the relationship between viruses and cancers. The early studies were focused on tumor viruses that do not cause cancers in their natural hosts. These studies provided the basis for the subsequent studies on the six known human oncogenic viruses. These human oncogenic viruses, which include hepatitis B virus, hepatitis C virus, human papillomavirus, Epstein-Barr virus, Kaposi's sarcoma-associated herpesvirus, and human T-cell leukemia virus 1 are associated with nearly 20% of the human cancer cases. In this chapter, we review the historical aspects of oncogenic virus research, human oncogenic viruses, and the molecular mechanisms of cellular transformation by viruses.

1. Introduction and Historical Aspects

Cancer develops from a succession of genetic changes, which cumulatively provide growth advantage for the cancerous cells. Despite the heterogeneity of human cancers in cellular origin, etiology and pathogenesis, they more or less share the same characteristics defined by Hanahan and Weinberg (Hanahan & Weinberg, 2000): self-sufficiency

*Department of Molecular Microbiology and Immunology, University of Southern California, Keck School of Medicine, Los Angeles, California.

in growth stimulation, insensitivity to antigrowth signals, evasion of apoptosis, infinite lifespan, sustained angiogenesis, tissue invasion and metastasis ability, and genetic instability (Hanahan & Weinberg, 2000). These cellular changes may be inherited genetically or acquired as a combinational aftermath of environmental mutagens and infectious agents such as viruses.

The initial observation that viruses may cause cancer was made in 1908 when Vilhelm Ellerman and Oluf Bang found that cell-free filtrates could transfer leukemia from one chicken to another (Ellerman & Bang, 1908). This observation was reinforced in 1911 when Peyton Rous demonstrated that healthy chickens injected with cell-free sarcoma filtrates, in which only viruses could be present, developed sarcoma (Peyton, 1911). It is now clear that the causative infectious agent in chicken leukemia and Rous sarcoma are both retroviruses, with the former named avian leukosis virus and the latter named Rous sarcoma virus. That viruses can induce tumors were reaffirmed in the 1950s and 1960s, when three additional DNA viruses, simian vacuolating virus 40 (SV40), mouse polyomavirus and adenovirus, were found to cause tumors in newborn rodents (Girardi *et al.*, 1962; Stewart *et al.*, 1958; Trentin *et al.*, 1962). These three different viruses, however, did not cause tumors in their natural hosts.

The early research on retroviruses and DNA tumor viruses, which include the aforementioned SV40, mouse polyomavirus and adenovirus, has generated much valuable information for understanding viral tumorigenesis and cancer biology. The discovery of transducing retroviruses, which carry an oncogene (*v-onc*) in their genome, led to the discovery of cellular homologues (*c-onc*) of these viral oncogenes (Stehelin *et al.*, 1976). Retroviruses are now known to induce tumors through three different mechanisms. The first mechanism involves transducing retroviruses. These viruses induce tumors at a high frequency and requires a short latency period. The second mechanism involves *cis*-acting retroviruses. These *cis*-acting retroviruses do not carry a cellular oncogene. However, they can activate cellular oncogenes through the insertion of the provirus into the cellular chromosomes (Hayward *et al.*, 1981). This mechanism induces tumors at an intermediate frequency and requires a longer latency period. The third mechanism involves *trans*-acting retroviruses. These viruses encode regulatory proteins to affect cell growth and death. These viruses induce tumors at a low frequency and often require a long latency period.

The research on DNA tumor viruses also led to a better understanding of viral oncogenesis and facilitated the later research on human oncogenic viruses. SV40 and mouse polyomavirus, which both belong to the *polyomaviridae* family, encode early gene products that are capable of causing tumors. These gene products were thus termed tumor (T) antigens. The large T antigen of SV40 and mouse polyomavirus is a multifunctional protein that can immortalize primary cells, bind to the tumor suppressor p53 to different degrees and to the retinoblastoma protein RB, and activate gene expressions to promote cell cycle progression (Conzen & Cole, 1995; Imperiale & Major, 2006). The mouse polyomavirus middle T-antigen, which is absent in SV40, possesses additional activities (Ichaso & Dilworth, 2001). This middle T-antigen can bind to and constitutively activate *c-src*, an important tyrosine kinase that activate cellular signaling pathways, and can also serve as a substrate of *c-src* to activate phosphotyrosine-binding proteins such as phosphoinositol-3-kinase and phospholipase C-γ (Dilworth, 2002). SV40 and mouse polyomavirus also produce a small t-antigen that can enhance the transformation activity of the virus (Khalili *et al.*, 2008). Similarly, the research on adenovirus led to the finding that its E1A and E1B proteins have oncogenic potential. These two proteins can bind to RB and p53, respectively. Of particular interest is the highly oncogenic Ad12 adenovirus strain. The E1A protein of this particular adenovirus strain can suppress the expression of the major histocompatibility (MHC) class I antigen and inhibit the cytotoxic T lymphocyte (CTL) response (Schrier *et al.*, 1983; Vasavada *et al.*, 1986). This indicates that the modulation of the immune system is also important for viral oncogenesis.

Despite the research progresses on animal tumor viruses, conclusive evidence on a similar viral etiology in human malignancies was not available until 1964, when Epstein-Barr virus (EBV) was identified in B-cell lines derived from Burkitt's lymphoma samples sarcoma samples using representational differential analysis (Chang *et al.*, 1994). The KSHV genome is a double-stranded DNA with a size of about 160 Kb that contains over 80 protein coding sequences. Similar to other herpesviruses, KSHV can cause either lytic infection or latent infection. During latency, the viral genome replicates as a closed circular episome in the nucleus; only a subset of viral genes are expressed and no progeny viral particles are produced. During lytic infection, the viral genome is linearized, nearly the entire genome is expressed, and progeny virions are produced and released upon the death of the host cell. The virus-encoded replication and transcription activator (RTA) protein plays an important role in inducing lytic replication from latency (Sun *et al.*, 1998).

The transmission route of KSHV is largely unknown. Sexual and other parenteral transmission pathways have been suggested. KHSV infection is not as the common as the other herpesviral infections. Epidemiological studies have shown great geographic variations of the KSHV prevalence rate. Low level infections (0–20%) occur in North America and northern Europe, intermediate level infections (10–25%) are observed in Mediterranean countries; and high seropositivity rates (>30%) are detected in Africa (Jarrett, 2001). Most KSHV infections are asymptomatic. However, co-infection by human immunodeficiency virus-1 can greatly increase the risk for Kaposi's sarcoma (KS), which is the leading cause of AIDS-associated morbidity and mortality (Ganem, 2006).

KS is a multifocal angioproliferative disorder that often presents as a cutaneous lesion. It is estimated that greater than 95% of Kaposi' sarcoma lesions are positive for KSHV DNA, indicating an association between Kaposi's sarcoma and KSHV infection. Besides Kaposi's sarcoma, primary effusion lymphoma (PEL) and multicentric Castleman's diseases (MCD), which are two types of B-cell lymphomas, are also associated with KSHV infection (Sullivan *et al.*, 2006). KSHV DNA is present in all PEL lesions, which may contain EBV as well. Nearly 100% of AIDS-associated MCD and 50% of non-AIDS-associated MCD are positive for KSHV DNA (Damania, 2007).

2.6. Human T-cell Leukemia Virus-1 (HTLV-1)

HTLV-1 was first discovered in 1980 from patients suffering from a disease at that time thought to be mycosis fungoides, a cutaneous T-cell lymphoma (Poiesz *et al.*, 1980). It is the only human oncogenic retrovirus known at present.

HTLV-1 is a member of the *deltaretrovirus* genus of the *Retroviridae* family and is closely related to HTLV-II, bovine leukemia virus and simian T-cell leukemia virus. The single-stranded RNA genome of HTLV-1 is composed of about 9000 nucleotides and contains several genes, including *env*, *gag*, *pol* and *tax* as well as two long terminal repeats (LTRs). HTLV-1 does not harbor any oncogenes derived from the host cells and thus is not a transducing retrovirus.

HTLV-1 infection is endemic in southern Japan, West Africa, the Caribbean Islands and South America, but rare in North America and Europe. About 10 to 20 million people worldwide have been infected by HTLV-1 (Pagano *et al.*, 2004). HTLV-1 is transmitted either directly from mother to infant, or through sexual contact and other parenteral routes. The ubiquitously expressed glucose transporter 1 protein (GLUT1) and heparin proteoglycans have been suggested to be the viral receptors (Manel *et al.*, 2003; Okuma *et al.*, 2003). Interestingly, this virus cannot be transmitted as free virions and it appears that cell-to-cell contact is required for HTLV-1 transmission.

HTLV-1 infection is causally associated with adult T-cell leukemia (ATL), a human malignancy with poor prognosis. Integrated proviral DNA are found in the majority of ATL and seropositivity is high among ATL patients. It has been estimated that the cumulative lifetime risk of ATL among HTLV-1 carriers is about 1–4.5% (Levine *et al.*, 1998).

3. Mechanisms of Virus-induced Cellular Transformation

The oncogenic mechanisms used by different viruses differ significantly. We will summarize some of the common mechanisms in this section and the more detailed descriptions of the mechanisms

CXCR1 and CXCR2, the cellular receptor for IL-8. However, it is constitutively active. Downstream cellular events activated by vGPCR include all three MAP kinase pathways (ERK, JNK and p38MAPK), the PI3K pathway, the NF-κB pathway as well as the JAK/STAT pathway (Sullivan *et al.*, 2006). vGPCR contributes to the pathogenesis of KS, PEL and MCD through its pro-angiogenesis and cytokine-inducing activities.

3.1.3. *Mimicking the intracellular signaling adaptors*

Several gamma herpesviruses, including KSHV, encode a viral FLICE inhibitory protein (vFLIP). vFLIP is another protein expressed in latently KSHV-infected KS and PEL cells (Sun *et al.*, 2003b). The primary function of vFLIP is to protect cells from both intrinsic and extrinsic apoptotic pathways. As its name suggests, the virus-encoded vFLIPs mimic the function of cellular FLIP (Ganem, 2006). vFLIP interacts with the IKK-γ (NEMO) complex and activates the anti-apoptotic NF-κB pathway. The NF-κB activation by vFLIP may also be mapped to even earlier signaling events such as binding to TARF2 and RIP (Ganem, 2006; Nicholas, 2007). This activation of NF-κB by vFLIP is important for the survival of leukemia cells after serum withdrawal (Sun *et al.*, 2003a) and it is the primary anti-apoptotic signal in latently infected PEL cells (Keller *et al.*, 2000).

3.1.4. *Activation of cell surface receptors*

The HPV E5 protein is a small membrane protein that can induce the dimerization and activation of growth factor receptors, including epidermal growth factor receptor (EGFR), platelet-derived growth factor receptor, and colony-stimulating factor-1 receptor. Overexpression of HPV E5 can result in elevated phosphorylation and decreased endosomal degradation of EGFR (Longworth & Laimins, 2004), possibly through inhibition of the vacuolar proton-ATPase on the endosomal membrane (Straight *et al.*, 1995). The HPV E5 protein moderately transforms rodent fibroblasts *in vitro* (Bedell *et al.*, 1989).

3.2. Deregulation of the Cell Cycle

With a few exceptions, somatic cells may enter terminally differentiated post-mitotic state by losing their proliferation ability permanently or may be quiescent and proliferate only upon stimulation by mitogenic signals. The cell cycle is divided into four phases named G1, S, G2 and M. Most of the extracellular signals induce cell proliferation by promoting the G1 to S phase transition. Once the cell enters the S phase, the cell cycle will proceed in an autonomous way, independent of extracellular signals. The critical step before the G1/S transition is referred to as the restriction point or R point.

The cell cycle is regulated by multiple protein complexes, each with a catalytic Ser/Thr protein kinase CDK and a regulatory unit of cyclin. Both the kinase activity and the substrate specificity of CDKs are determined by the cyclins associated with them. For example, CDK4 and CDK6 can bind to one of the three Gl cyclins, D1, D2 and D3 to form a functional complex for the progression of the cell cycle during the early-mid Gl phase. The cyclin E/CDK2 complex, in contrast, is critical for the cell to pass the R point. Similarly, cyclin A/CDC2 and cyclin B/CDC2 are important for the S phase and the G2/M phase, respectively. Consistent with the notion that cell cycle is regulated by extrinsic stimuli only during the Gl phase, the Gl cyclins accumulate in response to the extracellular mitogenic signals, leading to the activation of CDK4/6. The kinase activities of CDKs are also subject to negative regulation by inhibitors, which form a ternary complex with CDKs. $p16^{Ink4A}$, $p15^{Ink4B}$, $p18^{Ink4C}$, and $p19^{Ink4D}$ are the inhibitors specific for CDK4 and CDK6, whilst $p27^{Kip}$ and $p21^{Cip}$ are for all CDKs.

The activation of CDK4/6 can promote the cell cycle through the Gl phase just before the R point. For the cell cycle to progress further, it will need to remove the cell cycle blocks imposed by members of the RB protein family, which includes the closely related proteins RB, p107 and p130. RB is a tumor suppressor and is mutated in retinoblastoma, a tumor of the eye. In normal cells, RB is mainly regulated via phosphorylation by CDKs such as cyclinD-CDK4/6 and cyclinE-CDK2. Hypophosphorylated RB binds to E2F transcription factors

(E2F1 to E2F6) and inhibits their transcriptional regulatory activity. However, hyperphosphorylation of RB at the R point dissociates E2F from RB, leading to the functional activation of E2F.

RB is the molecular target of the large T antigen of SV40 and mouse polyomavirus and the E1A protein of adenovirus. For these DNA tumor viruses, their DNA replication requires enzymes and substrates that are produced in the S phase. Therefore, it is critical for these viruses to induce entry of their host cells into the S phase of the cell cycle. Human oncogenic viruses have also developed multiple levels of regulation to promote cell cycle progression and cell proliferation.

3.2.1. *Abrogation of the RB function*

The HPV E7 protein can bind to RB. This protein contains three conserved regions, termed CR1, CR2 and CR3. The LXCXE motif within the CR2 region mediates the interaction with RB and displaces E2F from the Rb/E2F complex to cause deregulation of the cell cycle. Although E7 from both high risk and low risk groups of HPV bind to RB, the affinity of the high-risk HPV E7 for RB can be 10-fold stronger than that of the low-risk HPV E7. Furthermore, the high-risk HPV E7 enhances the degradation of RB by proteasomes via a second low-affinity RB binding motif present in its C-terminus. Studies show that the loss of RB in stratified squamous epithelia in a mouse model is well correlated with the expression of E7 (Balsitis *et al.*, 2003).

3.2.2. *Enhancement of CDK activities*

The cell cycle is negatively regulated by CDK inhibitors. Therefore, several viruses have developed strategies to counteract these inhibitors. HPV E7 is reported to be able to bind to $p21^{Cip}$ and $p27^{Kip}$ (Funk *et al.*, 1997). Importantly, the interaction between E7 and p21 suppresses the $p21^{Cip}$ activity. This interaction with CDK inhibitors may serve as a failsafe mechanism to ensure the complete inactivation of RB to allow entry of the cell into the S phase.

A similar activity is also exhibited by the HTLV-1 *tax* protein, which physically interacts with p16^{Ink4A}/p15^{Ink4B} to suppress their CDK inhibitor activities (Matsuoka & Jeang, 2007). In addition, as a transcription factor, *tax* also suppresses the expression of p18^{Ink4C}, p19^{Ink4D} and p21^{Cip} genes.

3.2.3. *Targeting of cyclin*

The kinase activities of CDKs drive the progression of the cell cycle. However, the activation of CDKs requires cyclins. Viruses may target cyclins by transcriptional regulation, post-transcriptional modification or by expression of a viral version of cyclin.

Elevated expression of the G1-phase cyclin D2 is seen in HTLV-1 transformed cell. Further studies indicate that the HTLV-1 *tax* protein can transcriptionally activate the promoter of the cyclin D2 (*CCND2*) gene. In contrast, KSHV encodes a viral version of cyclin (*v-cyclin*) during both the latent infection and the lytic replication. The sequence of *v-cyclin* has 58% sequence homology with human cellular cyclin D2, and this protein binds predominantly to CDK6. Similar to its cellular counterpart, *v-cyclin*/CDK6 complex functions at the G1/S transition to promote entry into the S phase. However, this complex has a broader substrate range and is more resistant to the negative regulation by CDK inhibitors including p16^{Ink4a}, p21^{Cip} and p27^{Kip}. The resistance to p27^{Kip} is due to either the phosphorylation-coupled proteasomal degradation or enhanced cytoplasmic localization of p27^{Kip} (Jarviluoma *et al.*, 2004; Sarek *et al.*, 2006). The contribution of *v-cyclin* to cellular transformation seems to be context dependent. The expression of *v-cyclin* in mouse embryonic fibroblasts (MEFs) leads to multinucleation and polyploidy, and triggers apoptosis in the presence of p53. However, in the absence of p53, *v-cyclin* transgenic mice developed lymphomas (Verschuren *et al.*, 2002).

3.3. Escape of Apoptosis

Tissue homeostasis is a balance between cell proliferation and cell attrition. Metazoan organisms actively minimize the number of malfunctioning cells from their tissues through an important process known as apoptosis. Although uncoordinated growth is a key characteristic of cancer, numerous studies have indicated that proliferation alone is not sufficient to cause cancer. For example, deregulation of the cell cycle may allow cells to proliferate rapidly. However, unless other survival signals exist, these cells, by default, will be eliminated by apoptosis. Therefore, overriding the barrier created by such a failsafe mechanism is required for cellular transformation.

Apoptosis, also called programmed cell death, is executed through a process that involves sensors and effectors. Apoptosis can be provoked by extracellular and intracellular signals. Examples of extracellular death signals include those carried by TNF-α and Fas ligand, which are captured by their corresponding receptors on the cell surface. A wide range of stresses, such as DNA damage and hypoxia, can induce cell death from inside the cells. Regardless of the origin of the death signals, apoptotic pathway converges at the mitochondria, where the Bcl-2 family proteins, either pro-apoptotic or anti-apoptotic, coordinate with one another to decide on the release of cytochrome c from the mitochondria. This release of cytochrome c will activate an array of caspases, including caspases 8 and 9, which elicit the caspase-cleavage cascade to pass death signals to the downstream effector (executioner) caspases, which will target different cellular components such as chromatin, cellular membrane, cytoskeleton, etc. to cause their disintegration.

The infection by human oncogenic viruses imposes significant amount of stress to cells. To avoid premature cell death, these viruses use different ways to counteract apoptosis. These countermeasures play important roles in the eventual transformation of the infected cells.

3.3.1. *Inactivation of the "gatekeeper" p53*

p53 was discovered as a tumor suppressor in late 1970s during the studies on cellular transformation mediated by the SV40 T-antigen (Lane & Crawford, 1979; Linzer & Levine, 1979). Mutation of its gene exists in more than 50% of all human cancers (Hanahan & Weinberg, 2000). In human cancers without p53 mutations, the activity of p53 is frequently lost due to various indirect mechanisms. Up to date, more than 150 p53 target genes have been identified, most of which are implicated in cell-cycle arrest, senescence, DNA repair and apoptosis (Bode & Dong, 2004). Due to its important role in preventing oncogenesis, p53 is referred to as "gatekeeper" or "guardian" for cells.

Most of the p53 functions rely on its transcriptional regulatory activities. Tetrameric p53 binds to p53-specific DNA sequence present in the promoter regions of its target genes and functions either as a transcriptional activator or repressor. The steady state level of p53 within normal unstressed cells is very low due to its short half-life. The degradation of p53 is mediated through its ubiquitination by the ubiquitin E3-ligase MDM2, followed by degradation by the 26S proteasome. Upon sensing stress signals, p53 is stabilized by its dissociation from MDM2 and it activates the expression of proapoptotic genes such as Bax, which in turn triggers the release of cytochrome c and the activation of the caspase cascade. More recently, activated p53 has been shown to be able to translocate to mitochondria, where it directly interacts through its DNA binding domain with anti-apoptotic proteins, such as Bcl-2 and Bcl-XL, to induce apoptosis (Mihara *et al.*, 2003).

HPV E6 is a small protein with approximately 150 amino acids. Two zinc finger domains with four C-X-X-C motifs mediate most of the interactions of E6 with its cellular target proteins. E6 binds to p53 and a cellular ubiquitin E3-ligase, the E6-associating protein (E6-AP), to promote ubiquitination and the proteasomal degradation of p53 (Scheffner *et al.*, 1990). The activities of p53 can also be regulated by acetylation at its C-terminal lysine residues by coactivators such as p300/CBP and PCAF. HPV E6 can also be recruited to the promoter region of the $p21^{Cip}$ gene, where it will interact with both p53 and p300 to inhibit p300-mediated acetylation of p53 (Thomas & Chiang, 2005). This will suppress p53-dependent transcription. Moreover, HPV E6 may further suppress the normal functions of p53 through inhibition of p53 DNA-binding activity or by sequestering p53 in the cytoplasmic compartment (Wise-Draper & Wells, 2008).

3.3.2. *Expression of viral version of Bcl-2 (vBcl-2)*

The Bcl-2 protein family includes more than 20 closely related proteins. Each of these proteins contains up to four domains termed Bcl-2-homologous regions (BH) arranged in the order BH4-BH3-BH1-BH2. An additional transmembrane domain (TM) at the C-terminus mediates the membrane association. Depending on their structural organization and functions, these proteins can be grouped as pro-apoptotic, anti-apoptotic or BH3-only. The pro-apoptotic members BAX and BAK multimerize at the surface of mitochondria to form a channel to allow the release of cytochrome c and other pro-apoptotic factors. The anti-apoptotic members, such as Bcl-2, are thought to sequester the BH3 only members from interaction with the pro-apoptotic members and thus prevent the activation of these pro-apoptotic proteins. A virus encoded Bcl-2 homolog has been identified in all of the members of the gammaherpesvirus, including the human oncogenic viruses EBV and KSHV (D'Agostino *et al.*, 2005).

BHRF1, the Bcl-2 homolog encoded by EBV, is expressed during the early stage of the lytic replication cycle. It can protect cells from a broad array of extrinsic and intrinsic apoptotic stimuli, such as death factor signaling, DNA damaging factors including drugs and radiation, deprivation of growth signals, or the over-expression of BIK or BOK (Cuconati & White, 2002; D'Agostino *et al.*, 2005). Similarly, KSHV ORF-16 also encodes a viral homolog of Bcl-2. This homolog has about 15–20% sequence homology with its cellular counterpart (D'Agostino *et al.*, 2005).

Yeast two-hybrid screening has identified several cellular proteins that interact with vBcl-2. BHRF1 possibly interacts with the pro-apoptotic Bcl-2 members such as BAK, BAX, BIK, and BOK. KSHV vBcl-2 can bind to Bcl-2 (D'Agostino *et al.*, 2005). However, whether viral Bcl-2 functions through heterodimerizaion with other Bcl-2 members is still being debated.

Caspase-3 cleavage of anti-apoptotic Bcl-2 family members, such as Bcl-2 and Bcl-X_L, in their loop domain near the N-terminus converts them into potent pro-apoptotic factors upon receiving the right death signals. In contrast, such a negative regulation mechanism seems to be absent for the viral Bcl-2. They are either resistant to protease cleavage or their C-terminus cleavage products are not pro-apoptotic (Hardwick & Bellows, 2003).

3.4. Immortalization of Cells

Normal mammalian cells have limited propagation potentials, averaging about 60–70 cell divisions (Hanahan & Weinberg, 2000). Once their division numbers reach the "Hayflick limit," cells will become senescent. Loss of tumor suppressor genes such as p53 or RB may endow cells with additional replicative abilities. However, these cells will eventually enter a "crisis" state, featured by massive apoptotic cell deaths and end-to-end joining of chromosomes. The only exceptions are stem cells, which can self-renew infinitely.

This limited ability of cells to propagate is due to an autonomous cell generation counting device called telomere, which is an array of thousands of copies of a hexanucleotide repeat at the ends of chromosomes. This telomere will be shortened by 50–100 base pairs after each cell division. Telomerase, a ribonucleoprotein composed of an RNA component TERC (telomerase RNA component) and a protein component TERT (telomerase reverse transcriptase), can replenish the telomere repeats at the ends of chromosomes. The expression level of TERT is extremely low in somatic cells and high in stem cells, which explains the different replication potentials between these two types of cells. In contrast to most somatic cells, telomerase reactivation is frequently seen in malignantly transformed cells. Alternatively, telomere may also be maintained by a recombination-based mechanism called ALT (alternative lengthening of telomere). By these mechanisms, cancer cells obtain infinite multiplication potentials similar to that of stem cells.

Several human oncogenic viruses target the hTERT to immortalize their infected cells. Since the transcription rate of the hTERT gene is very low in normal somatic cells, most of the reactivation seen in virus infected cells is achieved by transcriptional activation. The hTERT core promoter region contains E and GC boxes, which can be bound by transcription factors such as myc, Sp1 and USF. Expression of HPV16 E6 in the early passages of human cell cultures leads to an elevated hTERT activity due to the activation of hTERT transcription (Katzenellenbogen *et al.*, 2007; Liu *et al.*, 2005; Veldman *et al.*, 2003). Several distinct mechanisms have been proposed for the E6-mediated hTERT reactivation. Interaction between myc and E6/E6AP will bring the latter to the promoter region and activate the myc-mediated transcription activation of hTERT (Veldman *et al.*, 2003). Alternatively, the E6/E6AP complex may remove the suppressive effect of NTX1, a transcriptional repressor for the hTERT promoter, by ubiquitination and destabilization of NFX1 (Gewin *et al.*, 2004). The functional interaction between E6/E6AP and p300/CBP increases histone acetylation at the hTERT promoter. Such an epigenetic modification can also activate hTERT transcription (James *et al.*, 2006). In a similar way, the LANA oncoprotein encoded by KSHV has also been reported to upregulate the gene transcription of hTERT through its interaction with the ubiquitous transcription factor Sp1 (Verma *et al.*, 2004).

3.5. Induction of Genetic Instability

One of the important hallmarks of cancer cells is their intrinsic genetic instability at either the gene level or the chromosome level. The former results in gene mutations and the latter leads to microsatellite instability (MIN) or chromosomal instability (CIN).

It is well accepted that tumorigenesis is a multi-step event, which requires the accumulation of multiple genetic/epigenetic alterations in the genome throughout the progression of tumors. However, although somatic cells are constantly exposed to mutagens from both outside and inside, they have evolved a wide array of ways to protect the genomic integrity. For instance, high-fidelity DNA polymerases ensure a low error rate during DNA replication. In additions, cells employ multiple mechanisms to monitor DNA damages and to restore the damaged genetic information using a variety of DNA repair systems. DNA alkyltransferase reverses base modifications. Base-excision repair (BER) and nucleotide-excision repair (NER) take care of DNA lesions originated from endogenous and exogenous sources, respectively. In addition, cells may undergo error-prone DNA repair when massive DNA damages occur. The mitotic check-point during cell cycle further scrutinizes any abnormality of chromosomal segregation during mitosis. The fact that tumors nonetheless occur argues that the genome of cancer cells are highly mutable (Hanahan & Weinberg, 2000; Weiberg, 2007). This elevated mutability provides the tumor-initiating cell a much greater chance to gather enough mutations to reach the stage of malignant transformation.

HCV infection causes a "mutator" phenotype in which higher mutation frequency are observed in multiple cellular genes in HCV-infected B cell lines, peripheral mononuclear cells and HCC tumor tissues (Machida *et al.,* 2004b). Consistent with this phenotype, higher activity of B-cell somatic mutation machinery and error-prone DNA polymerase, as well as increased amount of double strand DNA breaks (DSB) are observed in these samples (Machida *et al.,* 2004b). Further analysis reveals that the expression of HCV core and NS3 proteins leads to elevated level of reactive oxygen species (ROS), which contributes to the formation of DSB (Machida *et al.,* 2006; Machida *et al.,* 2004a). In addition, the binding of HCV E2 envelope protein to the viral receptor CD81 in B-cell lines induces the activation-induced cytidine deaminase (AID) and causes hypermutations in the immunoglobulin gene (Machida *et al.,* 2005). These findings highlight an important role of virus-induced genomic instability in tumorigenesis.

Expression of E6 and E7 protein in HPV infected cells are usually characterized by the loss of p53 and Rb and the deregulated cell cycle control, which in turn leads to the genomic instability of the host cell. High risk HPV E6-expressing cells usually show nuclear abnormality as a result of blockage of cytokinesis due to the loss of p53 (Duensing & Munger, 2003a). Expression of high risk E7 protein can also induce abnormal centrosome synthesis, which subsequently leads to numerical chromosomal instability (Duensing *et al.,* 2001). This activity of E7 is independent of its ability to abrogate the activity of RB (Duensing & Munger, 2003a; Duensing & Munger, 2003b).

Recently, viral replication has also been suggested to be another factor contributing to the genome instability. The replication of HPV DNA from the integrated viral replication origin may be extended to the adjacent cellular DNA. Removal of the replication intermediate by the host DNA repair system may cause recombination and rearrangement of the cellular DNA (Kadaja *et al.*, 2007).

DNA damage and chromosomal abnormality are frequently present in HTLV-1-associated ATL cells. Proper centrosome duplication and segregation are vital to preserve chromosomal integrity. HTLV-1 *tax* affects both by targeting TAX1BP2 and RanBP1 (Matsuoka & Jeang, 2007). HTLV-1 *tax* further engenders the formation of multinucleated cells by down-regulating the mitotic spindle assembly checkpoint (SAC) complex through its interaction with MAD-1 (Jin *et al.*, 1998). It has been shown that *tax* abrogates the DNA damage checkpoint during the G2/M phase. Further studies show that *tax* suppresses DNA damage pathways, including Chk1/Chk2, BER, NER and mismatch repair (Grassmann *et al.*, 2005; Matsuoka & Jeang, 2007).

3.6. Insertional Mutagenesis

The life cycle of retroviruses requires the integration of proviral DNA into the host genome. This integration may occur in the vicinity of or inside important cellular genes, leading to their mutations. The outcome of proviral insertions can be at multiple levels depending on where the integration occurs. For example, transcriptional regulatory elements in the long terminal repeats of the proviral genome may lead to transcriptional activation of cellular genes. Alternatively, the splicing donor sites in the viral genome may generate chimeric or truncated cellular gene transcripts (Uren *et al.*, 2005).

Although all of the human DNA tumor viruses, including HPV, EBV, KSHV and HBV are capable of maintaining their genomes as episomes, the integration of their genomes into the host chromosomes is frequently detected, particularly in tumor samples. The insertional mutagenesis caused by these viral DNA integrations likely do not play major roles in viral oncogenesis, as common integration sites in the host genome have not been identified. It is noteworthy, however, that the DNA of woodchuck hepatitis B virus (WHV), a virus that is closely related to HBV, is frequently found to integrate next to the cellular N-*myc* oncogene for its activation (Fourel *et al.*, 1990; Hansen *et al.*, 1993). Such an integration pattern is not detected for HBV. HBV DNA integrants are frequently found in the host chromosomes of HCC tissues (Matsubara & Tokino, 1990) and have been detected near cellular erb-A and cyclin A genes (Dejean *et al.*, 1986; Wang *et al.*, 1990). However, the integration of HBV DNA near genes that may regulate cell proliferation is a rare event. Nevertheless, the possibility that host chromosomal rearrangements and deletions caused by HBV DNA integrations may exert random mutagenic effects and contribute to the process of oncogenesis cannot be ruled out.

Viral DNA integration itself may help to preserve or enhance the expression of viral oncoproteins. The integration of the HBV DNA has been found to produce a truncated middle surface antigen protein (MHBst), which perturbs cellular signaling pathways and has been shown to have oncogenic potential (Meyer *et al.*, 1992). The integration of the HPV genome commonly results in the disruption of the E2 region and abolishes the expression of E2, which negatively regulates the transcription of E6 and E7 oncoproteins (Boccardo & Villa, 2007; Shirasawa *et al.*, 1987; Woodman *et al.*, 2007). It has also been reported that E6 and E7 transcripts derived from the DNA integrants have longer half-lives than those from the episome (Jeon & Lambert, 1995). Consequently, increased expression of E6 and E7 oncoproteins may provide cells with growth advantages (Jeon *et al.*, 1995).

3.7. Induction of Chronic Inflammation

A link between inflammation and tumorigenesis was proposed about 150 years ago, when Rudolf Virchow noted the development of cancers at the sites of chronic inflammation (Moss & Blaser, 2005). Indeed, inflammation, which precedes wound healing, may also lead to cancer. During inflammation, inflammatory cells (both leukocytes and mast cells) are recruited by cytokines as well as chemokines to the site of infection or irritation. A respiratory burst then follows, in which leukocytes release free radicals derived from the oxygen uptake.

The inflammation during wound-healing is "self-limiting," i.e. cell proliferation and inflammation stop after the tissue regenerates. For cancer development, however, the inflammatory response sustains and provides the initiated tumor cells with an environment rich in growth/survival factors, activated stroma and DNA-damaging agents, which together promote cell proliferation as well as neoplastic transformation (Coussens & Werb, 2002).

Many human cancers, for instance, smoking-associated lung cancers and inflammatory bowel disease-associated colon cancers, are usually preceded by chronic inflammation. Furthermore, epidemiology studies showed that long-term usage of non-steroid anti-inflammatory drugs, such as aspirin, protects people from colon cancer and pancreatic cancer (Baron & Sandler, 2000; Coussens & Werb, 2002). Chronic inflammation in response to viral infection can also lead to the development of cancer. HCC caused by HBV and HCV is one such example.

Chronic liver inflammation caused by HBV and HCV infections frequently precedes the development of HCC in patients. The most direct evidence to support the role of chronic inflammation in the development of HBV-associated HCC comes from the studies on transgenic mice that expressed a non-cytopathic amount of HBV envelope protein known as the surface antigen (HBsAg). Due to the congenital expression of HBsAg from the transgene, there was immunotolerance to this viral protein in the mice. Immune response against HBsAg was reintroduced into thymectomized and lethally irradiated transgenic mice by adoptive transfer of bone marrow and spleen cells from syngeneic nontransgenic mice that had been previously immunized with a recombinant vaccinia virus that expressed HBsAg. This reconstitution of the immune system in transgenic mice induced chronic liver inflammation and liver injury and eventually the development of HCC in these mice (Nakamoto *et al.*, 1998).

Leukocyte (especially macrophage) infiltration is frequently observed in neoplastic tissues. These tumor-associated leukocytes are important for the removal of neoplastic cells. However, these immune cells also secrete many pro-angiogenic factors, cytokines and extracellular proteases, which promote angiogenesis, cell proliferation and metastasis (Coussens & Werb, 2002).

Free radicals are other key carcinogenic factors produced during inflammation. These free radicals can be generated from either reactive oxygen intermediate or reactive nitrogen intermediate during inflammation (Federico *et al.*, 2007). Reactive free radicals, such as hydroxyl radicals ($OH^{\bullet}$), peroxynitrite ($ONOO^{-}$) and nitric oxide ($NO^{\bullet}$), can damage DNA directly to cause single- or double-stranded DNA breaks, nucleotide modifications, DNA adducts and DNA-protein crosslinks (Hussain *et al.*, 2003). Normal cells respond to these damages by arresting the cell cycle for DNA repair to complete or by eliminating themselves through apoptosis. However, if mutations occur in crucial cancer-causing genes during the repairing process, neoplasic transformation of the cell may follow.

Studies have also pointed to an association between p53 mutation and elevated expression of iNOS, the major inducible enzyme for the production of $NO^{\bullet}$ in ulcerative colitis, hemochromatosis, as well as cancers in stomach, brain and breast. Moreover, $NO^{\bullet}$ and its derivatives may promote angiogenesis through its regulation of VEGF expression in the absence of wild-type p53. Therefore, free radicals may function as both tumor initiator and promoter during carcinogenesis (Hussain *et al.*, 2003).

Over-expression of HBV large envelope protein in transgenic mice led to necroinflammatory diseases that progressed to HCC (Chisari *et al.*, 1987). Further analysis indicated that sustained hepatocyte proliferation was accompanied by elevated production of ROS as well as oxidative damage long before the development of HCC (Hagen *et al.*, 1994). These studies lend further support to a causal role of ROS in the development of HCC.

Free radicals and oxidative stress are clearly induced by HCV infection, which is evidenced by decreased levels of hepatic and plasmatic glutathione, an important reductant, and increased levels of 4′-hydroxynonenal and 8-hydroxyguanosine, markers for oxidative DNA damage (Choi & Ou, 2006). Interestingly, free radicals are not only generated during HCV infection as a consequence of chronic inflammation, but can also be generated by HCV core protein and NS5A, which can directly affect mitochondrial electron transport, or by a secondary effect of endoplasmic reticulum (ER) stress induced by

Bosch FX, Lorincz A, Munoz N, Meijer CJ, Shah KV (2002) The causal relation between human papillomavirus and cervical cancer. *J Clin Pathol* **55**(4): 244–265.

Boshart M, Gissmann L, Ikenberg H, Kleinheinz A, Scheurlen W, zur Hausen H (1984) A new type of papillomavirus DNA, its presence in genital cancer biopsies and in cell lines derived from cervical cancer. *Embo J* **3**(5): 1151–1157.

Cahir McFarland ED, Izumi KM, Mosialos G (1999) Epstein-barr virus transformation: involvement of latent membrane protein 1-mediated activation of NF-kappaB. *Oncogene* **18**(49): 6959–6964.

Chang MH, Chen CJ, Lai MS, Hsu HM, Wu TC, Kong MS, Liang DC, Shau WY, Chen DS (1997) Universal hepatitis B vaccination in Taiwan and the incidence of hepatocellular carcinoma in children. Taiwan Childhood Hepatoma Study Group. *N Engl J Med* **336**(26): 1855–1859.

Chang Y, Cesarman E, Pessin MS, Lee F, Culpepper J, Knowles DM, Moore PS (1994) Identification of herpesvirus-like DNA sequences in AIDS-associated Kaposi's sarcoma. *Science* **266**(5192): 1865–1869.

Chen D, Nicholas J (2006) Structural requirements for gp80 independence of human herpesvirus 8 interleukin-6 (vIL-6) and evidence for gp80 stabilization of gp130 signaling complexes induced by vIL-6. *J Virol* **80**(19): 9811–9821.

Chisari FV, Filippi P, Buras J, McLachlan A, Popper H, Pinkert CA, Palmiter RD, Brinster RL (1987) Structural and pathological effects of synthesis of hepatitis B virus large envelope polypeptide in transgenic mice. *Proc Natl Acad Sci USA* **84**(19): 6909–6913.

Choi J, Lee KJ, Zheng Y, Yamaga AK, Lai MM, Ou JH (2004) Reactive oxygen species suppress hepatitis C virus RNA replication in human hepatoma cells. *Hepatology* **39**(1): 81–89.

Choi J, Ou JH (2006) Mechanisms of liver injury. III. Oxidative stress in the pathogenesis of hepatitis C virus. *Am J Physiol Gastrointest Liver Physiol* **290**(5): G847–851.

Choi J, Xu Z, Ou JH (2003) Triple decoding of hepatitis C virus RNA by programmed translational frameshifting. *Mol Cell Biol* **23**(5): 1489–1497.

Choo QL, Kuo G, Weiner AJ, Overby LR, Bradley DW, Houghton M (1989) Isolation of a cDNA clone derived from a blood-borne non-A, non-B viral hepatitis genome. *Science* **244**(4902): 359–362.

Conzen SD, Cole CN (1995) The three transforming regions of SV40 T antigen are required for immortalization of primary mouse embryo fibroblasts. *Oncogene* **11**(11): 2295–2302.

Coussens LM, Werb Z (2002) Inflammation and cancer. *Nature* **420**(6917): 860–867.

Cuconati A, White E (2002) Viral homologs of BCL-2: role of apoptosis in the regulation of virus infection. *Genes Dev* **16**(19): 2465–2478.

D'Agostino DM, Bernardi P, Chieco-Bianchi L, Ciminale V (2005) Mitochondria as functional targets of proteins coded by human tumor viruses. *Adv Cancer Res* **94**: 87–142.

Damania B (2007) DNA tumor viruses and human cancer. *Trends Microbiol* **15**(1): 38–44.

Dane DS, Cameron CH, Briggs M (1970) Virus-like particles in serum of patients with Australia-antigen-associated hepatitis. *Lancet* **1**(7649): 695–698.

Dejean A, Bougueleret L, Grzeschik KH, Tiollais P (1986) Hepatitis B virus DNA integration in a sequence homologous to v-erb-A and steroid receptor genes in a hepatocellular carcinoma. *Nature* **322**(6074): 70–72.

Dilworth SM (2002) Polyoma virus middle T antigen and its role in identifying cancer-related molecules. *Nat Rev Cancer* **2**(12): 951–956.

Duensing S, Duensing A, Crum CP, Munger K (2001) Human papillomavirus type 16 E7 oncoprotein-induced abnormal centrosome synthesis is an early event in the evolving malignant phenotype. *Cancer Res* **61**(6): 2356–2360.

Duensing S, Munger K (2003a) Centrosome abnormalities and genomic instability induced by human papillomavirus oncoproteins. *Prog Cell Cycle Res* **5**: 383–391.

Duensing S, Munger K (2003b) Human papillomavirus type 16 E7 oncoprotein can induce abnormal centrosome duplication through a mechanism independent of inactivation of retinoblastoma protein family members. *J Virol* 77(22): 12331–12335.

Durst M, Gissmann L, Ikenberg H, zur Hausen H (1983) A papillomavirus DNA from a cervical carcinoma and its prevalence in cancer biopsy samples from different geographic regions. *Proc Natl Acad Sci USA* **80**(12): 3812–3815.

Eliopoulos AG, Blake SM, Floettmann JE, Rowe M, Young LS (1999a) Epstein-Barr virus-encoded latent membrane protein 1 activates the

JNK pathway through its extreme C terminus via a mechanism involving TRADD and TRAF2. *J Virol* **73**(2): 1023–1035.

Eliopoulos AG, Dawson CW, Mosialos G, Floettmann JE, Rowe M, Armitage RJ, Dawson J, Zapata JM, Kerr DJ, Wakelam MJ, Reed JC, Kieff E, Young LS (1996) CD40-induced growth inhibition in epithelial cells is mimicked by Epstein-Barr Virus-encoded LMP1: involvement of TRAF3 as a common mediator. *Oncogene* **13**(10): 2243–2254.

Eliopoulos AG, Gallagher NJ, Blake SM, Dawson CW, Young LS (1999b) Activation of the p38 mitogen-activated protein kinase pathway by Epstein-Barr virus-encoded latent membrane protein 1 coregulates interleukin-6 and interleukin-8 production. *J Biol Chem* **274**(23): 16085–16096.

Eliopoulos AG, Stack M, Dawson CW, Kaye KM, Hodgkin L, Sihota S, Rowe M, Young LS (1997) Epstein-Barr virus-encoded LMP1 and CD40 mediate IL-6 production in epithelial cells via an NF-kappaB pathway involving TNF receptor-associated factors. *Oncogene* **14**(24): 2899–2916.

Ellerman V, Bang O (1908) Experimentelle Leukämie bei Hühnern. *Zentralbl Bakteriol Parasitenkd Infectionskr Hyg Abt Orig* **46**: 595–609.

Epstein MA, Achong BG, Barr YM (1964) Virus particles in cultured lymphoblasts from Burkitt's lymphoma. *Lancet* **1**: 702–703.

Farrell PJ (2002) Tumour viruses — could they be an Achilles' heel of cancer? *Eur J Cancer* **38**(14): 1815–1816.

Fattovich G (2003) Natural history and prognosis of hepatitis B. *Semin Liver Dis* **23**(1): 47–58.

Federico A, Morgillo F, Tuccillo C, Ciardiello F, Loguercio C (2007) Chronic inflammation and oxidative stress in human carcinogenesis. *Int J Cancer* **121**(11): 2381–2386.

Feng H, Shuda M, Chang Y, Moore PS (2008) Clonal integration of a polyomavirus in human Merkel cell carcinoma. *Science* **319**(5866): 1096–1100.

Fiorucci M, Boulant S, Fournillier A, Abraham JD, Lavergne JP, Paranhos-Baccala G, Inchauspe G, Bain C (2007) Expression of the alternative reading frame protein of Hepatitis C virus induces cytokines involved in hepatic injuries. *J Gen Virol* **88**(Pt 4): 1149–1162.

Fourel G, Trepo C, Bougueleret L, Henglein B, Ponzetto A, Tiollais P, Buendia MA (1990) Frequent activation of N-myc genes by hepadnavirus insertion in woodchuck liver tumours. *Nature* **347**(6290): 294–298.

Funk JO, Waga S, Harry JB, Espling E, Stillman B, Galloway DA (1997) Inhibition of CDK activity and PCNA-dependent DNA replication by p21 is blocked by interaction with the HPV-16 E7 oncoprotein. *Genes Dev* **11**(16): 2090–2100.

Galibert F, Mandart E, Fitoussi F, Tiollais P, Charnay P (1979) Nucleotide sequence of the hepatitis B virus genome (subtype ayw) cloned in *E. coli. Nature* **281**(5733): 646–650.

Ganem D (2006) KSHV infection and the pathogenesis of Kaposi's sarcoma. *Annu Rev Pathol* **1**: 273–296.

Gewin L, Myers H, Kiyono T, Galloway DA (2004) Identification of a novel telomerase repressor that interacts with the human papillomavirus type-16 E6/E6-AP complex. *Genes Dev* **18**(18): 2269–2282.

Girardi AJ, Sweet BH, Slotnick VB, Hilleman MR (1962) Development of tumors in hamsters inoculated in the neonatal period with vacuolating virus, SV-40. *Proc Soc Exp Biol Med* **109**: 649–660.

Grassmann R, Aboud M, Jeang KT (2005) Molecular mechanisms of cellular transformation by HTLV-1 Tax. *Oncogene* **24**(39): 5976–5985.

Hagen TM, Huang S, Curnutte J, Fowler P, Martinez V, Wehr CM, Ames BN, Chisari FV (1994) Extensive oxidative DNA damage in hepatocytes of transgenic mice with chronic active hepatitis destined to develop hepatocellular carcinoma. *Proc Natl Acad Sci USA* **91**(26): 12808–12812.

Hanahan D, Weinberg RA (2000) The hallmarks of cancer. *Cell* **100**(1): 57–70.

Hansen LJ, Tennant BC, Seeger C, Ganem D (1993) Differential activation of myc gene family members in hepatic carcinogenesis by closely related hepatitis B viruses. *Mol Cell Biol* **13**(1): 659–667.

Hardwick JM, Bellows DS (2003) Viral versus cellular BCL-2 proteins. *Cell Death Differ* **10**(1): S68–76.

Hayward WS, Neel BG, Astrin SM (1981) Activation of a cellular onc gene by promoter insertion in ALV-induced lymphoid leukosis. *Nature* **290**(5806): 475–480.

Hebner CM, Laimins LA (2006) Human papillomaviruses: basic mechanisms of pathogenesis and oncogenicity. *Rev Med Virol* **16**(2): 83–97.

Henderson BE (1989) Establishment of an association between a virus and a human cancer. *J Natl Cancer Inst* **81**(5): 320–321.

Hussain SP, Hofseth LJ, Harris CC (2003) Radical causes of cancer. *Nat Rev Cancer* **3**(4): 276–285.

Ichaso N, Dilworth SM (2001) Cell transformation by the middle T-antigen of polyoma virus. *Oncogene* **20**(54): 7908–7916.

Imperiale MJ, Major EO (2006) Polyomaviruses. In: Knipe DM, Howley PM (eds), *Fields Virology*, 5th edn, Vol. 61, pp. 2263–2298. Philadelphia: Lippincott Williams & Wilkins.

James MA, Lee JH, Klingelhutz AJ (2006) HPV16-E6 associated hTERT promoter acetylation is E6AP dependent, increased in later passage cells and enhanced by loss of p300. *Int J Cancer* **119**(8): 1878–1885.

Jarrett RF (2001) Human Herpesvirus-8. In: Grand RJA (ed), *Viruses, Cell Transformation and Cancer*, Vol. 5, pp. 253–290. Elsevier.

Jarviluoma A, Koopal S, Rasanen S, Makela TP, Ojala PM (2004) KSHV viral cyclin binds to p27KIP1 in primary effusion lymphomas. *Blood* **104**(10): 3349–3354.

Jeon S, Allen-Hoffmann BL, Lambert PF (1995) Integration of human papillomavirus type 16 into the human genome correlates with a selective growth advantage of cells. *J Virol* **69**(5): 2989–2997.

Jeon S, Lambert PF (1995) Integration of human papillomavirus type 16 DNA into the human genome leads to increased stability of E6 and E7 mRNAs: implications for cervical carcinogenesis. *Proc Natl Acad Sci USA* **92**(5): 1654–1658.

Jin DY (2007) Molecular pathogenesis of hepatitis C virus-associated hepatocellular carcinoma. *Front Biosci* **12**: 222–233.

Jin DY, Spencer F, Jeang KT (1998) Human T cell leukemia virus type 1 oncoprotein Tax targets the human mitotic checkpoint protein MAD1. *Cell* **93**(1): 81–91.

Kadaja M, Sumerina A, Verst T, Ojarand M, Ustav E, Ustav M (2007) Genomic instability of the host cell induced by the human papillomavirus replication machinery. *Embo J* **26**(8): 2180–2191.

Kane M (1995) Global programme for control of hepatitis B infection. *Vaccine* **13**(1): S47–49.

Katzenellenbogen RA, Egelkrout EM, Vliet-Gregg P, Gewin LC, Gafken PR, Galloway DA (2007) NFX1-123 and poly(A) binding proteins synergistically augment activation of telomerase in human papillomavirus type 16 E6-expressing cells. *J Virol* **81**(8): 3786–3796.

Keller SA, Schattner EJ, Cesarman E (2000) Inhibition of NF-kappaB induces apoptosis of KSHV-infected primary effusion lymphoma cells. *Blood* **96**(7): 2537–2542.

Kenney JL, Guinness ME, Curiel T, Lacy J (1998) Antisense to the epstein-barr virus (EBV)-encoded latent membrane protein 1 (LMP-1) suppresses LMP-1 and bcl-2 expression and promotes apoptosis in EBV-immortalized B cells. *Blood* **92**(5): 1721–1727.

Khalili K, Del Valle L, Wang JY, Darbinian N, Lassak A, Safak M, Reiss K (2003) T-antigen of human polyomavirus JC cooperates with IGF-IR signaling system in cerebellar tumors of the childhood-medulloblastomas. *Anticancer Res* **23**(3A): 2035–2041.

Khalili K, Sariyer IK, Safak M (2008) Small tumor antigen of polyomaviruses: role in viral life cycle and cell transformation. *J Cell Physiol* **215**(2): 309–319.

Kiyosawa K, Sodeyama T, Tanaka E, Gibo Y, Yoshizawa K, Nakano Y, Furuta S, Akahane Y, Nishioka K, Purcell RH, *et al.* (1990) Interrelationship of blood transfusion, non-A, non-B hepatitis and hepatocellular carcinoma: analysis by detection of antibody to hepatitis C virus. *Hepatology* **12**(4 Pt 1): 671–675.

Kuppers R (2003) B cells under influence: transformation of B cells by Epstein-Barr virus. *Nat Rev Immunol* **3**(10): 801–812.

Lane DP, Crawford LV (1979) T antigen is bound to a host protein in SV40-transformed cells. *Nature* **278**(5701): 261–263.

Levine P, Strickler H, Manns A, Diamondstone L (1998) Epidemiology of viruses associated with human cancer. In: McCane D (ed), *Human Tumor Viruses*, American Society for Microbiology.

Linzer DI, Levine AJ (1979) Characterization of a 54K dalton cellular SV40 tumor antigen present in SV40-transformed cells and uninfected embryonal carcinoma cells. *Cell* **17**(1): 43–52.

Liu C, Okruzhnov Y, Li H, Nicholas J (2001) Human herpesvirus 8 (HHV-8)-encoded cytokines induce expression of and autocrine signaling by vascular endothelial growth factor (VEGF) in HHV-8-infected primary-effusion lymphoma cell lines and mediate VEGF-independent antiapoptotic effects. *J Virol* **75**(22): 10933–10940.

Liu X, Yuan H, Fu B, Disbrow GL, Apolinario T, Tomaic V, Kelley ML, Baker CC, Huibregtse J, Schlegel R (2005) The E6AP ubiquitin ligase is required for transactivation of the hTERT promoter by the human papillomavirus E6 oncoprotein. *J Biol Chem* **280**(11): 10807–10816.

Longworth MS, Laimins LA (2004) Pathogenesis of human papillomaviruses in differentiating epithelia. *Microbiol Mol Biol Rev* **68**(2): 362–372.

Lowe DB, Shearer MH, Jumper CA, Kennedy RC (2007) SV40 association with human malignancies and mechanisms of tumor immunity by large tumor antigen. *Cell Mol Life Sci* **64**(7–8): 803–814.

Machida K, Cheng KT, Lai CK, Jeng KS, Sung VM, Lai MM (2006) Hepatitis C virus triggers mitochondrial permeability transition with production of reactive oxygen species, leading to DNA damage and STAT3 activation. *J Virol* **80**(14): 7199–7207.

Machida K, Cheng KT, Pavio N, Sung VM, Lai MM (2005) Hepatitis C virus E2-CD81 interaction induces hypermutation of the immunoglobulin gene in B cells. *J Virol* **79**(13): 8079–8089.

Machida K, Cheng KT, Sung VM, Lee KJ, Levine AM, Lai MM (2004a) Hepatitis C virus infection activates the immunologic (type II) isoform of nitric oxide synthase and thereby enhances DNA damage and mutations of cellular genes. *J Virol* **78**(16): 8835–8843.

Machida K, Cheng KT, Sung VM, Shimodaira S, Lindsay KL, Levine AM, Lai MY, Lai MM (2004b) Hepatitis C virus induces a mutator phenotype: enhanced mutations of immunoglobulin and protooncogenes. *Proc Natl Acad Sci USA* **101**(12): 4262–4267.

Manel N, Kim FJ, Kinet S, Taylor N, Sitbon M, Battini JL (2003) The ubiquitous glucose transporter GLUT-1 is a receptor for HTLV. *Cell* **115**(4): 449–459.

Matsubara K, Tokino T (1990) Integration of hepatitis B virus DNA and its implications for hepatocarcinogenesis. *Mol Biol Med* 7(3): 243–260.

Matsuoka M, Jeang KT (2007) Human T-cell leukaemia virus type 1 (HTLV-1) infectivity and cellular transformation. *Nat Rev Cancer* 7(4): 270–280.

Melartin L, Blumberg BS (1966) Production of antibody against "Australia antigen" in rabbits. *Nature* **210**(5043): 1340–1341.

Meyer M, Caselmann WH, Schluter V, Schreck R, Hofschneider PH, Baeuerle PA (1992) Hepatitis B virus transactivator MHBst: activation of NF-kappa B, selective inhibition by antioxidants and integral membrane localization. *Embo J* **11**(8): 2991–3001.

Mihara M, Erster S, Zaika A, Petrenko O, Chittenden T, Pancoska P, Moll UM (2003) p53 has a direct apoptogenic role at the mitochondria. *Mol Cell* **11**(3): 577–590.

Milich DR, Jones JE, Hughes JL, Price J, Raney AK, McLachlan A (1990) Is a function of the secreted hepatitis B e antigen to induce immunologic tolerance in utero? *Proc Natl Acad Sci USA* **87**(17): 6599–6603.

Moore PS, Boshoff C, Weiss RA, Chang Y (1996) Molecular mimicry of human cytokine and cytokine response pathway genes by KSHV. *Science* **274**(5293): 1739–1744.

Moss SF, Blaser MJ (2005) Mechanisms of disease: inflammation and the origins of cancer. *Nat Clin Pract Oncol* **2**(2): 90–97; quiz 91 p following 113.

Nakamoto Y, Guidotti LG, Kuhlen CV, Fowler P, Chisari FV (1998) Immune pathogenesis of hepatocellular carcinoma. *J Exp Med* **188**(2): 341–350.

Nicholas J (2007) Human herpesvirus 8-encoded proteins with potential roles in virus-associated neoplasia. *Front Biosci* **12**: 265–281.

Okuma K, Dalton KP, Buonocore L, Ramsburg E, Rose JK (2003) Development of a novel surrogate virus for human T-cell leukemia virus type 1: inhibition of infection by osteoprotegerin. *J Virol* 77(15): 8562–8569.

Pagano JS, Blaser M, Buendia MA, Damania B, Khalili K, Raab-Traub N, Roizman B (2004) Infectious agents and cancer: criteria for a causal relation. *Semin Cancer Biol* **14**(6): 453–471.

Peyton R (1911) Transmission of a Malignant New Growth by means of a Cell-free Filtrate. *Journal of the American Medical Association* **56**: 198.

Poiesz BJ, Ruscetti FW, Gazdar AF, Bunn PA, Minna JD, Gallo RC (1980) Detection and isolation of type C retrovirus particles from fresh and cultured lymphocytes of a patient with cutaneous T-cell lymphoma. *Proc Natl Acad Sci USA* 77(12): 7415–7419.

Poulin DL, DeCaprio JA (2006) Is there a role for SV40 in human cancer? *J Clin Oncol* **24**(26): 4356–4365.

Sarek G, Jarviluoma A, Ojala PM (2006) KSHV viral cyclin inactivates p27KIP1 through Ser10 and Thr187 phosphorylation in proliferating primary effusion lymphomas. *Blood* **107**(2): 725–732.

Scheffner M, Werness BA, Huibregtse JM, Levine AJ, Howley PM (1990) The E6 oncoprotein encoded by human papillomavirus types 16 and 18 promotes the degradation of p. 53. *Cell* **63**(6): 1129–1136.

Schrier PI, Bernards R, Vaessen RT, Houweling A, van der Eb AJ (1983) Expression of class I major histocompatibility antigens switched off by highly oncogenic adenovirus 12 in transformed rat cells. *Nature* **305**(5937): 771–775.

Shirasawa H, Tomita Y, Sekiya S, Takamizawa H, Simizu B (1987) Integration and transcription of human papillomavirus type 16 and 18 sequences in cell lines derived from cervical carcinomas. *J Gen Virol* **68**(Pt 2): 583–591.

Shope RE (1932) A filtrable virus causing a tumor-like condition in rabbits and its relationship to virus myxomatosum. *J Exp Med* **56**: 803–822.

Sisk EA, Robertson ES (2002) Clinical implications of human papillomavirus infection. *Front Biosci* 7: e77–84.

Stehelin D, Varmus HE, Bishop JM, Vogt PK (1976) DNA related to the transforming gene(s) of avian sarcoma viruses is present in normal avian DNA. *Nature* **260**(5547): 170–173.

Stevens CE (1994) In utero and perinatal transmission of hepatitis viruses. *Pediatr Ann* **23**(3): 152, 155–158.

Stevens CE, Beasley RP, Tsui J, Lee WC (1975) Vertical transmission of hepatitis B antigen in Taiwan. *N Engl J Med* **292**(15): 771–774.

Stewart SE, Eddy BE, Borgese N (1958) Neoplasms in mice inoculated with a tumor agent carried in tissue culture. *J Natl Cancer Inst* **20**(6): 1223–1243.

Straight SW, Herman B, McCance DJ (1995) The E5 oncoprotein of human papillomavirus type 16 inhibits the acidification of endosomes in human keratinocytes. *J Virol* **69**(5): 3185–3192.

Sullivan R, Dezube BJ, Koon HB (2006) Signal transduction targets in Kaposi's sarcoma. *Curr Opin Oncol* **18**(5): 456–462.

Sun Q, Matta H, Chaudhary PM (2003a) The human herpes virus 8-encoded viral FLICE inhibitory protein protects against growth factor withdrawal-induced apoptosis via NF-kappa B activation. *Blood* **101**(5): 1956–1961.

Sun Q, Zachariah S, Chaudhary PM (2003b) The human herpes virus 8-encoded viral FLICE-inhibitory protein induces cellular transformation via NF-kappaB activation. *J Biol Chem* **278**(52): 52437–52445.

Sun R, Lin SF, Gradoville L, Yuan Y, Zhu F, Miller G (1998) A viral gene that activates lytic cycle expression of Kaposi's sarcoma-associated herpesvirus. *Proc Natl Acad Sci USA* **95**(18): 10866–10871.

Szmuness W (1978) Hepatocellular carcinoma and the hepatitis B virus: evidence for a causal association. *Prog Med Virol* **24**: 40–69.

Takeshita H, Yoshizaki T, Miller WE, Sato H, Furukawa M, Pagano JS, Raab-Traub N (1999) Matrix metalloproteinase 9 expression is induced by Epstein-Barr virus latent membrane protein 1 C-terminal activation regions 1 and 2. *J Virol* **73**(7): 5548–5555.

Thomas MC, Chiang CM (2005) E6 oncoprotein represses p53-dependent gene activation via inhibition of protein acetylation independently of inducing p53 degradation. *Mol Cell* **17**(2): 251–264.

Trentin JJ, Yabe Y, Taylor G (1962) The quest for human cancer viruses. *Science* **137**: 835–841.

Uchida J, Yasui T, Takaoka-Shichijo Y, Muraoka M, Kulwichit W, Raab-Traub N, Kikutani H (1999) Mimicry of CD40 signals by Epstein-Barr virus LMP1 in B lymphocyte responses. *Science* **286**(5438): 300–303.

Uren AG, Kool J, Berns A, van Lohuizen M (2005) Retroviral insertional mutagenesis: past, present and future. *Oncogene* **24**(52): 7656–7672.

Vasavada R, Eager KB, Barbanti-Brodano G, Caputo A, Ricciardi RP (1986) Adenovirus type 12 early region 1A proteins repress class I HLA expression in transformed human cells. *Proc Natl Acad Sci USA* **83**(14): 5257–5261.

Vassilaki N, Mavromara P (2003) Two alternative translation mechanisms are responsible for the expression of the HCV ARFP/F/core+1 coding open reading frame. *J Biol Chem* **278**(42): 40503–40513.

Veldman T, Liu X, Yuan H, Schlegel R (2003) Human papillomavirus E6 and Myc proteins associate *in vivo* and bind to and cooperatively activate the telomerase reverse transcriptase promoter. *Proc Natl Acad Sci USA* **100**(14): 8211–8216.

Verma SC, Borah S, Robertson ES (2004) Latency-associated nuclear antigen of Kaposi's sarcoma-associated herpesvirus up-regulates transcription of human telomerase reverse transcriptase promoter through interaction with transcription factor Sp1. *J Virol* **78**(19): 10348–10359.

Verschuren EW, Klefstrom J, Evan GI, Jones N (2002) The oncogenic potential of Kaposi's sarcoma-associated herpesvirus cyclin is exposed by p53 loss *in vitro* and *in vivo*. *Cancer Cell* **2**(3): 229–241.

Walewski JL, Keller TR, Stump DD, Branch AD (2001) Evidence for a new hepatitis C virus antigen encoded in an overlapping reading frame. *Rna* 7(5): 710–721.

Wang J, Chenivesse X, Henglein B, Brechot C (1990) Hepatitis B virus integration in a cyclin A gene in a hepatocellular carcinoma. *Nature* **343**(6258): 555–557.

Weiberg RA (2007) *The Biology of Cancer*. Garland Science, Taylor & Francis Group, LLC.

Wise-Draper TM, Wells SI (2008) Papillomavirus E6 and E7 proteins and their cellular targets. *Front Biosci* **13**: 1003–1017.

Woodman CB, Collins SI, Young LS (2007) The natural history of cervical HPV infection: unresolved issues. *Nat Rev Cancer* 7(1): 11–22.

Xu Z, Choi J, Yen TS, Lu W, Strohecker A, Govindarajan S, Chien D, Selby MJ, Ou J (2001) Synthesis of a novel hepatitis C virus protein by ribosomal frameshift. *Embo J* **20**(14): 3840–3848.

Young LS (2001) Epstein-Barr virus and oncogenesis: from tumors to transforming genes. In: Grand RJA (ed), *Viruses, Cell Tranformation and Cancer*, Vol. 5, pp. 229–251. Elsevier Science B.V.

Zhang L, Pagano JS (2000) Interferon regulatory factor 7 is induced by Epstein-Barr virus latent membrane protein 1. *J Virol* **74**(3): 1061–1068.

Zheng ZM, Baker CC (2006) Papillomavirus genome structure, expression, and post-transcriptional regulation. *Front Biosci* **11**: 2286–2302.

Chapter 2

Hepatitis B Virus and Hepatocellular Carcinogenesis

T. S. Benedict Yen*

Abstract: Hepatitis B virus (HBV) infection is the major cause of hepatocellular carcinoma (HCC), the fifth most common cancer in the world and the third most common cause of cancer death. HBV-mediated carcinogenesis is a complex process, with both virus-specific and non-specific factors playing important roles. The former include viral proteins such as the X protein, as well as insertion of fragments of the viral DNA into the host chromosome. Non-specific factors include inflammation, hepatocellular damage, and cirrhosis. Aflatoxins and perhaps other environmental carcinogens also synergize with HBV to cause HCC. The data regarding the mechanism of action of these factors, as well as the many still unknown aspects of HBV-associated carcinogenesis, are presented and discussed in this chapter.

1. Hepatitis B Virus and Hepatocellular Carcinoma

Hepatitis B virus (HBV) is one of three viruses listed as known human carcinogens in the Eleventh Report on Carcinogens prepared by the US National Institute of Environmental Health and Safety in 2004

*Pathology Service, San Francisco VA Medical Center and Department of Pathology, University of California, San Francisco, San Francisco, California.

(http://ntp.niehs.nih.gov/ntp/roc/toc11.html), with the others being hepatitis C virus (HCV) and human papillomaviruses (HPVs). Several cross-sectional studies in the 1970s found a strong association of primary liver cell cancer (hepatocellular carcinoma or HCC) with serum positivity for HBV surface antigen (HBsAg), which is a marker of infection by HBV. In 1981, Beasley and colleagues (Beasley *et al.*, 1981) published a landmark cohort study of 22,707 men in Taiwan, which showed that the relative risk for HCC development in HBsAg-seropositive men was 223 times that for seronegative men. The 95% confidence interval was large (28–1479), since only one subject with HCC was negative for HBsAg. Subsequent studies have shown a range of somewhat smaller relative risks. Part of the variation in the results may be explained by the fact that the relative risk of HCC varies widely, depending on patient parameters such as the sex, the age, and the level of viral replication. For example, the relative risk is large (95.5) for HBsAg-positive men over the age of 55 who have active HBV replication as indicated by positivity for the viral early antigen (HBeAg), while the relative risk is much smaller (6.1) for men up to the age of 55 who are HBeAg negative (Yang *et al.*, 2002). Thus, the relative risk for HCC development calculated for HBV-infected people in any particular study would depend heavily on the mix of patients.

Because HCV is also strongly associated with HCC (Chap. 3), and HCV was as yet unknown at the time of many of the early studies, co-infection by the latter virus could have been a confounding factor. However, subsequent studies have shown that these two viruses are independent factors in hepatocarcinogenesis. For example, a meta-analysis of 32 case-control studies from four continents revealed that, compared with patients without serum markers for either infection, the odds ratio of HCC for HBV-positive and HCV-negative people was 22.5, while the odds ratio for HBV-negative and HCV-positive people was 17.3 (Donato *et al.*, 1998). Interestingly, the same study revealed that the odds ratio for people with double-positive for both viruses was 191, leading the authors to conclude that the two viruses synergize in carcinogenesis. More direct evidence for the causal role of HBV in HCC has come in recent years, as both vaccination to prevent infection and drug therapy to block viral replication have been shown to decrease HCC incidence in the general population or chronic hepatitis B patients, respectively (Chang *et al.*, 1997; Liaw *et al.*, 2004). Furthermore, woodchucks and ground squirrels experimentally infected by closely related viruses also show increased risk of HCC (Tennant, 2001). HBV is now recognized as the most common cause of HCC (Pisani *et al.*, 1997), which is the third leading cause of cancer death in the world (Pisani *et al.*, 1997). Specifically, approximately 330,000 people each year are conservatively estimated to die from HBV-associated HCC (Goldstein *et al.*, 2005). This number is expected to increase substantially over the next few decades because of population growth and ageing (Goldstein *et al.*, 2005).

2. Biology and Epidemiology of HBV

HBV is one of a group of closely related small enveloped DNA viruses known as the hepadnaviruses that infect various species of mammals and birds (Ganem & Schneider, 2001) and the only one in this family known to infect human beings. It is a common infectious agent in the world, as it is estimated that one-third of the 6.7 billion people in the world has been exposed to this virus. It is transmitted by blood and blood products. In East and Southeast Asia, mother-to-infant transmission during the birthing process is the main route. In Africa, the age of infection is slightly older and is associated with transmission within close family members. The exact means of transmission remains unclear but possibly involves shared toothbrushes, razor blades, and other household items that come into contact with blood. In Northwestern Europe, Australia, and North America, the mode of transmission is mainly through sexual contact and sharing of contaminated needles and syringes, and hence young adults are most at risk.

Upon acute infection, HBV usually causes no specific symptoms or causes only mild hepatitis, and most people successfully clear the virus and enjoy lifelong immunity to a second infection. However, between 5 and 10% of infected adults, and a large proportion of infected children, fail to mount a protective immune response and do not clear the virus from their hepatocytes (Hollinger & Liang, 2001). These chronically infected people (estimated 350 million worldwide) then constitute a reservoir for horizontal and vertical transmission, since viral particles circulate in their sera. More importantly, a sizable proportion of them develop chronic hepatitis of variable severity, sometimes with ensuing cirrhosis. If severe enough, this can be debilitating or life-threatening. Furthermore, chronically infected people are those at risk for HCC. Owing to these complications, HBV is estimated by the U.S. Department of Health & Human Services to cause approximately 700,000 deaths annually (http://www.omhrc.gov/templates/content.aspx?ID=7240&lvl=2&lvlid=190) and it is recognized to be the second most deadly human virus, after the human immunodeficiency virus (HIV).

The distribution of chronically infected people, and hence of HBV-related diseases, is uneven in the world. Because of high infection rates during infancy or early childhood, there is a high rate of HBV chronicity in sub-Saharan Africa and East and Southeast Asia. At the other extreme are Northwestern Europe, Australia, and North America, where infection largely takes place during adulthood and hence rates of chronicity are low. HBV is nevertheless an important cause of morbidity and mortality in the latter regions. Specifically, the US Centers for Disease Control and Prevention (http://www.cdc.gov/hepatitis/HBV/HBVfaq.htm#overview) estimates that there are as many as 1.4 million people with chronic HBV infection in the United States. The rate is particularly high among many minority groups, such as African Americans, Asian Americans, and Native Americans. The prevalence of HBV infection in African Americans is more than four times higher than in non-Hispanic whites (Rawls & Vega, 2005), and in New York City, the prevalence in Asian Americans is approximately 35 times that in the general population (Pollack *et al.*, 2006). Not surprisingly, then, HCC was the second leading cause of cancer deaths among Asian American men in California from 1998 to 2002, according to the Cancer Registry of the California Department of Health Services (http://ccrcal.org/Cancer05/Tables1-6-05.pdf).

3. HBV Virology

HBV has been well studied at the molecular level in recent years (Ganem & Schneider, 2001; Yen, 2001), although many details remain unknown because of the lack of robust cell culture or small animal models. The HBV virion has a partially double-stranded circular DNA genome of approximately 3.2 kilobasepairs (kb), enclosed in a capsid composed of the viral core protein (Fig. 1). The positive-strand DNA is slightly greater than full-length and is attached at its 5′-end to the viral polymerase, while the negative strand is less than full-length. This unusual genomic arrangement results from the use of reverse transcription for HBV DNA replication (see next paragraph). The virion has an outer envelope, comprising host lipids and three forms of viral surface (envelope) protein. After the virus attaches to and penetrates the host cell via unknown mechanisms, the genomic DNA enters the nucleus, within which it becomes converted into a supercoiled, fully double-stranded form (Fig. 2). This episomal DNA is then transcribed by host factors into several major species of mRNA, which are in turn translated into viral proteins.

There are four major open reading frames (ORF) in the HBV genome that are all conserved in the mammalian hepadnaviruses (Fig. 3) (Yen, 1993). The core ORF codes for two forms of the core protein

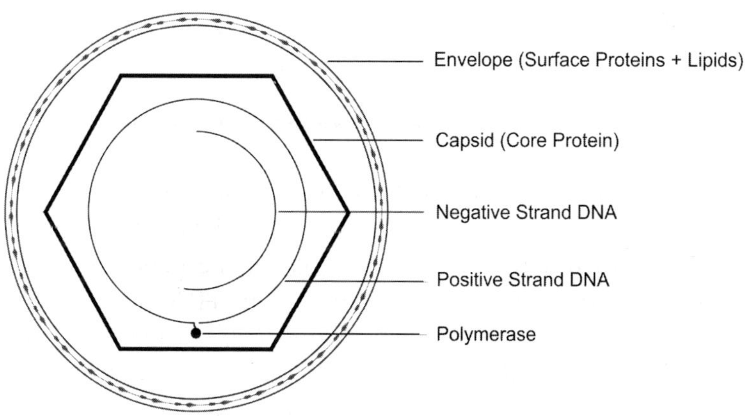

Fig. 1 Schematic diagram of the HBV virion.

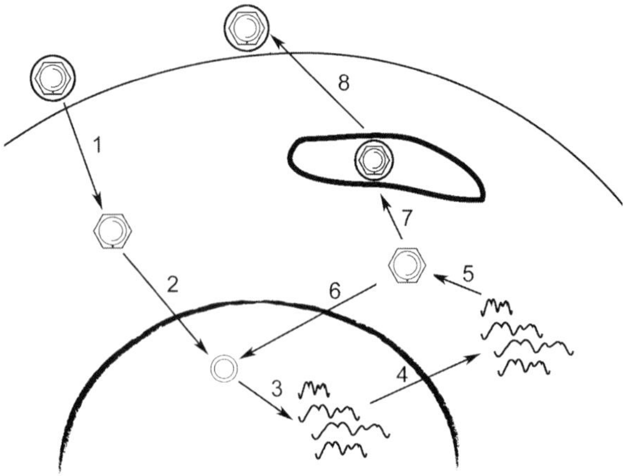

Fig. 2 HBV life cycle. 1. Incoming virion binds to cell surface and is taken up into the cytosol after losing the envelope. 2. The nucleocapsid travels to the nuclear envelope, and the genome goes into the nucleus and is repaired into covalently closed circular form. 3. The episomal DNA is transcribed into 4 classes of mRNA. 4. The transcripts are exported to the cytosol and translated. 5. The pregenomic RNA is encapsidated together with the polymerase by the core protein and reverse transcribed. 6. Early in infection, DNA-containing (mature) nucleocapsids are recycled into the nucleus. 7. The majority of mature nucleocapsids interact with surface proteins in the endoplasmic reticulum (ER) and bud into the lumen to form complete viral particles. 8. Progeny viral particle is exported via the constitutive secretory pathway. (See Ganem and Schneider (2001) for details.)

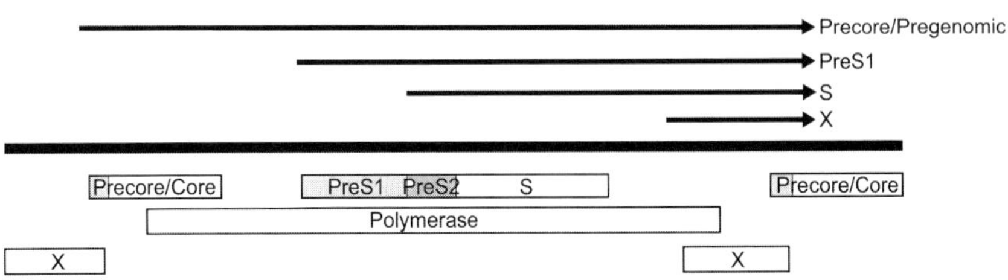

Fig. 3 **Gene map of HBV.** The central thick line represents the DNA (linearized and with the ends shown duplicated, since the precore mRNA and the pregenomic RNA are greater than one genome length). The precore region of the precore/core gene and the preS1 and preS2 regions of the surface gene are shaded in gray. (See Yen [1993, 2001] for details.)

(including the secreted HBeAg that is a proteolytic product of the so-called precore protein); the surface ORF codes for three forms of the surface protein (known collectively as HBsAg); the pol ORF codes for the polymerase protein, which has reverse transcriptase and other enzymatic activities necessary for viral replication; and the X ORF codes for as many as three forms of a regulatory factor (see Sec. 5.2.1). When enough viral proteins accumulate, one of the core mRNA species (pregenomic RNA) and the polymerase protein are co-packaged into cytosolic capsid particles by the core protein. The RNA is reverse transcribed into partially double-stranded DNA by the polymerase and degraded. These mature nucleocapsid particles then become competent to either recycle into the nucleus to maintain the number of episomal HBV genomes at approximately 20 copies per cell or bud through the membrane of the endoplasmic reticulum (ER), where they pick up the outer envelope, comprising all three forms of the viral surface protein embedded in host lipids. The viral particles are then released via the constitutive secretory pathway, without lysis of the host cell. Thus, despite having a DNA genome, HBV exclusively utilizes reverse transcription for its genomic replication and is distantly related to the retroviruses. Notably, with prolonged infection, there is random integration of HBV DNA fragments into the host genome (Hino *et al.*, 1989). These integrants are not replication competent and represent dead-end side products for the virus, but can still give rise, frequently, to some viral gene products, usually the surface proteins and a truncated X protein.

One unusual feature of HBV infection is that there is secretion of empty subviral (HBsAg) particles into the serum of infected people at a ratio of up to several orders of magnitude higher than actual virion particles. In fact, it is the high levels of these particles that allowed the early development of a sensitive serum immunoassay for HBV infection. These particles comprise mostly the small and middle surface proteins (MSPs) complexed with lipids. Thus, these viral proteins are synthesized at vastly greater quantities than necessary for virion morphogenesis. In contrast, the large surface protein (LSP) is found largely in virions, and hence it is not "over expressed." Indeed, subviral particles that are composed exclusively of LSP, or just comprise a greater than usual percentage of LSP, are retained in a distal ER component and cannot be secreted (Xu *et al.*, 1997a). This unusual feature will be discussed in more detail later, in Secs. 5.2.2.2 and 5.3.

The production of progeny HBV virions does not require lysis of the host cell. Indeed, it is clear from multiple lines of evidence that HBV is generally non-cytopathic. A substantial number of chronically infected people have high titers of HBV in their serum but show no evidence of liver injury by either serum chemistry or liver pathology (Hollinger & Liang, 2001). Cultured cells that have been transfected with the entire HBV genome produce infectious HBV particles but grow indefinitely with no signs of cytopathology (Sureau *et al.*, 1986). Finally, transgenic mice containing the entire HBV genome also produce infectious HBV particles without showing any signs of liver injury (Guidotti *et al.*, 1995). Thus, it is widely accepted that the hepatitis seen in chronic hepatitis B results largely from the host immune response to viral antigens, which is sufficient to cause injury but, for unknown reasons, ineffective in clearing the virus. It should be noted, however, that there is increasing evidence from both patients and experimental models that high-level HBV replication in the liver may be directly cytopathic (Foo *et al.*, 2002; Lau *et al.*, 1992; Mason *et al.*, 1993; Meuleman *et al.*, 2006; Sugiyama *et al.*, 2008).

4. Prevention and Treatment of HBV

Effective vaccines against HBV have been available for more than two decades. The original vaccine was derived from the non-infectious HBsAg particles that circulate in large amounts in the serum of many infected people. Later, recombinant vaccines derived from yeast-expressed small surface protein (SSP) became available. However, large numbers of people in the world still do not have access to these vaccines, and hence HBV will not be eliminated for the near future. Furthermore, vaccination does not help those who are already infected, and hence in many countries that recently instituted universal vaccination, such as Vietnam, the incidence of HBV-associated disease is not expected to decrease in the coming decade or two (Nguyen *et al.*, 2008).

There are two types of drugs commonly used against HBV (Pardo *et al.*, 2007). Type I interferons, such as interferon-α2, are thought to have direct antiviral effects and also boost the host immune response to HBV. As a result, a small proportion of treated patients respond well and can even clear the virus. However, most patients do not show such a dramatic response. Furthermore, interferons must be injected intravenously, and many people cannot tolerate the severe side effects. The other class of drugs comprises inhibitors of the viral polymerase (reverse transcriptase). Lamivudine was the first such drug approved for HBV, and it can dramatically decrease the serum viral load in most patients. Unfortunately, resistant viruses arise within a few years in many patients, thereby limiting its usefulness. Several other polymerase inhibitors have been approved in recent years, and it appears that resistance to these drugs may develop more slowly. Thus, drug therapy for HBV is slowly improving albeit still far from universally effective.

5. Mechanisms of HBV Carcinogenesis

5.1. Overview

While HBV infection is clearly a major risk factor for hepatic carcinogenesis, the molecular mechanisms are as yet incompletely understood (Cougot *et al.*, 2005; Farazi & DePinho, 2006). Two major theories, which are not mutually exclusive, have been proposed (Robinson, 1994). One possibility is that the virus plays a specific role in malignant transformation. For example, it may carry an oncogene in its genome, and/or viral DNA can disrupt a tumor-suppressing gene or it can activate a proto-oncogene by virtue of integrating within or nearby one of those host genes. Incontrovertible experimental evidence for either situation has been difficult to obtain (see Sec. 5.2), thus leading investigators to propose a second possibility, namely that HBV plays no role other than as an inciter of inflammation and hepatocyte damage. It is presumed that long-term stimulation of hepatocyte proliferation renders their DNA susceptible to mutagenesis by endogenous and/or exogenous carcinogens, and these mutations as well as errors in replication become "fixed" because successive rounds of rapid DNA synthesis do not allow adequate time for complete repair (Ames & Gold, 1990). Hepatocyte turnover *per se* is likely insufficient for carcinogenesis, as serial transplantation experiments in mice have revealed that hepatocytes can undergo a minimum of 69 cell doublings (7.3×10^{20}-fold expansion) without malignant transformation (Overturf *et al.*, 1997). Therefore, inflammatory cells must also contribute to carcinogenesis, by releasing genotoxic reactive oxygen species, cytokines, and/or other factors (Hofseth & Ying, 2005). Liver fibrosis resulting from chronic damage may also contribute by altering the extracellular environment of the hepatocyte (Cutroneo *et al.*, 2006). In support of this model, inflammation has been recently appreciated to play an important role in carcinogenesis in other models. For example, inflammation promotes colon carcinogenesis induced by azoxymethane (Greten *et al.*, 2004), apparently by activating NF-κB in both the inflammatory cells and the colonic epithelial cells, while both B- and T-lymphocytes promote skin carcinogenesis induced by HPV oncogenes (Daniel *et al.*, 2003). Even diethylnitrosamine-induced hepatocarcinogenesis is delayed or mitigated if macrophage activation is blocked by knocking out the receptor for interferon-γ (Matsuda *et al.*, 2005) or by knocking out IκB kinase β (Maeda *et al.*, 2005). Direct evidence for a role of inflammatory damage in HBV carcinogenesis has also been demonstrated by Chisari and colleagues in transgenic mice, although the results are complicated by the presence of viral gene products in their model (see Sec. 5.3).

However, it is noteworthy that although inflammation clearly plays an important role in the various animal models of liver, colon, and skin carcinogenesis discussed previously, in all of those cases, few or no cancer is observed unless there is the presence of chemical carcinogens or viral oncogenes in addition to inflammation (Greten *et al.*, 2004; Maeda *et al.*, 2005; Matsuda *et al.*, 2005). Conversely, transgenic mouse lines that suffer from chronic hepatitis because of abnormal cytokeratin production (Ku *et al.*, 1997), ectopic expression of osteopontin (Mochida *et al.*, 2004), or overexpression of interferon-γ (Toyonaga *et al.*, 1994) are not known to have increased incidence of spontaneous HCC. The only apparent counter-example in the literature is a knockout mouse line lacking the transporter that pumps bile out of hepatocytes (Pikarsky *et al.*, 2004). These mice suffer from chronic hepatitis and eventually develop HCC without the need for an exogenous carcinogen. However, it turns out that bile acids are themselves pro-carcinogenic (Mahmoud *et al.*, 1999; Reddy *et al.*, 1977), and thus HCC in this model may result from a combination of bile acids and chronic inflammation acting cooperatively.

Indeed, clinical data indicate that it is unlikely that chronic hepatitis constitutes the sole carcinogenic factor during chronic hepatitis B. For if such were the case, then all people with chronic hepatitis, of whatever cause, should have an equal risk for HCC that is determined by the severity of the liver injury rather than by the inciting agent. Yet this is not the case. In one large study, it was shown that among all people with chronic hepatitis, those with HBV infection had a seven-fold greater risk for HCC than those without HBV infection (Tsukuma *et al.*, 1993). Unlike the situation for HCV, HCC not uncommonly occurs in HBV-infected people in the absence of prolonged severe liver injury or cirrhosis (Hsu *et al.*, 1987). One study showed that the incidence of HCC in non-cirrhotic HBV-infected people is 0.4–0.6% per year, which is much higher than the incidence in non-cirrhotic HCV-infected people (<0.1% per year) (Bruix *et al.*, 2004). Another prospective study revealed that in an 11-year follow-up period, 40% of the HBV-associated HCC cases developed in a non-cirrhotic liver, but only 7.7% of the HCV-associated cases developed in a non-cirrhotic liver (Takano *et al.*, 1995). Even in patients with full-blown cirrhosis due to hepatitis C, HBV infection further increases the risk for HCC (Ikeda *et al.*, 2007; Shetty *et al.*, 2008). Interestingly, the molecular pathology of HCC also differs between hepatitis B and hepatitis C, in that the HCC arising in the former tend to show genomic instability while those arising in the latter more commonly show β-catenin mutations (Hsu *et al.*, 2000; Huang *et al.*, 1999; Kawai *et al.*, 2000). HBV-related HCC also differ from non-viral HCC in terms of their genetic changes (Marchio *et al.*, 2000). These findings support the idea that HBV provides virus-specific factor(s) in carcinogenesis.

Furthermore, recent studies have shown that the serum titer of HBV is directly correlated with the risk of HCC development in a dose-dependent manner. Multivariate analysis reveals that while HBV titer is an independent risk factor for HCC, hepatocyte injury, as measured by elevation of serum alanine aminotransferase (ALT) levels, is not (Chen *et al.*, 2006; Yang *et al.*, 2008). This observation is difficult to reconcile with the idea that liver injury alone constitutes the carcinogenic factor, as an inflammatory response to HBV would be expected to limit viral titers in the serum but induce higher ALT levels.

The presence of clonally integrated HBV genomes in the majority of HBV-associated HCC also suggests a direct role of the virus in carcinogenesis. A recent large-scale study was able to clone out integrated HBV DNA in 56 of 60 HCC samples (Murakami *et al.*, 2005). Although the percentage of hepatocytes with integrated viral DNA in human HBV infection is unknown, the fraction in woodchucks chronically infected with woodchuck hepatitis virus (WHV) has been estimated at less than 5% (Summers & Mason, 2004). Assuming that HBV integration in human livers is not a significantly more frequent event, then the almost universal presence of HBV integration in HCC would suggest that the minority of hepatocytes with integrated viral sequences constitute the main or perhaps sole population at risk of carcinogenesis. This inference is incompatible with liver inflammation and injury being the only impetus for oncogenic transformation, as in that case presumably all hepatocytes in the liver would be similarly exposed to these factors. It should be noted that although the data cited here would on face value suggest that HBV DNA integration constitutes the oncogenic factor, such may not necessarily be the case, as the presence of HBV integration may simply be a marker for a cell that has supported HBV replication for an extended period. In any case, it would be important to quantify the percentage of human hepatocytes that contain integrated HBV DNA during chronic hepatitis B.

In summary, it is likely that in human infections, HBV causes cancer by a combination of HBV-specific and non-specific factors. The various factors, both specific and non-specific to HBV, will be discussed in detail in the following sections.

5.2. HBV-specific Factors

Although the evidence cited above strongly suggests that HBV contributes one or more specific factors to carcinogenesis, the identity of the factor(s) remains unsettled. HBV clearly does not express an acutely transforming oncogene, as several independently derived transgenic mice containing and expressing the entire viral genome produce infectious virions without suffering from HCC (Chisari, 1991; Zheng *et al.*, 2007a). Nevertheless, it remains possible that HBV produces a weakly oncogenic factor. The other possibility suggested by studies of animal retroviruses is the insertional mutagenesis mechanism. There is evidence in favor of both scenarios, which are discussed in detail below.

5.2.1. *X protein*

The X protein has received considerable attention as a possible oncogenic factor ever since the HBV genome was sequenced, since it is not a structural protein and the position of its gene, at the downstream end of the genome, is analogous to that of Tax and other oncoproteins of retroviruses (see Chap. 7). Furthermore, the X protein is conserved in all mammalian hepadnaviruses but not avian ones, and mammalian but not avian hepadnaviruses are associated with HCC (Tennant, 2001). Although incontrovertible evidence in favor of X protein being an oncoprotein is still lacking, it is probable that X protein plays an accessory role in carcinogenesis. Indeed, expression of the viral X gene alone in transgenic mice has been reported to lead to atypical hyperplasia and subsequent malignant transformation of hepatocytes (Kim *et al.*, 1991). However, HCC is seen only with overexpression of X protein in a mouse strain that is already susceptible to spontaneous hepatic carcinogenesis. HCC has not been observed in other transgenic mice expressing the X protein (Billet *et al.*, 1995; Lee *et al.*, 1990), although these mice do show an increased susceptibility to liver carcinogenesis caused by either *c-myc* overexpression or carcinogen exposure (Madden *et al.*, 2001; Terradillos *et al.*, 1997). Furthermore, transgenic mice containing the entire wild-type HBV genome and expressing the X protein have not been reported to develop HCC spontaneously (Guidotti *et al.*, 1995; Xu *et al.*, 2002). Therefore, X protein probably acts only as a cofactor in hepatic carcinogenesis, via one or more mechanisms, as discussed below. It is also notable that HBV-transgenic mice with the X gene inactivated are just as susceptible to chemical carcinogenesis as mice with the wild-type HBV genome (Zheng *et al.*, 2007a), indicating the presence of additional oncogenic factor(s) encoded by the HBV genome.

5.2.1.1. Function of X protein in the HBV life cycle

Knocking out the X ORF in the woodchuck virus results in greatly diminished or no viral replication in exposed animals (Chen *et al.*, 1993; Zhang *et al.*, 2001; Zoulim *et al.*, 1994), establishing the importance of this protein *in vivo*. However, initial experiments using HBV in transfection experiments failed to reveal any consistent effect of X protein on viral gene expression or replication (Blum *et al.*, 1992). Later, it became clear that X protein did affect these processes, but only in quiescent (non-dividing) cells (Bouchard *et al.*, 2001b; Keasler *et al.*, 2007). X protein was found to increase viral mRNA levels modestly (~4 fold), while viral replication showed a much larger increase when X protein is present (>15 fold) (Bouchard *et al.*, 2001b). Both defects could be rescued with X protein supplied in *trans* by an expression plasmid. The difference in the magnitudes of these two effects suggested that X protein impacted two different processes: viral transcription and DNA replication. However, because there may not be a linear relationship between viral protein levels and efficiency of pregenomic RNA encapsidation, it could be argued that the amount of core protein and perhaps other structural components does not reach a critical level needed for efficient replication unless X protein is present to boost transcription. Indeed, mutants of X protein show a correlation between the ability of supporting HBV replication and transcription (Tang *et al.*, 2005). On the other hand, studies using kinase inhibitors in cultured cells argue against this possibility, as some inhibitors can block viral replication without affecting viral transcription in an X-protein-dependent manner (Bouchard *et al.*, 2003).

Comparison of HBV-transgenic mouse lines with or without an intact X gene confirms that there is a 3–5-fold decrease in viral mRNA levels with the loss of X protein (Xu *et al.*, 2002). However, the decrease in intracellular replicative HBV DNA as well as in circulating virion levels in the serum was of a similar magnitude, suggesting that, in this model, X protein had little or no direct effect on replication. Interestingly, the X-protein effect on mRNA levels was the strongest in fully grown mature mice, suggesting that the function of X protein *in vivo* was not evident in the dividing hepatocytes of young mice, similar to the situation in cultured cells. Experiments in mouse liver acutely transfected with the HBV genome using the hydrodynamic injection method showed yet again a different set of results (Keasler *et al.*, 2007). Viral transcript levels dropped by ~4 fold, but the amount of circulating HBV virion DNA in the serum dropped by almost two orders of magnitude. Unlike the situation in transfected cultured cells, however, the amount of intracellular encapsidated HBV DNA dropped only 4–5 fold.

In summary, there is general agreement that the absence of X protein causes a 4–5-fold decrease in HBV mRNA levels, regardless of the model system used, although this effect was seen only in non-dividing cells. However, there are conflicting data on whether X protein has an additional effect on viral replication, and the exact step in replication involved. Some of these differences undoubtedly result from use of host cells with various extents of differentiation and different cell cycle kinetics. Acute versus chronic expression of X protein may also influence the results, as cells may adapt to the presence of X protein. Yet another possible source of variations is the expression of short forms of X protein. In cultured cells, it has been shown that two N-terminally truncated forms of X protein can be expressed, either via initiation at internal ATG codons or production of mRNAs from weak promoters downstream of the canonical X promoter (Kwee *et al.*, 1992; Zheng *et al.*, 1994). These short forms of X protein appear functional in at least some transcription and replication assays, but their expression has not been studied in any of the publications reporting the role of X protein in the viral life cycle. Thus, it is possible that different host cells, different expression systems, and/or different mutations to knock out the X gene may lead to different levels of expression of the shorter forms of X protein and hence variable outcomes. In any case, the strong dependence of WHV infection on the X protein suggests an effect beyond a modest increase in viral transcription.

5.2.1.2. Effect of X protein on transcription

X protein can *trans*-activate cellular as well as HBV genes. Transient transfection experiments have repeatedly demonstrated that X protein can increase transcription from a variety of promoters to a modest degree (less than 10 fold) (Yen, 1996). However, X protein clearly does not bind to DNA, and many different *cis*-acting elements appear to respond to X protein. Two general models, that are not mutually exclusive, have been proposed for how X protein can have such pleiotropic effects. In the first model, X protein binds to cellular transcription factors and enhances the function of the latter. Many different such factors have been proposed, ranging from sequence-specific factors such as AP2 and members of the basic leucine zipper family of proteins including CREB and c/EBPα (Maguire *et al.*, 1991; Qadri *et al.*, 1995; Seto *et al.*, 1990), to co-activators and general transcription factors such as CBP, TBP, TFIIB, TFIIH, and the RPB5 subunit of RNA polymerase II (Cheong *et al.*, 1995; Choi *et al.*, 1999; Haviv *et al.*, 1998; Qadri *et al.*, 1996). X-protein binding to many such factors has been shown *in vitro* or *in vivo* with the two-hybrid assay in yeast cells or transient overexpression in mammalian cells, but because of the extremely low levels of X protein that accumulate in cells replicating the HBV genome, demonstration of interaction in a situation mimicking the environment of an infected hepatocyte has not been possible. Perhaps the most relevant of this kind of nuclear function for X protein is the interaction of X protein with the basic leucine zipper family of transcription factors. The interaction of X protein with CREB or c/EBPα has been shown to increase binding of these factors to their respective *cis*-acting sites *in vitro*, either by directly affecting the DNA binding affinity or by increasing dimer formation (Maguire *et al.*, 1991; Williams & Andrisani, 1995).

As the HBV enhancers contain binding sites for these and related factors (Yen, 1993), such an interaction can potentially lead to an increase in transcription from the HBV enhancers.

In the other model of how X protein might in an indirect way affect multiple transcriptional pathways, the X protein is proposed to act in the cytoplasm to increase cytoplasmic calcium levels, by interacting with the mitochondria and causing calcium release from this organelle (McClain *et al.*, 2007; Rahmani *et al.*, 2000). The modulation of calcium levels then leads to activation of two tyrosine kinases, i.e. focal adhesion kinase and the proline-rich tyrosine kinase 2 (Bouchard *et al.*, 2003). These two related kinases are upstream of c-Src, which itself is upstream of the Ras-Raf-MAP kinase pathway. The latter pathway in turn can then activate transcription from a wide variety of *cis*-acting elements. Such a scheme would nicely explain the pleiotropic effects of X protein on cellular transcription. However, although there is good evidence that this pathway is involved in the X-protein activation of AP1, NFκB, and NFAT, there is as yet no evidence that this pathway is involved in activating HBV transcription. Therefore, it is tempting to speculate that X protein acts in the nucleus to increase HBV transcription, but it acts in the cytoplasm to increase transcription via other factors.

Yet another possible target of the X protein is the ubiquitin proteasome system (UPS). Using the yeast two-hybrid screening method, X protein has been shown to bind to a subunit of the 20S proteasome as well as a subunit of the 19S proteasome (Fischer *et al.*, 1995; Huang *et al.*, 1996). Apparently, because of this interaction, proteasomal function is adversely affected (Hu *et al.*, 1999). As many transcription factors or their regulators are degraded by the UPS, this direct effect of the X protein on the proteasome can potentially explain the numerous *cis*-acting elements through which X protein can act. Indeed, microarray analysis has revealed that the transcript levels for many cellular proteins can be modulated by X protein (Hu *et al.*, 2006), perhaps reflecting changes in the amount of the transcription factors regulating these genes. However, the downstream targets of proteasomal dysregulation by X protein relevant for viral gene expression have not been identified.

5.2.1.3. Effect of X protein on viral replication

The mechanism by which X protein increases HBV replication is also murky. As discussed above, some but not all experiments point to a role for X protein in augmenting HBV replication that is independent of its ability to activate HBV transcription. One possibility is that X protein increases transcription of a cellular factor that is limiting for HBV replication, but such a factor has not been identified. Another possibility is that X protein has an activity entirely independent of transcriptional activation. Indeed, there is good evidence that Src, which has little effect on HBV transcription, is important for HBV replication (Bouchard *et al.*, 2001b, 2003). Melegari and colleagues (Melegari *et al.*, 2005) have shown that X protein can affect the phosphorylation pattern of HBV core protein. As core protein phosphorylation is a dynamic process that is intimately connected with the different phases of HBV genomic replication, this finding can explain the effect of X protein on HBV replication. However, the precise pathway by which X protein may affect core protein phosphorylation is not defined yet.

5.2.1.4. X protein and DDB1

The X protein can also potentially interact with the UPS in a manner apart from or in addition to direct binding to the proteasome that may be highly relevant to the functions of X protein. Several groups have shown that X protein interacts with the DNA damage binding protein 1 (DDB1) (Bergametti *et al.*, 2002; Bontron *et al.*, 2002; Wentz *et al.*, 2000). Originally DDB1 was described as the binding partner of DDB2 in the recognition of DNA damage, while more recently DDB1 has been recognized to be an adapter protein in an ubiquitin ligase E3 complex, which may have a variety of functions (Higa & Zhang, 2007). Although the effect of X protein on this E3 ligase is yet unclear, it is certainly possible that X protein could affect the function of DDB1 and hence modulate the amount of protein degraded by DDB1-containing E3 ligases. Intriguingly, DDB1 function is hijacked by three other families of viruses in this manner for their own purposes. The paramyxoviruses code for the V protein, which binds to DDB1 to redirect it toward degradation of members of the STAT family of transcription factors (Ulane *et al.*, 2005). As these proteins are critical for the cellular type I interferon response, this action effectively blocks a major cellular antiviral pathway to facilitate viral replication. V-minus mutants of paramyxoviruses behave as attenuated viruses in infected animals, showing a shorter duration and lower level of viral replication (Devaux *et al.*, 2008). The human lentiviruses HIV I and II code for a protein known as either Vpr or Vpx, respectively, that also interacts with DDB1 (Dehart & Planelles, 2008; Le Rouzic *et al.*, 2007). Recent evidence showed that Vpr/Vpx counteracts a powerful innate antiviral response in macrophages that restricts viral reverse transcription, although the molecular target is as yet uncharacterized (Sharova *et al.*, 2008; Srivastava *et al.*, 2008). Finally, the latency-associated M2 protein of murine gamma herpes virus 68, a close relative of Kaposi's sarcoma herpes virus, has been found to bind DDB1 and cause the degradation of STAT1 and STAT2 (Liang *et al.*, 2006; Liang *et al.*, 2004). Given these precedents, it is quite possible that X protein modifies DDB1 function to either induce or decrease the degradation of one or more cellular proteins to increase viral transcription and/or replication, perhaps by blocking an innate antiviral response. This scenario would also explain the observation that X-minus WHV apparently can replicate at an extremely low level for a brief period and efficiently produce protective immunity (Zhang *et al.*, 2001), somewhat similar to V-minus paramyxoviruses. Therefore, it would be of great interest to identify the cellular protein(s) targeted by the X-DDB1 complex, as this may point to a novel means to control HBV infection.

5.2.1.5. X-protein carcinogenesis

The precise mechanism by which X protein may cause HCC is as yet unknown. Several possibilities can be entertained, based on its various activities. Since X protein can increase transcription from a variety of promoters, it could increase the expression of one or more cellular proto-oncogenes. One such example would be CREB, which has been implicated in carcinogenesis in various cell types (Aggarwal *et al.*, 2008; Shankar *et al.*, 2005; Xie *et al.*, 1997), although its role in liver carcinogenesis is unknown. X protein has been shown to increase the binding of CREB to its cognate DNA element and to increase the loading of the co-activators CBP and p300 onto CREB (Cougot *et al.*, 2007). Thus, these activities of X protein would mimic overexpression of CREB and potentially lead to oncogenesis. However, there is no experimental evidence to show that the level of X protein expressed from the HBV genome is sufficient to augment CREB activity in the normal hepatocyte (e.g. by looking at transcript levels of genes downstream of CREB) or that CREB is necessary for X-protein-associated hepatocarcinogenesis.

Another possibility is that X protein, by virtue of its ability to stimulate the c-Src kinase, activates oncogenic pathways downstream of the latter protein (Cha *et al.*, 2004; Lara-Pezzi *et al.*, 2001). Indeed, overexpression of c-Src causes HCC in transgenic mice (Kline *et al.*, 2008). Again, however, there is no experimental evidence to show that the level of X protein expressed from the HBV genome is sufficient to activate c-Src in the hepatocytes of an intact animal or that c-Src is necessary for X-protein-associated hepatocarcinogenesis.

The interaction of DDB1 with X protein raises the question whether DNA damage repair may be impaired in cells expressing X protein, since DDB1 in complex with DDB2 is important for nucleotide excision repair, which corrects DNA lesions induced by chemical carcinogens (Li *et al.*, 2006; Wakasugi *et al.*, 2008). Indeed, transgenic mice expressing low levels of X protein have been shown to suffer a very modest increase in hepatocyte DNA mutations, as well as a specific increase in transversions, upon exposure to the liver carcinogen aflatoxin B1 (Madden *et al.*, 2002). Because mice are resistant to aflatoxin-induced hepatic carcinogenesis, it could not be determined whether this effect actually leads to increased HCC incidence. However, X-transgenic mice do show increased mutation frequency and develop more preneoplastic lesions and HCC after treatment with diethylnitrosamine (Madden *et al.*, 2001; Slagle *et al.*, 1996), which is a widespread food-borne carcinogen. In contrast, transgenic mice not treated with carcinogens did not show an increase in mutation frequency (Madden *et al.*, 2000). Therefore, although X-protein-induced defect in DNA repair likely mediates the ability of HBV to enhance carcinogen-induced HCC, it may not be important for spontaneous HBV carcinogenesis.

Finally, X protein has been demonstrated to induce aberrations of the cell cycle in cultured cells. There is agreement that X protein causes multipolar spindle formation, chromosome segregation defects, and aneuploidy (Forgues *et al.*, 2003; Kim *et al.*, 2008; Lee *et al.*, 2002; Livezey *et al.*, 2002; Martin-Lluesma *et al.*, 2008; Rakotomalala *et al.*, 2008; Wen *et al.*, 2008; Yun *et al.*, 2004), hallmarks of cancer that are believed to be of pathogenic importance (Pihan & Doxsey, 2003). Multiple mechanisms have been proposed to explain how X protein may directly interfere with normal mitosis, including activation of the Ras-MEK-MAPK pathway (Yun *et al.*, 2004), binding to and cytosolic sequestration of Crm1 with resultant abnormal centriole genesis (Forgues *et al.*, 2003), dysfunction of HBXIP, a protein that binds X protein and is needed for proper spindle formation (Wen *et al.*, 2008), and disruption of the mitotic checkpoint by binding to BubR1 (Kim *et al.*, 2008). However, there is also evidence that X protein causes prolongation of the S phase (Bouchard *et al.*, 2001a; Lee *et al.*, 2002; Martin-Lluesma *et al.*, 2008), which would not be caused by the mitotic defects mentioned above. Therefore, an alternative possibility is that X protein primarily interferes with proper DNA synthesis, with mitotic abnormalities accumulating as a secondary phenomenon. Recently, it was shown that a point mutant of X protein that does not bind DDB1 also does not cause prolongation of the S phase and mitotic abnormalities (Martin-Lluesma *et al.*, 2008). Since DDB1 is essential for preventing DNA re-replication and maintaining genomic integrity (Lee & Zhou, 2007), this finding raises the possibility that X protein interferes with the normal function of DDB1 by binding to it. The regulated degradation of Cdt1 is believed to be a key mechanism by which DDB1 performs these functions (Lovejoy *et al.*, 2006). However, the degradation of Cdt1 appears to be normal in cells expressing X protein (Martin-Lluesma *et al.*, 2008). It is possible that X protein dysregulates a different function of DDB1 or redirects DDB1 to a different substrate that is important for normal S phase progression. Alternatively, Cdt1 expression can be activated by X protein (Rakotomalala *et al.*, 2008). Intriguingly, the other viral proteins discussed in Sec. 5.2.1.4 that bind DDB1 also perturb the cell cycle (Dehart & Planelles, 2008; Liang *et al.*, 2006; Lin & Lamb, 2000).

One question raised by the finding that X protein causes abnormal mitoses, whatever the mechanism, is why there are not gross liver abnormalities in transgenic mice expressing X protein in hepatocytes. In these mice, X protein is believed to be expressed from birth, and the liver is known to undergo postnatal expansion by cell division. A possible explanation is that the level of X protein may be much higher in the transfected cells than in the transgenic hepatocytes, which thus may exhibit only subtle mitotic defects. Up to now, there are conflicting data in the literature regarding the effect of X protein on hepatocyte replication following partial hepatectomy, with both delay and acceleration of the cell cycle being found (Hodgson *et al.*, 2008; Tralhao *et al.*, 2002; Wu *et al.*, 2006). These discrepant results may be attributed to the fact that these studies have been done using very different mouse models and methodologies. Furthermore, cell culture studies have shown that although S phase progression is slowed by X protein, entry into and progression through G1 is actually promoted by X protein (Bouchard *et al.*, 2001a; Lee *et al.*, 2002); therefore, apparently conflicting results can potentially be obtained, depending on the methods used. Clearly, it will be important to perform additional experiments using standardized mouse strains and conditions. Another possibility is that chronic expression of X protein may allow the host cell to adapt. Acute expression of X protein in the liver by hydrodynamic transfection or other methods in the intact animal may provide useful insights.

5.2.2. *Other viral proteins potentially involved in carcinogenesis*

X protein is not the only virally encoded protein implicated in carcinogenesis. In particular, aberrant products of mutated surface genes have been found to have possibly oncogenic effects on the host. Two such products are described below.

5.2.2.1. Truncated MSP

Some HCCs contain fragments of HBV that result in potential expression of a truncated MSP. This protein (usually called MHBs^t) apparently does not interact normally with the ER, resulting in a cytosolic disposition of its N-terminus, in contrast with the luminal orientation of the full-length protein (Hildt *et al.*, 1995). The N-terminus can then activate the protein kinase C pathway, with resultant c-Raf-1/Erk2 signaling (Hildt *et al.*, 2002). Expression of MHBs^t in the liver of transgenic mice leads to formation of tumors, likely representing hyperplastic nodules, in both male and female mice at a higher frequency than non-transgenic controls (Hildt *et al.*, 2002). The equal incidence of nodules in both sexes is different from the situation in people with hepatitis B, wherein male sex is strongly associated with carcinogenesis (Giannitrapani *et al.*, 2006). It is also worth noting that MHBs^t is likely greatly overexpressed in these mice, as the strong albumin promoter was used to drive transcription, and the β-globin intron was used to substitute for the posttranscriptional regulatory element (Huang & Yen, 1994, 1995), which is a downstream RNA element that is needed for efficient export of the mRNA and is missing in the naturally occurring truncated HBV genomes that express MHBs^t. Thus, further study of this protein in a more natural context is needed to confirm its role in carcinogenesis during human infections. In any case, presumably only a minority of HCC arise from hepatocytes with HBV fragments capable of expressing MHBs^t.

5.2.2.2. preS2 mutants

Several groups have independently demonstrated that patients with advanced HBV-related disease (cirrhosis and especially HCC) show a markedly increased incidence of circulating viruses with mutations in the preS2 region of the genome (Chen *et al.*, 2008; Fang *et al.*, 2008; Huy *et al.*, 2003; Raimondo *et al.*, 2004; Tai *et al.*, 2002). Typically, these viruses contain in-frame deletions of the N-terminus of the preS2 region, associated with a missense mutation of the ATG start codon of the preS2 region, although some patients have only one or the other mutation. As a result of these mutations, there is expression of an internally deleted LSP, lack of expression of MS protein, and slightly decreased expression of small S protein because of the deletion of a small portion of the S promoter. These viruses likely arise because of immune pressure, and they appear to be infectious, since a prototypical preS2 mutant virus can infect hepatocytes in culture (Fernholz *et al.*, 1993) and since in rare cases, patients with acute hepatitis B have been found to have only preS2 mutants detectably circulating in the serum (Pollicino *et al.*, 1997; Sterneck *et al.*, 1998).

Cultured cells transfected with preS2 mutants show a mild defect in the export of surface proteins, as reflected by a small increase in the ratio of intracellular versus secreted surface proteins (Fan *et al.*, 2001). This phenotype is likely a result of the synthesis of an abnormal ratio of large to small S proteins, since increased levels of LSP in subviral particles lead to retention of these particles in the distal ER (Xu *et al.*, 1997a). Presumably because of this retention, ER stress ensues (Xu *et al.*, 1997b). This type of stress induces a signaling pathway from the ER to the cytosol and nucleus called the unfolded protein response (UPR), which either allows the host cell to eliminate or adapt to the stress, or causes the cell to undergo apoptosis (Lin *et al.*, 2008). Some of the proteins induced by the UPR, such as the chaperone GRP78 (BiP) and the transcription factor XBP1, have been linked to malignancies (Ma & Hendershot, 2004). These proteins are not only more highly expressed in cancer cells than in non-transformed cells, knocking down their expression prevents growth of fibrosarcoma cells xenografted into nude mice (Jamora *et al.*, 1996; Romero-Ramirez *et al.*, 2004). Furthermore, transgenic mice engineered to overexpress XBP1 in B-lymphocytes develop a B-cell derived malignancy similar to multiple myeloma (Carrasco *et al.*, 2007). Therefore, XBP1 appears to be a *bona fide* proto-oncogene. Other carcinogenic pathways have also been proposed to be activated by preS2 mutants via additional mechanisms (Wang *et al.*, 2005). Thus, based on the clinical and laboratory observations, it has been suggested that preS2 mutations may play a causative role in carcinogenesis (Fang *et al.*, 2008). Indeed, a single transgenic mouse line containing a fragment of the HBV genome with a typical preS2 mutation has been generated, and the livers of the mice show hepatocyte dysplasia (Su *et al.*, 2008). Further study on these mutants is clearly warranted, although again it is unlikely that all HCC patients are infected by these mutants.

5.2.2.3. Core gene mutants

Two types of mutations commonly arise in the core gene during chronic hepatitis B. The first, known as precore mutation, contains a premature termination codon in the precore coding region and hence leads to an inability of the mutant to synthesize the precore protein and its degradation product, HBeAg (Carman *et al.*, 1989). The precore gene products are believed to suppress host immunity and/or viral replication (Chen *et al.*, 2004; Ou, 1997), and hence precore mutants may be predicted to have a greater pathogenic potential than the wild-type virus. However, although some early studies have shown an association of these mutants with more aggressive disease and higher incidence of HCC, other studies have either come to the opposite conclusion or found no difference in clinical outcomes with wild-type virus (Mendy *et al.*, 2008; Tong *et al.*, 2006; Yang *et al.*, 2008; Yuen *et al.*, 2008). Hence, the role of these mutants, if any, in carcinogenesis is unknown.

The other type of core gene mutants contains point mutations in the basal promoter and the upstream enhancer II. The most common of these show linked double mutations at nucleotide positions 1762 and 1764. Remarkably, several recent studies have consistently shown an association of this double mutant with HCC, independent of serum HBV viral load and ALT levels (Kao *et al.*, 2003; Liu *et al.*, 2006; Tong *et al.*, 2006; Yang *et al.*, 2008; Yuen *et al.*, 2008). The mechanism by which this mutant may have increased oncogenic potential is unclear. One possibility is suggested by the observation that, because the double mutation changes the spectrum of host transcription factors that bind in this region of the core promoter

(Li *et al.*, 1999; Zheng *et al.*, 2004), there is a decrease in precore gene expression and hence this mutant would behave similarly to the precore mutant discussed above. However, given that the precore mutant does not have a strong association with HCC and that the association of the core promoter double mutant with HCC is independent of viral load and liver injury, altered precore protein expression is likely not the major explanation for the increased oncogenic potential of this mutant. The more intriguing possibility comes from the observation that the double mutation is actually within the X coding region and hence leads to sequence changes in the X protein. The resulting mutant X protein is known to have more potent transcriptional activity in cultured cells (Li *et al.*, 2002; Zheng *et al.*, 2004) and thus may well have increased oncogenic functions, as well. It will be important to test this hypothesis in transgenic mice.

5.2.3. *Insertional mutagenesis*

Fragments of HBV genome commonly integrate randomly into the host chromosome and almost all HBV-associated HCC contain clonally integrated HBV DNA (Ganem & Schneider, 2001), raising the possibility that such an insertion could specifically activate a host proto-oncogene or inactivate a tumor suppressor gene to cause HCC. Indeed, the related WHV has been shown to integrate frequently within or near the *c-Myc*, *N-Myc*, or, most frequently, *N-Myc2* proto-oncogene, resulting in its transcriptional activation in woodchuck HCC (Hsu *et al.*, 1988). In contrast, early studies revealed that no common HBV integration site could be found in the case of human HCC (Nagaya *et al.*, 1987). Recent analyses confirmed the absence of a single common integration site but found that the telomerase gene and the mixed-lineage leukemia (MLL) 4 proto-oncogene were repeatedly targeted, albeit still in a small minority of tumors (Murakami *et al.*, 2005; Saigo *et al.*, 2008). Other cancer-related genes, such as those for cyclin A and retinoid acid receptor, have been shown to be targeted in a single HCC each (Benbrook *et al.*, 1988; Wang *et al.*, 1990). These findings suggest that, even though HBV integration does not target a single specific gene for oncogenesis, it is possible that in a subset of HCC the integration event contributes to carcinogenesis via multiple different mechanisms, depending on the specific host gene affected by HBV integration. In support of this view, one study showed that, among the HCCs without HBV integration near MLL 4, approximately 2/3 showed translocation of MLL 4 on chromosome 19 to a specific region of chromosome 17 (Saigo *et al.*, 2008). These data suggest that MLL 4 deregulation commonly plays a role in HCC oncogenesis and that in a minority of HCC HBV integration is the means of this deregulation.

However, it is important to note that as yet there is no experimental proof of a role for HBV integration in liver carcinogenesis. For the WHV, such evidence is extremely strong, as transgenic mice containing a viral/*N-myc2* fusion gene isolated from a woodchuck HCC develop HCC at a high frequency (Renard *et al.*, 2000). No similar experiment has been performed for HBV. It is also relevant to note that the woodchuck virus causes HCC in almost all chronically infected woodchucks within 2–4 years, while HBV causes HCC in a minority of people and usually over a time span of several decades, yet viral genomic integration is as common in human as in woodchuck HCCs. Thus, it seems unlikely that HBV integration plays a consistent role in human carcinogenesis, unlike the situation in woodchucks.

Another possible mechanism by which integrated HBV DNA may contribute to carcinogenesis has been proposed. It has been noted that HBV integrants are sometimes present in sites of gross chromosomal rearrangements, such as translocations (Rogler *et al.*, 1987). This observation led to the suggestion that integrated HBV can induce chromosomal instability by inducing recombination between different HBV integrants. Indeed, a small region of the HBV genome has been shown to facilitate *in-vitro* recombination (Kajino *et al.*, 1994). However, as the number of integrants in a single HCC is limited, it is unlikely that this mechanism can account for the generalized chromosomal instability found in HBV-induced HCC.

A final possibility is that HBV DNA integration leads to deregulation of a viral gene that is oncogenic. This would be similar to the situation for HPV, whose E6–E7 oncoproteins become overexpressed upon integration of the viral DNA into random sites in the host chromosome (Chap. 4). Many HBV integrants show truncation of the downstream end of the X gene (Poussin *et al.*, 1999; Takada & Koike, 1990), and it has been suggested that truncated X proteins may have increased oncogenic potential, based on cell culture studies (Tu *et al.*, 2001; Wang *et al.*, 2004; Xu *et al.*, 2007). However, no transgenic mice containing a truncated X gene have been described.

5.3. Role of Liver Injury and Inflammation

Based on clinical observations, chronic liver injury and inflammation are clearly risk factors for HCC, whatever the inciting cause (Sec. 5.1). Chisari and colleagues were able to confirm the role of these factors in a mouse model of HCC (Chisari *et al.*, 1989). They generated transgenic mice that express the HBV LSP under the control of the strong albumin promoter, whose activity is largely restricted to hepatocytes. As discussed in Sec. 5.2.2.2, surface protein particles made up mostly or purely of LSP cannot be secreted but remain in the lumen of the distal ER. This accumulation, if severe enough, results in cellular injury that eventually kills the host cell (Foo *et al.*, 2002). Therefore, some strains of the albumin-LSP transgenic mice suffer from chronic liver injury. After a latency period of approximately one year, many of these male mice develop HCC (Chisari *et al.*, 1989). In contrast, albumin-LSP transgenic mouse lines that express relatively low levels of LSP do not suffer from chronic hepatitis and do not develop HCC (Chisari *et al.*, 1989). Remarkably, if chronic hepatitis is induced in these latter mice by adoptive transfer of lymphocytes from non-transgenic mice immunized against surface proteins, they become highly susceptible to HCC, albeit at a relatively late age (almost two years old) (Nakamoto *et al.*, 1998).

These data clearly show an important role for liver injury and inflammation in HCC pathogenesis. However, it should be noted that these mice express HBV gene products, and hence a cofactor role for one or more viral factors cannot be excluded. Although the amount of 0.8 kb X mRNA is apparently undetectable in the liver by Northern blotting in these mice (Chisari *et al.*, 1989), the X protein may nevertheless be one such factor as a low level of expression cannot be ruled out. Furthermore, a significant amount of X protein may be translated from a 4-kb transcript that results from read-through of the polyadenylation signal at the first pass (Guo *et al.*, 1991); this mRNA was not specifically examined in these mice. More importantly, because LSP is a strong activator of the UPR in cultured cells (Xu *et al.*, 1997b), a role for the UPR in liver carcinogenesis in these mice cannot be excluded (see Sec. 5.2.2.2 for a discussion of UPR and carcinogenesis). Although it is not clear if the UPR is activated in the hepatocytes of the albumin-LSP mice, this possibility clearly needs to be investigated. Indeed, there is already indirect evidence that LSP may play a role in carcinogenesis in these mice. The HCC in these mice do not show expression of LSP, despite the presence of the intact transgene (Chisari *et al.*, 1989). Initially, this finding was taken to indicate that the LSP-expressing cells stop proliferating and/or die, leading to selective proliferation and eventual malignant transformation of a minor population of non-expressing cells. However, subsequent analysis revealed that nodules of non-LSP-expressing but non-malignant hepatocytes also arise in these livers, starting at a time prior to HCC development (Crawford *et al.*, 2006). Detailed genetic studies revealed that these non-transformed, non-expressing hepatocytes contain inactivating somatic mutations in the LSP gene, while, in agreement with the previous study, the malignant hepatocytes do not show such mutations (Crawford *et al.*, 2006). The lack of LSP expression in the fully transformed cells probably results from the dedifferentiation of these cells, since the HBV enhancers and the LSP promoter all depend on hepatocyte-enriched transcription factors for maximal expression (Yen, 1993). Apparently, loss of LSP expression due to somatic mutation of the transgene leads to the loss (or a marked decrease) of the ability of the host hepatocyte to become malignantly transformed. These results suggest that hepatocytes expressing LSP are actually the ones most likely to undergo transformation; in other words, LSP provides a cell-intrinsic component to oncogenesis. In any case, it appears premature to conclude from these mice that chronic liver injury, inflammation, and hepatocyte turnover are sufficient to cause HCC, even though these factors are clearly necessary in this model.

5.4. Dietary Carcinogens

Aflatoxins are metabolites of *Aspergillus flavus* and related fungi that grow on heat- and drought-stressed grain and nut plants and can contaminate improperly stored grain and nuts in warm, humid climates (Smela *et al.*, 2001). They have been experimentally proven to cause HCC in animals (Wogan & Pong, 1970), and epidemiological studies suggest a similar effect in people (Smela *et al.*, 2001). Aflatoxins form DNA adducts that lead to G:C to T:A transversions (Smela *et al.*, 2001), and it is presumed that it is this mutagenic property that leads to carcinogenesis.

More recent studies using molecular markers confirm the role of aflatoxins in HCC pathogenesis and further show a synergistic effect with HBV infection. A hallmark of aflatoxin exposure is the presence of aflatoxin–nucleotide or aflatoxin–protein adducts in urine, serum, and other bodily fluids. A study in China showed that, compared with controls, the presence of these adducts alone caused a 3.4 increase in HCC risk and the presence of chronic hepatitis B alone caused a 7.3 increase, while the presence of both dramatically increased the risk to 59.4 (Qian *et al.*, 1994). Studies conducted in Taiwan and the Gambia similarly revealed a strong synergism between aflatoxins and HBV in hepatic carcinogenesis (Kirk *et al.*, 2005b; Wang *et al.*, 1996). Another footprint of aflatoxin exposure is the presence of an inactivating G to T transversion at codon 249 of the tumor suppressor gene *p53*. This mutation has been repeatedly shown to be much more frequent in HCC and even non-tumorous liver tissues of people in high aflatoxin-exposure regions (Aguilar *et al.*, 1994; Kirk *et al.*, 2005a; Pineau *et al.*, 2008), confirming that aflatoxin exposure can indeed lead to DNA mutations in hepatocytes. TP53 mutation has been found to be present mostly in more advanced and aggressive hepatic neoplasms, suggesting that it plays a role in tumor progression (Lunn *et al.*, 1997; Su *et al.*, 2000; Teramoto *et al.*, 1994). A plausible molecular mechanism by which HBV and aflatoxins can synergize is that, as discussed in Sec. 5.2.1.5, the X protein may decrease the ability of the cell to repair aflatoxin-induced mutations. In any case, reducing environmental aflatoxin exposure appears to be a relatively straightforward and inexpensive way to reduce HCC risk among people with chronic hepatitis B (Turner *et al.*, 2005).

Nitrosamines are found in foods such as cured meats, preserved vegetables, and beer, as well as in cigarette smoke (Mitacek *et al.*, 1999), and they are DNA alkylating agents that have been clearly shown to be hepatic carcinogens in animals (Schoeffner & Thorgeirsson, 2000). Whether the levels ingested by people are sufficient to cause a significant number of HCC is unknown, since there is no reliable biomarker for nitrosamine exposure. Notably, transgenic mice expressing either the entire HBV genome or only the X gene, that normally do not develop HCC, show increased susceptibility to HCC induction by nitrosamines (Madden *et al.*, 2001; Zheng *et al.*, 2007a). Thus, it is possible that nitrosamines such as aflatoxins can synergize with HBV in carcinogenesis.

Prolonged alcohol consumption in high doses moderately increases the risk of HCC, but the risk appears to be additive with that of chronic hepatitis B (Chen *et al.*, 1991; Kuper *et al.*, 2000; Wang *et al.*, 2003), indicating a lack of interaction between these factors. Smoking is also now generally believed to be a weak hepatic carcinogen (Chuang *et al.*, 2008), but contradictory results have been obtained as to whether it may synergize with HBV in causing HCC (Chen *et al.*, 1991; Kuper *et al.*, 2000; Wang *et al.*, 2003).

5.5. Other Aspects of HBV Oncogenesis

5.5.1. *Role of genotypes*

Eight genotypes of HBV have been characterized, and some differences in the biology among them have been noted, although because there is geographic variation in the prevalence of the genotypes, in many cases it is not clear if the differences are due to the virus or to the host and/or environment (McMahon, 2005). However, genotype C has recently been shown to be more strongly associated with HCC than genotype B in relatively homogenous populations in Taiwan and Hong Kong (Yang *et al.*, 2008; Yu *et al.*, 2005; Yuen *et al.*, 2004). Initially, it appeared that this may have been due to the increased occurrence of the double core promoter mutation (see Sec. 5.2.2.3) in genotype C (Yu *et al.*, 2005), but a large study subsequently showed that genotype C and the core promoter mutation are independent risk factors for HCC (Yang *et al.*, 2008). The increased pathogenicity of genotype C also cannot be accounted for by greater viral load or ALT levels. The mechanism of increased oncogenicity by genotype C has not been characterized.

5.5.2. *Role of sex hormones*

HCC, whether due to hepatitis B or other causes, is more common in men than women (El-Serag & Rudolph, 2007; Giannitrapani *et al.*, 2006). It has long been known that, upon exposure, men have higher average levels of serum HBV particles and a stronger propensity to develop chronic liver diseases than women, possibly because of activation of HBV transcription by androgen (Breidbart *et al.*, 1993), but even after taking these differences into consideration, male sex is an independent risk factor for HCC (Yuen *et al.*, 2009). Recently, two groups have shown that the X protein interacts with the androgen receptor and increases the transcriptional activity of the latter (Chiu *et al.*, 2007; Zheng *et al.*, 2007b). Since the androgen receptor appears to play a direct role in hepatocarcinogenesis (Ma *et al.*, 2008), this function of X protein may be important in the increased incidence of HCC in HBV-infected men. On the other hand, androgen receptor knockout mice still show a male predominance in carcinogen-induced HCC incidence (Ma *et al.*, 2008), implying the importance of additional sex-specific factors, such as differences in cytokine responses (Naugler *et al.*, 2007). Once a good mouse model of HBV-induced HCC has been established, it will be important to determine if the androgen receptor is necessary for the sexual dimorphism of HCC development, as the results, if positive, may well have implications for the prevention of HCC in HBV-infected men.

6. Summary

In common with the other oncogenic viruses discussed in this book, the mechanism of HBV-induced carcinogenesis is clearly complex and incompletely understood. As detailed above, multiple factors are almost surely involved. That is, viral factors (acting in *trans* by one or more protein products and in *cis* by chromosomal insertion) and cellular damage and regeneration induced by chronic hepatitis act synergistically to induce HCC, with a further contribution from endogenous and ingested carcinogens. In any individual patient, many but not necessarily all of these factors would probably be at play. This scenario is consistent with all existing literature and would explain why not all causes of chronic hepatitis show an equally strong association with HCC, and why HCC in people with chronic HBV infection frequently but not invariably arises in the setting of long-standing chronic hepatitis. Clearly, better animal models of HBV infection and carcinogenesis are needed to prove this inference and clarify the mechanistic details. Only then can new and rational means of predicting and treating HCC during chronic hepatitis B be developed.

Note

A recent paper by Keasler *et al.* has demonstrated that nuclear but not cytosolic X protein increases HBV replication in a mouse model. Thus, it is very likely that X protein has separate functions in both the nucleus and cytosol.

References

Aggarwal S, Kim SW, Ryu SH, Chung WC, Koo JS (2008) Growth suppression of lung cancer cells by targeting cyclic AMP response element-binding protein. *Cancer Res* **68**: 981–988.

Aguilar F, Harris CC, Sun T, Hollstein M, Cerutti P (1994) Geographic variation of *p53* mutational profile in nonmalignant human liver. *Science* **264**: 1317–1319.

Ames BN, Gold LS (1990) Too many rodent carcinogens: mitogenesis increases mutagenesis. *Science* **249**: 970–971.

Beasley RP, Hwang LY, Lin CC, Chien CS (1981) Hepatocellular carcinoma and hepatitis B virus. A prospective study of 22,707 men in Taiwan. *Lancet* **2**: 1129–1133.

Benbrook D, Lernhardt E, Pfahl M (1988) A new retinoic acid receptor identified from a hepatocellular carcinoma. *Nature* **333**: 669–672.

Bergametti F, Sitterlin D, Transy C (2002) Turnover of hepatitis B virus X protein is regulated by damaged DNA-binding complex. *J Virol* **76**: 6495–6501.

Billet O, Grimber G, Levrero M, Seye KA, Briand P, Joulin V (1995) *In vivo* activity of the hepatitis B virus core promoter: tissue specificity and temporal regulation. *J Virol* **69**: 5912–5916.

Blum HE, Zhang ZS, Galun E, von Weizsacker F, Garner B, Liang TJ, Wands JR (1992) Hepatitis B virus X protein is not central to the viral life cycle *in vitro*. *J Virol* **66**: 1223–1227.

Bontron S, Lin-Marq N, Strubin M (2002) Hepatitis B virus X protein associated with UV-DDB1 induces cell death in the nucleus and is functionally antagonized by UV-DDB2. *J Biol Chem* **277**: 38847–38854.

Bouchard M, Giannakopoulos S, Wang EH, Tanese N, Schneider RJ (2001a) Hepatitis B virus HBx protein activation of cyclin A-cyclin-dependent kinase 2 complexes and G1 transit via a Src kinase pathway. *J Virol* **75**: 4247–4257.

Bouchard MJ, Wang LH, Schneider RJ (2001b) Calcium signaling by HBx protein in hepatitis B virus DNA replication. *Science* **294**: 2376–2378.

Bouchard MJ, Puro RJ, Wang L, Schneider RJ (2003) Activation and inhibition of cellular calcium and tyrosine kinase signaling pathways identify targets of the HBx protein involved in hepatitis B virus replication. *J Virol* **77**: 7713–7719.

Breidbart S, Burk RD, Saenger P (1993) Hormonal regulation of hepatitis B virus gene expression: influence of androgen receptor. *Pediatr Res* **34**: 300–302.

Bruix J, Boix L, Sala M, Llovet JM (2004) Focus on hepatocellular carcinoma. *Cancer Cell* **5**: 215–219.

Carman WF, Jacyna MR, Hadziyannis S, Karayiannis P, McGarvey MJ, Makris A, Thomas HC (1989) Mutation preventing formation of hepatitis B e antigen in patients with chronic hepatitis B infection. *Lancet* **2**: 588–591.

Carrasco DR, Sukhdeo K, Protopopova M, Sinha R, Enos M, Carrasco DE, Zheng M, Mani M, Henderson J, Pinkus GS, Munshi N, Horner J, Ivanova EV, Protopopov A, Anderson KC, Tonon G, DePinho RA (2007) The differentiation and stress response factor XBP-1 drives multiple myeloma pathogenesis. *Cancer Cell* **11**: 349–360.

Cha MY, Kim CM, Park YM, Ryu WS (2004) Hepatitis B virus X protein is essential for the activation of Wnt/beta-catenin signaling in hepatoma cells. *Hepatology* **39**: 1683–1693.

Chang MH, Chen CJ, Lai MS, Hsu HM, Wu TC, Kong MS, Liang DC, Shau WY, Chen DS (1997) Universal hepatitis B vaccination in Taiwan and the incidence of hepatocellular carcinoma in children. Taiwan Childhood Hepatoma Study Group. *N Engl J Med* **336**: 1855–1859.

Chen CH, Changchien CS, Lee CM, Hung CH, Hu TH, Wang JH, Wang JC, Lu SN (2008) Combined mutations in pre-s/surface and core promoter/precore regions of hepatitis B virus increase the risk of hepatocellular carcinoma: a case-control study. *J Infect Dis* **198**: 1634–1642.

Chen CJ, Liang KY, Chang AS, Chang YC, Lu SN, Liaw YF, Chang WY, Sheen MC, Lin TM (1991) Effects of hepatitis B virus, alcohol drinking, cigarette smoking and familial tendency on hepatocellular carcinoma. *Hepatology* **13**: 398–406.

Chen CJ, Yang HI, Su J, Jen CL, You SL, Lu SN, Huang GT, Iloeje UH (2006) Risk of hepatocellular carcinoma across a biological gradient of serum hepatitis B virus DNA level. *JAMA* **295**: 65–73.

Chen HS, Kaneko S, Girones R, Anderson RW, Hornbuckle WE, Tennant BC, Cote PJ, Gerin JL, Purcell RH, Miller RH (1993) The woodchuck hepatitis virus X gene is important for establishment of virus infection in woodchucks. *J Virol* **67**: 1218–1226.

Chen MT, Billaud JN, Sallberg M, Guidotti LG, Chisari FV, Jones J, Hughes J, Milich DR (2004) A function of the hepatitis B virus precore protein is to regulate the immune response to the core antigen. *Proc Natl Acad Sci USA* **101**: 14913–14918.

Cheong JH, Yi M, Lin Y, Murakami S (1995) Human RPB5, a subunit shared by eukaryotic nuclear RNA polymerases, binds human hepatitis B virus X protein and may play a role in X transactivation. *Embo J* **14**: 143–150.

Chisari FV (1991) Analysis of hepadnavirus gene expression, biology, and pathogenesis in the transgenic mouse. *Curr Top Microbiol Immunol* **168**: 85–101.

Chisari FV, Klopchin K, Moriyama T, Pasquinelli C, Dunsford HA, Sell S, Pinkert CA, Brinster RL, Palmiter RD (1989) Molecular pathogenesis of hepatocellular carcinoma in hepatitis B virus transgenic mice. *Cell* **59**: 1145–1156.

Chiu CM, Yeh SH, Chen PJ, Kuo TJ, Chang CJ, Chen PJ, Yang WJ, Chen DS (2007) Hepatitis B virus X protein enhances androgen receptor-responsive gene expression depending on androgen level. *Proc Natl Acad Sci USA* **104**: 2571–2578.

Choi BH, Park GT, Rho HM (1999) Interaction of hepatitis B viral X protein and CCAAT/enhancer-binding protein alpha synergistically activates the hepatitis B viral enhancer II/pregenomic promoter. *J Biol Chem* **274**: 2858–2865.

Chuang SC, Vecchia CL, Boffetta P (2008) Liver cancer: descriptive epidemiology and risk factors other than HBV and HCV infection. *Cancer Lett* in press.

Cougot D, Neuveut C, Buendia MA (2005) HBV induced carcinogenesis. *J Clin Virol* **34**(1): S75–S78.

Cougot D, Wu Y, Cairo S, Caramel J, Renard CA, Levy L, Buendia MA, Neuveut C (2007) The hepatitis B virus X protein functionally interacts with CREB-binding protein/p300 in the regulation of CREB-mediated transcription. *J Biol Chem* **282**: 4277–4287.

Crawford DR, Ostrowski S, Vakharia D, Ilic Z, Sell S (2006) Separate origins of hepatitis B virus surface antigen-negative foci and hepatocellular carcinomas in transgenic HBsAg (alb/psx) mice. *Am J Pathol* **169**: 223–232.

Cutroneo KR, White SL, Chiu JF, Ehrlich HP (2006) Tissue fibrosis and carcinogenesis: divergent or successive pathways dictate multiple molecular therapeutic targets for oligo decoy therapies. *J Cell Biochem* **97**: 1161–1174.

Daniel D, Meyer-Morse N, Bergsland EK, Dehne K, Coussens LM, Hanahan D (2003) Immune enhancement of skin carcinogenesis by CD4+ T cells. *J Exp Med* **197**: 1017–1028. Epub 2003 Apr 14.

Dehart JL, Planelles V (2008) Human immunodeficiency virus type 1 Vpr links proteasomal degradation and checkpoint activation. *J Virol* **82**: 1066–1072.

Devaux P, Hodge G, McChesney MB, Cattaneo R (2008) Attenuation of V- or C-defective measles viruses: infection control by the inflammatory and interferon responses of rhesus monkeys. *J Virol* **82**: 5359–5367.

Donato F, Boffetta P, Puoti M (1998) A meta-analysis of epidemiological studies on the combined effect of hepatitis B and C virus infections in causing hepatocellular carcinoma. *Int J Cancer* **75**: 347–354.

El-Serag HB, Rudolph KL (2007) Hepatocellular carcinoma: epidemiology and molecular carcinogenesis. *Gastroenterology* **132**: 2557–2576.

Fan YF, Lu CC, Chen WC, Yao WJ, Wang HC, Chang TT, Lei HY, Shiau AL, Su IJ (2001) Prevalence and significance of hepatitis B virus (HBV) pre-S mutants in serum and liver at different replicative stages of chronic HBV infection. *Hepatology* **33**: 277–286.

Fang ZL, Sabin CA, Dong BQ, Wei SC, Chen QY, Fang KX, Yang JY, Huang J, Wang XY, Harrison TJ (2008) Hepatitis B virus pre-S deletion mutations are a risk factor for hepatocellular carcinoma: a matched nested case-control study. *J Gen Virol* **89**: 2882–2890.

Farazi PA, DePinho RA (2006) Hepatocellular carcinoma pathogenesis: from genes to environment. *Nat Rev Cancer* **6**: 674–687.

Fernholz D, Galle PR, Stemler M, Brunetto M, Bonino F, Will H (1993) Infectious hepatitis B virus variant defective in pre-S2 protein expression in a chronic carrier. *Virology* **194**: 137–148.

Fischer M, Runkel L, Schaller H (1995) HBx protein of hepatitis B virus interacts with the C-terminal portion of a novel human proteasome alpha-subunit. *Virus Genes* **10**: 99–102.

Foo NC, Ahn BY, Ma X, Hyun W, Yen TS (2002) Cellular vacuolization and apoptosis induced by hepatitis B virus large surface protein. *Hepatology* **36**: 1400–1407.

Forgues M, Difilippantonio MJ, Linke SP, Ried T, Nagashima K, Feden J, Valerie K, Fukasawa K, Wang XW (2003) Involvement of Crm1 in hepatitis B virus X protein-induced aberrant centriole replication and abnormal mitotic spindles. *Mol Cell Biol* **23**: 5282–5292.

Ganem D, Schneider R (2001) Hepadnaviridae: the viruses and their replication. In Fields BN, Knipe DM, Howley PM (eds.), *Fields Virology*, pp. 2923–2969. Philadelphia: Lippincott-Raven.

Giannitrapani L, Soresi M, La Spada E, Cervello M, D'Alessandro N, Montalto G (2006) Sex hormones and risk of liver tumor. *Ann NY Acad Sci* **1089**: 228–236.

Goldstein ST, Zhou F, Hadler SC, Bell BP, Mast EE, Margolis HS (2005) A mathematical model to estimate global hepatitis B disease burden and vaccination impact. *Int J Epidemiol* **34**: 1329–1339.

Greten FR, Eckmann L, Greten TF, Park JM, Li ZW, Egan LJ, Kagnoff MF, Karin M (2004) IKKbeta links inflammation and tumorigenesis in a mouse model of colitis-associated cancer. *Cell* **118**: 285–296.

Guidotti LG, Matzke B, Schaller H, Chisari FV (1995) High-level hepatitis B virus replication in transgenic mice. *J Virol* **69**: 6158–6169.

Guo WT, Wang J, Tam G, Yen TS, Ou JS (1991) Leaky transcription termination produces larger and smaller than genome size hepatitis B virus X gene transcripts. *Virology* **181**: 630–636.

Haviv I, Shamay M, Doitsh G, Shaul Y (1998) Hepatitis B virus pX targets TFIIB in transcription coactivation. *Mol Cell Biol* **18**: 1562–1569.

Higa LA, Zhang H (2007) Stealing the spotlight: CUL4-DDB1 ubiquitin ligase docks WD40-repeat proteins to destroy. *Cell Div* **2**: 5.

Hildt E, Munz B, Saher G, Reifenberg K, Hofschneider PH (2002) The PreS2 activator MHBs(t) of hepatitis B virus activates c-raf-1/Erk2 signaling in transgenic mice. *Embo J* **21**: 525–535.

Hildt E, Urban S, Hofschneider PH (1995) Characterization of essential domains for the functionality of the MHBst transcriptional activator and identification of a minimal MHBst activator. *Oncogene* **11**: 2055–2066.

Hino O, Ohtake K, Rogler CE (1989) Features of two hepatitis B virus (HBV) DNA integrations suggest mechanisms of HBV integration. *J Virol* **63**: 2638–2643.

Hodgson AJ, Keasler VV, Slagle BL (2008) Premature cell cycle entry induced by hepatitis B virus regulatory HBx protein during compensatory liver regeneration. *Cancer Res* **68**: 10341–10348.

Hofseth LJ, Ying L (2005) Identifying and defusing weapons of mass inflammation in carcinogenesis. *Biochim Biophys Acta* **1765**: 76–84.

Hollinger FB, Liang TJ (2001) Hepatitis B virus. In Fields BN, Knipe DM, Howley PM (eds.), *Fields Virology*, pp. 2971–3036. Philadelphia: Lippincott-Raven.

Hsu HC, Jeng YM, Mao TL, Chu JS, Lai PL, Peng SY (2000) Beta-catenin mutations are associated with a subset of low-stage hepatocellular carcinoma negative for hepatitis B virus and with favorable prognosis. *Am J Pathol* **157**: 763–770.

Hsu HC, Wu MZ, Chang MH, Su IJ, Chen DS (1987) Childhood hepatocellular carcinoma develops exclusively in hepatitis B surface antigen carriers in three decades in Taiwan. *J Hepatol* **5**: 260–267.

Hsu T, Moroy T, Etiemble J, Louise A, Trepo C, Tiollai P, Buendia MA (1988) Activation of *c-myc* by woodchuck hepatitis virus insertion in hepatocellular carcinoma. *Cell* **55**: 627–635.

Hu Z, Zhang Z, Doo E, Coux O, Goldberg AL, Liang TJ (1999) Hepatitis B virus X protein is both a substrate and a potential inhibitor of the proteasome complex. *J Virol* **73**: 7231–7240.

Hu Z, Zhang Z, Kim JW, Huang Y, Liang TJ (2006) Altered proteolysis and global gene expression in hepatitis B virus X transgenic mouse liver. *J Virol* **80**: 1405–1413.

Huang H, Fujii H, Sankila A, Mahler-Araujo BM, Matsuda M, Cathomas G, Ohgaki H (1999) Beta-catenin mutations are frequent in human hepatocellular carcinomas associated with hepatitis C virus infection. *Am J Pathol* **155**: 1795–1801.

Huang J, Kwong J, Sun EC, Liang TJ (1996) Proteasome complex as a potential cellular target of hepatitis B virus X protein. *J Virol* **70**: 5582–5591.

Huang ZM, Yen TS (1994) Hepatitis B virus RNA element that facilitates accumulation of surface gene transcripts in the cytoplasm. *J Virol* **68**: 3193–3199.

Huang ZM, Yen TS (1995) Role of the hepatitis B virus posttranscriptional regulatory element in export of intronless transcripts. *Mol Cell Biol* **15**: 3864–3869.

Huy TT, Ushijima H, Win KM, Luengrojanakul P, Shrestha PK, Zhong ZH, Smirnov AV, Taltavull TC, Sata T, Abe K (2003) High prevalence of hepatitis B virus pre-s mutant in countries where it is endemic and its relationship with genotype and chronicity. *J Clin Microbiol* **41**: 5449–5455.

Ikeda K, Marusawa H, Osaki Y, Nakamura T, Kitajima N, Yamashita Y, Kudo M, Sato T, Chiba T (2007) Antibody to hepatitis B core antigen and risk for hepatitis C-related hepatocellular carcinoma: a prospective study. *Ann Intern Med* **146**: 649–656.

Jamora C, Dennert G, Lee AS (1996) Inhibition of tumor progression by suppression of stress protein GRP78/BiP induction in fibrosarcoma B/C10ME. *Proc Natl Acad Sci USA* **93**: 7690–7694.

Kajino K, Hotta Y, Hino O (1994) Determination of a putative recombinogenic human hepatitis B virus sequence and its binding cellular protein. *Cancer Res* **54**: 3971–3973.

Kao JH, Chen PJ, Lai MY, Chen DS (2003) Basal core promoter mutations of hepatitis B virus increase the risk of hepatocellular carcinoma in hepatitis B carriers. *Gastroenterology* **124**: 327–334.

Kawai H, Suda T, Aoyagi Y, Isokawa O, Mita Y, Waguri N, Kuroiwa T, Igarashi M, Tsukada K, Mori S, Shimizu T, Suzuki Y, Abe Y, Takahashi T,

Nomoto M, Asakura H (2000) Quantitative evaluation of genomic instability as a possible predictor for development of hepatocellular carcinoma: comparison of loss of heterozygosity and replication error. *Hepatology* **31**: 1246–1250.

Keasler VV, Hodgson AJ, Madden CR, Slagle BL (2007) Enhancement of hepatitis B virus replication by the regulatory X protein *in vitro* and *in vivo*. *J Virol* **81**: 2656–2662.

Keasler VV, Hodgson AJ, Madden CR, Slagle BL (2009) Hepatitis B virus HBx protein localized to the nucleus restores HBx-deficient virus replication in HepG2 cells and *in vivo* in hydrodynamically-injected mice. *Virology*, in press.

Kim CM, Koike K, Saito I, Miyamura T, Jay G (1991) HBx gene of hepatitis B virus induces liver cancer in transgenic mice. *Nature* **351**: 317–320.

Kim S, Park SY, Yong H, Famulski JK, Chae S, Lee JH, Kang CM, Saya H, Chan GK, Cho H (2008) HBV X protein targets hBubR1, which induces dysregulation of the mitotic checkpoint. *Oncogene* **27**: 3457–3464.

Kirk GD, Lesi OA, Mendy M, Szymanska K, Whittle H, Goedert JJ, Hainaut P, Montesano R (2005a) 249(ser) TP53 mutation in plasma DNA, hepatitis B viral infection, and risk of hepatocellular carcinoma. *Oncogene* **24**: 5858–5867.

Kirk GD, Turner PC, Gong Y, Lesi OA, Mendy M, Goedert JJ, Hall AJ, Whittle H, Hainaut P, Montesano R, Wild CP (2005b) Hepatocellular carcinoma and polymorphisms in carcinogen-metabolizing and DNA repair enzymes in a population with aflatoxin exposure and hepatitis B virus endemicity. *Cancer Epidemiol Biomarkers Prev* **14**: 373–379.

Kline CL, Jackson R, Engelman R, Pledger WJ, Yeatman TJ, Irby RB (2008) Src kinase induces tumor formation in the c-SRC C57BL/6 mouse. *Int J Cancer* **122**: 2665–2673.

Ku NO, Wright TL, Terrault NA, Gish R, Omary MB (1997) Mutation of human keratin 18 in association with cryptogenic cirrhosis. *J Clin Invest* **99**: 19–23.

Kuper H, Tzonou A, Kaklamani E, Hsieh CC, Lagiou P, Adami HO, Trichopoulos D, Stuver SO (2000) Tobacco smoking, alcohol consumption and their interaction in the causation of hepatocellular carcinoma. *Int J Cancer* **85**: 498–502.

Kwee L, Lucito R, Aufiero B, Schneider RJ (1992) Alternate translation initiation on hepatitis B virus X mRNA produces multiple polypeptides that differentially transactivate class II and III promoters. *J Virol* **66**: 4382–4389.

Lara-Pezzi E, Roche S, Andrisani OM, Sanchez-Madrid F, Lopez-Cabrera M (2001) The hepatitis B virus HBx protein induces adherens junction disruption in a src-dependent manner. *Oncogene* **20**: 3323–3331.

Lau JY, Bain VG, Davies SE, O'Grady JG, Alberti A, Alexander GJ, Williams R (1992) High-level expression of hepatitis B viral antigens in fibrosing cholestatic hepatitis. *Gastroenterology* **102**: 956–962.

Le Rouzic E, Belaidouni N, Estrabaud E, Morel M, Rain JC, Transy C, Margottin-Goguet F (2007) HIV1 Vpr arrests the cell cycle by recruiting DCAF1/VprBP, a receptor of the Cul4-DDB1 ubiquitin ligase. *Cell Cycle* **6**: 182–188.

Lee J, Zhou P (2007) DCAFs, the missing link of the CUL4-DDB1 ubiquitin ligase. *Mol Cell* **26**: 775–780.

Lee S, Tarn C, Wang WH, Chen S, Hullinger RL, Andrisani OM (2002) Hepatitis B virus X protein differentially regulates cell cycle progression in X-transforming versus nontransforming hepatocyte (AML12) cell lines. *J Biol Chem* **277**: 8730–8740.

Lee TH, Finegold MJ, Shen RF, Demayo JL, Woo SL, Butel JS (1990) Hepatitis-B virus transactivator X-protein is not tumorigenic in transgenic mice. *J Virol* **64**: 5939–5947.

Li J, Buckwold VE, Hon MW, Ou JH (1999) Mechanism of suppression of hepatitis B virus precore RNA transcription by a frequent double mutation. *J Virol* **73**: 1239–1244.

Li J, Wang QE, Zhu Q, El-Mahdy MA, Wani G, Praetorius-Ibba M, Wani AA (2006) DNA damage binding protein component DDB1 participates in nucleotide excision repair through DDB2 DNA-binding and cullin 4A ubiquitin ligase activity. *Cancer Res* **66**: 8590–8597.

Li J, Xu Z, Zheng Y, Johnson DL, Ou JH (2002) Regulation of hepatocyte nuclear factor 1 activity by wild-type and mutant hepatitis B virus X proteins. *J Virol* **76**: 5875–5881.

Liang X, Pickering MT, Cho NH, Chang H, Volkert MR, Kowalik TF, Jung JU (2006) Deregulation of DNA damage signal transduction by herpesvirus latency-associated M2. *J Virol* **80**: 5862–5874.

Liang X, Shin YC, Means RE, Jung JU (2004) Inhibition of interferon-mediated antiviral activity by murine gammaherpesvirus 68 latency-associated M2 protein. *J Virol* **78**: 12416–12427.

Liaw YF, Sung JJ, Chow WC, Farrell G, Lee CZ, Yuen H, Tanwandee T, Tao QM, Shue K, Keene ON, Dixon JS, Gray DF, Sabbat J (2004) Lamivudine for patients with chronic hepatitis B and advanced liver disease. *N Engl J Med* **351**: 1521–1531.

Lin GY, Lamb RA (2000) The paramyxovirus simian virus 5 V protein slows progression of the cell cycle. *J Virol* **74**: 9152–9166.

Lin JH, Walter P, Yen TS (2008) Endoplasmic reticulum stress in disease pathogenesis. *Annu Rev Pathol* **3**: 399–425.

Liu CJ, Chen BF, Chen PJ, Lai MY, Huang WL, Kao JH, Chen DS (2006) Role of hepatitis B viral load and basal core promoter mutation in hepatocellular carcinoma in hepatitis B carriers. *J Infect Dis* **193**: 1258–1265.

Livezey KW, Negorev D, Simon D (2002) Increased chromosomal alterations and micronuclei formation in human hepatoma HepG2 cells transfected with the hepatitis B virus HBX gene. *Mutat Res* **505**: 63–74.

Lovejoy CA, Lock K, Yenamandra A, Cortez D (2006) DDB1 maintains genome integrity through regulation of Cdt1. *Mol Cell Biol* **26**: 7977–7990.

Lunn RM, Zhang YJ, Wang LY, Chen CJ, Lee PH, Lee CS, Tsai WY, Santella RM (1997). *p*53 mutations, chronic hepatitis B virus infection, and aflatoxin exposure in hepatocellular carcinoma in Taiwan. *Cancer Res* **57**: 3471–3477.

Ma WL, Hsu CL, Wu MH, Wu CT, Wu CC, Lai JJ, Jou YS, Chen CW, Yeh S, Chang C (2008) Androgen receptor is a new potential therapeutic target for the treatment of hepatocellular carcinoma. *Gastroenterology* **135**: 947–955, 955.e1–5. Epub 2008 May 22.

Ma Y, Hendershot LM (2004) The role of the unfolded protein response in tumour development: friend or foe? *Nat Rev Cancer* **4**: 966–977.

Madden CR, Finegold MJ, Slagle BL (2000) Expression of hepatitis B virus X protein does not alter the accumulation of spontaneous mutations in transgenic mice. *J Virol* **74**: 5266–5272.

Madden CR, Finegold MJ, Slagle BL (2001) Hepatitis B virus X protein acts as a tumor promoter in development of diethylnitrosamine-induced preneoplastic lesions. *J Virol* **75**: 3851–3858.

Madden CR, Finegold MJ, Slagle BL (2002) Altered DNA mutation spectrum in aflatoxin b1-treated transgenic mice that express the hepatitis B virus X protein. *J Virol* **76**: 11770–11774.

Maeda S, Kamata H, Luo JL, Leffert H, Karin M (2005) IKKbeta couples hepatocyte death to cytokine-driven compensatory proliferation that promotes chemical hepatocarcinogenesis. *Cell* **121**: 977–990.

Maguire HF, Hoeffler JP, Siddiqui A (1991) HBV X protein alters the DNA binding specificity of CREB and ATF-2 by protein-protein interactions. *Science* **252**: 842–844.

Mahmoud NN, Dannenberg AJ, Bilinski RT, Mestre JR, Chadburn A, Churchill M, Martucci C, Bertagnolli MM (1999) Administration of an unconjugated bile acid increases duodenal tumors in a murine model of familial adenomatous polyposis. *Carcinogenesis* **20**: 299–303.

Marchio A, Pineau P, Meddeb M, Terris B, Tiollais P, Bernheim A, Dejean A (2000) Distinct chromosomal abnormality pattern in primary liver cancer of non-B, non-C patients. *Oncogene* **19**: 3733–3738.

Martin-Lluesma S, Schaeffer C, Robert EI, van Breugel PC, Leupin O, Hantz O, Strubin M (2008) Hepatitis B virus X protein affects S phase progression leading to chromosome segregation defects by binding to damaged DNA binding protein 1. *Hepatology* **48**: 1467–1476.

Mason AL, Wick M, White HM, Benner KG, Lee RG, Regenstein F, Riely CA, Bain VG, Campbell C, Perrillo RP (1993) Increased hepatocyte expression of hepatitis B virus transcription in patients with features of fibrosing cholestatic hepatitis. *Gastroenterology* **105**: 237–244.

Matsuda M, Nakamoto Y, Suzuki S, Kurata T, Kaneko S (2005) Interferon-gamma-mediated hepatocarcinogenesis in mice treated with diethylnitrosamine. *Lab Invest* **85**: 655–663.

McClain SL, Clippinger AJ, Lizzano R, Bouchard MJ (2007) Hepatitis B virus replication is associated with an HBx-dependent mitochondrion-regulated increase in cytosolic calcium levels. *J Virol* **81**: 12061–12065.

McMahon BJ (2005) Epidemiology and natural history of hepatitis B. *Semin Liver Dis* **25**(1): 3–8.

Melegari M, Wolf SK, Schneider RJ (2005) Hepatitis B virus DNA replication is coordinated by core protein serine phosphorylation and HBx expression. *J Virol* **79**: 9810–9820.

Mendy ME, Kaye S, Le Roux E, Kirk GD, Jeng-Barry A, McConkey S, Cotten M, Kuniholm MH, Leligdowicz A, Hainaut P, Rowland-Jones S, Whittle H (2008) Application of a novel, rapid, and sensitive oligonucleotide ligation assay for detection of cancer-predicting mutations in the precore and basal core promoter of hepatitis B virus. *J Clin Microbiol* **46**: 2723–2730.

Meuleman P, Libbrecht L, Wieland S, De Vos R, Habib N, Kramvis A, Roskams T, Leroux-Roels G (2006) Immune suppression uncovers endogenous cytopathic effects of the hepatitis B virus. *J Virol* **80**: 2797–2807.

Mitacek EJ, Brunnemann KD, Suttajit M, Martin N, Limsila T, Ohshima H, Caplan LS (1999) Exposure to N-nitroso compounds in a population of high liver cancer regions in Thailand: volatile nitrosamine (VNA) levels in Thai food. *Food Chem Toxicol* **37**: 297–305.

Mochida S, Yoshimoto T, Mimura S, Inao M, Matsui A, Ohno A, Koh H, Saitoh E, Nagoshi S, Fujiwara K (2004) Transgenic mice expressing osteopontin in hepatocytes as a model of autoimmune hepatitis. *Biochem Biophys Res Commun* **317**: 114–120.

Murakami Y, Saigo K, Takashima H, Minami M, Okanoue T, Brechot C, Paterlini-Brechot P (2005) Large scaled analysis of hepatitis B virus (HBV) DNA integration in HBV related hepatocellular carcinomas. *Gut* **54**: 1162–1168.

Nagaya T, Nakamura T, Tokino T, Tsurimoto T, Imai M, Mayumi T, Kamino K, Yamamura K, Matsubara K (1987) The mode of hepatitis B virus DNA integration in chromosomes of human hepatocellular carcinoma. *Genes Dev* **1**: 773–782.

Nakamoto Y, Guidotti LG, Kuhlen CV, Fowler P, Chisari FV (1998) Immune pathogenesis of hepatocellular carcinoma. *J Exp Med* **188**: 341–350.

Naugler WE, Sakurai T, Kim S, Maeda S, Kim K, Elsharkawy AM, Karin M (2007) Gender disparity in liver cancer due to sex differences in MyD88-dependent IL-6 production. *Science* **317**: 121–124.

Nguyen VT, Law MG, Dore GJ (2008) An enormous hepatitis B virus-related liver disease burden projected in Vietnam by 2025. *Liver Int* **28**: 525–531.

Ou JH (1997) Molecular biology of hepatitis B virus e antigen. *J Gastroenterol Hepatol* **12**: S178–S187.

Overturf K, al-Dhalimy M, Ou CN, Finegold M, Grompe M (1997) Serial transplantation reveals the stem-cell-like regenerative potential of adult mouse hepatocytes. *Am J Pathol* **151**: 1273–1280.

Pardo M, Bartolome J, Carreno V (2007) Current therapy of chronic hepatitis B. *Arch Med Res* **38**: 661–677.

Pihan G, Doxsey SJ (2003) Mutations and aneuploidy: co-conspirators in cancer? *Cancer Cell* **4**: 89–94.

Pikarsky E, Porat RM, Stein I, Abramovitch R, Amit S, Kasem S, Gutkovich-Pyest E, Urieli-Shoval S, Galun E, Ben-Neriah Y (2004) NF-kappaB functions as a tumour promoter in inflammation-associated cancer. *Nature* **431**: 461–466. Epub 2004 Aug 25.

Pineau P, Marchio A, Battiston C, Cordina E, Russo A, Terris B, Qin LX, Turlin B, Tang ZY, Mazzaferro V, Dejean A (2008) Chromosome

Slagle BL, Lee TH, Medina D, Finegold MJ, Butel JS (1996) Increased sensitivity to the hepatocarcinogen diethylnitrosamine in transgenic mice carrying the hepatitis B virus X gene. *Mol Carcinog* **15**: 261–269.

Smela ME, Currier SS, Bailey EA, Essigmann JM (2001) The chemistry and biology of aflatoxin B(1): from mutational spectrometry to carcinogenesis. *Carcinogenesis* **22**: 535–545.

Srivastava S, Swanson SK, Manel N, Florens L, Washburn MP, Skowronski J (2008) Lentiviral Vpx accessory factor targets VprBP/DCAF1 substrate adaptor for cullin 4 E3 ubiquitin ligase to enable macrophage infection. *PLoS Pathog* **4**: e1000059.

Sterneck M, Kalinina T, Otto S, Gunther S, Fischer L, Burdelski M, Greten H, Broelsch CE, Will H (1998) Neonatal fulminant hepatitis B: structural and functional analysis of complete hepatitis B virus genomes from mother and infant. *J Infect Dis* **177**: 1378–1381.

Su IJ, Wang HC, Wu HC, Huang WY (2008) Ground glass hepatocytes contain pre-S mutants and represent preneoplastic lesions in chronic hepatitis B virus infection. *J Gastroenterol Hepatol* **23**: 1169–1174.

Su Q, Schroder CH, Otto G, Bannasch P (2000) Overexpression of *p53* protein is not directly related to hepatitis B X protein expression and is associated with neoplastic progression in hepatocellular carcinomas rather than hepatic preneoplasia. *Mutat Res* **462**: 365–380.

Sugiyama M, Tanaka Y, Kurbanov F, Maruyama I, Shimada T, Takahashi S, Shirai T, Hino K, Sakaida I, Mizokami M (2008) Direct cytopathic effects of particular hepatitis B virus genotypes in severe combined immunodeficiency transgenic with urokinase-type plasminogen activator mouse with human h. *Gastroenterology* **29**: 29.

Summers J, Mason WS (2004) Residual integrated viral DNA after hepadnavirus clearance by nucleoside analog therapy. *Proc Natl Acad Sci USA* **101**: 638–640. Epub 2003 Dec 29.

Sureau C, Romet-Lemonne JL, Mullins JI, Essex M (1986) Production of hepatitis B virus by a differentiated human hepatoma cell line after transfection with cloned circular HBV DNA. *Cell* **47**: 37–47.

Tai PC, Suk FM, Gerlich WH, Neurath AR, Shih C (2002) Hypermodification and immune escape of an internally deleted middle-envelope (M) protein of frequent and predominant hepatitis B virus variants. *Virology* **292**: 44–58.

Takada S, Koike K (1990) *Trans*-activation function of a 3′ truncated X gene-cell fusion product from integrated hepatitis B virus DNA in chronic hepatitis tissues. *Proc Natl Acad Sci USA* **87**: 5628–5632.

Takano S, Yokosuka O, Imazeki F, Tagawa M, Omata M (1995) Incidence of hepatocellular carcinoma in chronic hepatitis B and C: a prospective study of 251 patients. *Hepatology* **21**: 650–655.

Tang H, Delgermaa L, Huang F, Oishi N, Liu L, He F, Zhao L, Murakami S (2005) The transcriptional transactivation function of HBx protein is important for its augmentation role in hepatitis B virus replication. *J Virol* **79**: 5548–5556.

Tennant BC (2001) Animal models of hepadnavirus-associated hepatocellular carcinoma. *Clin Liver Dis* **5**: 43–68.

Teramoto T, Satonaka K, Kitazawa S, Fujimori T, Hayashi K, Maeda S (1994) *p*53 gene abnormalities are closely related to hepatoviral infections and occur at a late stage of hepatocarcinogenesis. *Cancer Res* **54**: 231–235.

Terradillos O, Billet O, Renard CA, Levy R, Molina T, Briand P, Buendia, MA (1997) The hepatitis B virus X gene potentiates *c-myc*-induced liver oncogenesis in transgenic mice. *Oncogene* **14**: 395–404.

Tong MJ, Blatt LM, Kao JH, Cheng JT, Corey WG (2006) Precore/basal core promoter mutants and hepatitis B viral DNA levels as predictors for liver deaths and hepatocellular carcinoma. *World J Gastroenterol* **12**: 6620–6626.

Toyonaga T, Hino O, Sugai S, Wakasugi S, Abe K, Shichiri M, Yamamura K (1994) Chronic active hepatitis in transgenic mice expressing interferon-gamma in the liver. *Proc Natl Acad Sci USA* **91**: 614–618.

Tralhao JG, Roudier J, Morosan S, Giannini C, Tu H, Goulenok C, Carnot F, Zavala F, Joulin V, Kremsdorf D, Brechot C (2002) Paracrine *in vivo* inhibitory effects of hepatitis B virus X protein (HBx) on liver cell proliferation: an alternative mechanism of HBx-related pathogenesis. *Proc Natl Acad Sci USA* **99**: 6991–6996.

Tsukuma H, Hiyama T, Tanaka S, Nakao M, Yabuuchi T, Kitamura T, Nakanishi K, Fujimoto I, Inoue A, Yamazaki H *et al.* (1993) Risk factors for hepatocellular carcinoma among patients with chronic liver disease [see comments]. *N Engl J Med* **328**: 1797–1801.

Tu H, Bonura C, Giannini C, Mouly H, Soussan P, Kew M, Paterlini-Brechot P, Brechot C, Kremsdorf D (2001) Biological impact of natural COOH-terminal deletions of hepatitis B virus X protein in hepatocellular carcinoma tissues. *Cancer Res* **61**: 7803–7810.

Turner PC, Sylla A, Gong YY, Diallo MS, Sutcliffe AE, Hall AJ, Wild CP (2005) Reduction in exposure to carcinogenic aflatoxins by postharvest intervention measures in West Africa: a community-based intervention study. *Lancet* **365**: 1950–1956.

Ulane CM, Kentsis A, Cruz CD, Parisien JP, Schneider KL, Horvath CM (2005) Composition and assembly of STAT-targeting ubiquitin ligase complexes: paramyxovirus V protein carboxyl terminus is an oligomerization domain. *J Virol* **79**: 10180–10189.

Wakasugi M, Kasashima H, Fukase Y, Imura M, Imai R, Yamada S, Cleaver JE, Matsunaga T (2008) Physical and functional interaction between DDB and XPA in nucleotide excision repair. *Nucleic Acids Res* **8**: 8.

Wang HC, Chang WT, Chang WW, Wu HC, Huang W, Lei HY, Lai MD, Fausto N, Su IJ (2005) Hepatitis B virus pre-S2 mutant upregulates cyclin A expression and induces nodular proliferation of hepatocytes. *Hepatology* **41**: 761–770.

Wang J, Chenivesse X, Henglein B, Brechot C (1990) Hepatitis B virus integration in a cyclin A gene in a hepatocellular carcinoma. *Nature* **343**: 555–557.

Wang LY, Hatch M, Chen CJ, Levin B, You SL, Lu SN, Wu MH, Wu WP, Wang LW, Wang Q, Huang GT, Yang PM, Lee HS, Santella RM (1996) Aflatoxin exposure and risk of hepatocellular carcinoma in Taiwan. *Int J Cancer* **67**: 620–625.

Wang LY, You SL, Lu SN, Ho HC, Wu MH, Sun CA, Yang HI, Chien-Jen C (2003) Risk of hepatocellular carcinoma and habits of alcohol drinking, betel quid chewing and cigarette smoking: a cohort of 2416 HBsAg-seropositive and 9421 HBsAg-seronegative male residents in Taiwan. *Cancer Causes Control* **14**: 241–250.

Wang Y, Lau SH, Sham JS, Wu MC, Wang T, Guan XY (2004) Characterization of HBV integrants in 14 hepatocellular carcinomas: association of truncated X gene and hepatocellular carcinogenesis. *Oncogene* **23**: 142–148.

Wen Y, Golubkov VS, Strongin AY, Jiang W, Reed JC (2008) Interaction of hepatitis B viral oncoprotein with cellular target HBXIP dysregulates centrosome dynamics and mitotic spindle formation. *J Biol Chem* **283**: 2793–2803.

Wentz MJ, Becker SA, Slagle BL (2000) Dissociation of DDB1-binding and transactivation properties of the hepatitis B virus X protein. *Virus Res* **68**: 87–92.

Williams JS, Andrisani OM (1995) The hepatitis B virus X protein targets the basic region-leucine zipper domain of CREB. *Proc Natl Acad Sci USA* **92**: 3819–3823.

Wogan GN, Pong RS (1970) Aflatoxins. *Ann NY Acad Sci* **174**: 623–635.

Wu BK, Li CC, Chen HJ, Chang JL, Jeng KS, Chou CK, Hsu MT, Tsai TF (2006) Blocking of G1/S transition and cell death in the regenerating liver of Hepatitis B virus X protein transgenic mice. *Biochem Biophys Res Commun* **340**: 916–928.

Xie S, Price JE, Luca M, Jean D, Ronai Z, Bar-Eli M (1997) Dominant-negative CREB inhibits tumor growth and metastasis of human melanoma cells. *Oncogene* **15**: 2069–2075.

Xu R, Zhang X, Zhang W, Fang Y, Zheng S, Yu XF (2007) Association of human APOBEC3 cytidine deaminases with the generation of hepatitis virus B X antigen mutants and hepatocellular carcinoma. *Hepatology* **46**: 1810–1820.

Xu Z, Bruss V, Yen TS (1997a) Formation of intracellular particles by hepatitis B virus large surface protein. *J Virol* **71**: 5487–5494.

Xu Z, Jensen G, Yen TS (1997b) Activation of hepatitis B virus S promoter by the viral large surface protein via induction of stress in the endoplasmic reticulum. *J Virol* **71**: 7387–7392.

Xu Z, Yen TS, Wu L, Madden CR, Tan W, Slagle BL, Ou JH (2002) Enhancement of hepatitis B virus replication by its X protein in transgenic mice. *J Virol* **76**: 2579–2584.

Yang HI, Lu SN, Liaw YF, You SL, Sun CA, Wang LY, Hsiao CK, Chen PJ, Chen DS, Chen CJ (2002) Hepatitis B e antigen and the risk of hepatocellular carcinoma. *N Engl J Med* **347**: 168–174.

Yang HI, Yeh SH, Chen PJ, Iloeje UH, Jen CL, Su J, Wang LY, Lu SN, You SL, Chen DS, Liaw YF, Chen CJ (2008) Associations between hepatitis B virus genotype and mutants and the risk of hepatocellular carcinoma. *J Natl Cancer Inst* **100**: 1134–1143.

Yen TS (1996) Hepadnaviral X protein: review of recent progress. *J Biomed Sci* **3**: 20–30.

Yen TSB (1993) Regulation of hepatitis B virus gene expression. *Seminars Virol* **4**: 33–42.

Yen TSB (2001) The molecular biology of hepatitis B virus. In Ou JH (ed.), *Hepatitis Viruses*, pp. 51–79. Boston: Kluwer Academic Publishers.

Yu MW, Yeh SH, Chen PJ, Liaw YF, Lin CL, Liu CJ, Shih WL, Kao JH, Chen DS, Chen CJ (2005) Hepatitis B virus genotype and DNA level and hepatocellular carcinoma: a prospective study in men. *J Natl Cancer Inst* **97**: 265–272.

Yuen MF, Tanaka Y, Fong DY, Fung J, Wong DK, Yuen JC, But DY, Chan AO, Wong BC, Mizokami M, Lai CL (2009) Independent risk factors and predictive score for the development of hepatocellular carcinoma in chronic hepatitis B. *J Hepatol* **50**: 80–88.

Yuen MF, Tanaka Y, Mizokami M, Yuen JC, Wong DK, Yuan HJ, Sum SM, Chan AO, Wong BC, Lai CL (2004) Role of hepatitis B virus genotypes Ba and C, core promoter and precore mutations on hepatocellular carcinoma: a case control study. *Carcinogenesis* **25**: 1593–1598.

Yuen MF, Tanaka Y, Shinkai N, Poon RT, But DY, Fong DY, Fung J, Wong DK, Yuen JC, Mizokami M, Lai CL (2008) Risk for hepatocellular carcinoma with respect to hepatitis B virus genotypes B/C, specific mutations of enhancer II/core promoter/precore regions and HBV DNA levels. *Gut* **57**: 98–102.

Yun C, Cho H, Kim SJ, Lee JH, Park SY, Chan GK, Cho H (2004) Mitotic aberration coupled with centrosome amplification is induced by hepatitis B virus X oncoprotein via the Ras-mitogen-activated protein/extracellular signal-regulated kinase-mitogen-activated protein pathway. *Mol Cancer Res* **2**: 159–169.

Zhang Z, Torii N, Hu Z, Jacob J, Liang TJ (2001) X-deficient woodchuck hepatitis virus mutants behave like attenuated viruses and induce protective immunity *in vivo*. *J Clin Invest* **108**: 1523–1531.

Zheng Y, Chen WL, Louie SG, Yen TS, Ou JH (2007a) Hepatitis B virus promotes hepatocarcinogenesis in transgenic mice. *Hepatology* **45**: 16–21.

Zheng Y, Chen WL, Ma WL, Chang C, Ou JH (2007b) Enhancement of gene transactivation activity of androgen receptor by hepatitis B virus X protein. *Virology* **363**: 454–461.

Zheng Y, Li J, Ou JH (2004) Regulation of hepatitis B virus core promoter by transcription factors HNF1 and HNF4 and the viral X protein. *J Virol* **78**: 6908–6914.

Zheng YW, Riegler J, Wu J, Yen TS (1994) Novel short transcripts of hepatitis B virus X gene derived from intragenic promoter. *J Biol Chem* **269**: 22593–22598.

Zoulim F, Saputelli J, Seeger C (1994) Woodchuck hepatitis virus X protein is required for viral infection *in vivo*. *J Virol* **68**: 2026–2030.

Chapter 3

Molecular Mechanism of Hepatitis C Virus Carcinogenesis

Keigo Machida*, Jing-hsiung James Ou* and Michael M. C. Lai*

Abstract: Hepatitis C virus (HCV) persistently infects 170 million people in the world and is a major cause of hepatocellular carcinoma (HCC). It can also induce B-cell proliferative disorders including B-cell lymphoma. HCV may induce cellular transformation by the induction of chronic liver inflammation mediated by the immune cells. This chronic liver inflammation leads to cell death, hepatocellular regeneration, and emergence of mutated cells that may be premalignant. In addition, HCV may also induce cellular transformation directly via the induction of oxidative stress and gene mutations as well as the alteration of cellular physiology, processes that may also lead to malignant cellular transformation. This chapter discusses the oncogenic pathways of HCV.

1. Introduction

Hepatitis C virus (HCV) persistently infects 170 million people worldwide and causes a spectrum of liver diseases, including chronic hepatitis, liver cirrhosis, and hepatocellular carcinoma (HCC) (Takeda *et al.*, 1992). It can also cause B-lymphocyte proliferative disorders, including mixed cryoglobulinemia (MC), a disorder

*Department of Molecular Microbiology and Immunology, University of Southern California, Keck School of Medicine, Los Angeles, California.

characterized by oligoclonal proliferation of B-lymphocytes, and B-cell lymphoma (Ferri *et al.*, 1994; Saito *et al.*, 1990; Silvestri *et al.*, 1997). In addition, HCV patients may also develop other diseases, including Sjögren's syndrome, lichen planus, disturbance in lipid metabolism, and diabetes or insulin resistance.

HCC is the third leading cause of cancer deaths and the fifth most frequent cancer in the world, with more than 600,000 deaths in 2007. The high mortality rate of HCC is due in part to its unresponsiveness to treatment, and in part to the lack of sensory fibers in the noncapsular part of the liver. The latter often leads to its detection in the late stage when surgical removal of the tumor is no longer an option. The 5-year survival rate of HCC is less than 5% with or without therapeutic intervention (El-Serag & Mason, 1999). The major cause of HCC is hepatitis B virus (HBV), followed by HCV. Other nonviral factors account for about 20% of the HCC cases (El-Serag & Mason, 1999). The lifetime risk of HCC in chronically infected HCV patients is 2–7% (Di Bisceglie *et al.*, 2003), and it may take 30–40 years for HCC to develop in these patients. HCC caused by HCV may be an indirect result of chronic liver inflammation, which causes liver injury and compensatory hepatocellular proliferation. This chronic liver inflammation can lead to liver cirrhosis and HCC. Various factors such as mutations in tumor-suppressor genes or proto-oncogenes or the activity of specific growth factors during the course of chronic HCV infection may enhance hepatocellular transformation (Simonetti *et al.*, 1992). The prolonged liver inflammation coupled with the repeated liver regeneration is an important factor in the multi-step process of hepatocarcinogenesis (Simonetti *et al.*, 1992).

HCV infection can also cause chronic, benign B-lymphocyte proliferation, which may evolve to a malignant non-Hodgkin's lymphoma (NHL). Approximately 22–50% of idiopathic NHL patients have HCV infection (Ferri *et al.*, 1997). The association between HCV and NHL, largely demonstrated in Italian patients, has also been supported by studies in the United States and Japan (Izumi *et al.*, 1996; Izumi *et al.*, 1997; Zuckerman *et al.*, 1997). These studies showed a significantly higher prevalence rate of HCV infection in patients with B-cell NHL than with other hematological malignancies such as Hodgkin's lymphoma, T-cell lymphoma, chronic lymphocytic leukemia, and multiple myeloma. The geographical distribution of HCV-positive NHL patients suggests that genetic and environmental factors may also be involved in lymphomagenesis.

The HCV genome is a single-stranded, positive-sense RNA of 9.6 Kbp. This genome codes for a polyprotein, which is proteolytically cleaved by viral and cellular proteases to generate 10 mature protein products. The structural proteins are located at the N-terminus of this polyprotein sequence. These structural proteins are the core protein and E1 and E2 envelope proteins. The structural proteins are followed by nonstructural proteins, including p7, NS2, NS3, NS4A, NS4B, NS5A, and NS5B. These nonstructural proteins are required for viral replication. In addition, the HCV genome also encodes a separate protein named the F protein or the alternative reading frame protein using a different reading frame. Based on the nucleotide sequences, HCV has been grouped into six major genotypes and many subtypes. The analysis of HCV genotypes indicates that genotype 1b is the most prevalent genotype associated with HCC (Simonetti *et al.*, 1992), and genotype 2a is more frequently found in HCV patients with complicating NHL (Ferri *et al.*, 1995). In the following sections, the molecular mechanisms of HCV-induced carcinogenesis will be discussed.

2. Molecular Carcinogenesis of HCV

2.1. Induction of Mutator Phenotype

The infection of B-cell lines and peripheral blood mononuclear cells (PBMC) with HCV *in vitro* can lead to a mutator phenotype, which involves enhanced mutations in many somatic genes, including immunoglobulin (*Ig*) genes, proto-oncogenes, and tumor suppressor genes (Machida *et al.*, 2004b). By comparing the nucleotide substitution patterns of these mutations with those of the predominant proto-oncogene mutations observed in HCV-associated B-cell lymphomas and HCC, the authors found that the mutations observed in HCV-infected B-cell lines or PBMC had nucleotide substitution patterns similar to those found in HCV-associated lymphoma (Machida *et al.*, 2004b). Furthermore, the mutations detected in the HCV-associated lymphomas, but not in the unselected HCV-infected cells, had a replacement/silent mutation ratio higher than the expected ratio in the absence of selection. Similarly, both the tumor and neighboring non-tumor tissues of HCV-associated HCC have similar nucleotide substitution patterns, but, interestingly, the tumor tissues have three to five times higher mutation rates than the non-tumor tissues. Moreover, the ratio of replacement/silent mutations in the tumors, but not the neighboring non-tumor tissues, was significantly higher than the ratio expected in the absence of selection (Machida *et al.*, 2004b). These findings together suggest that certain HCV-induced somatic mutations, which include mutations in proto-oncogenes and tumor suppressor genes such as *β-catenin*, *BCL-6*, and *p53*, may be selected as they confer a growth advantage on the cell during tumorigenesis. It is striking that other types of tumors, including lymphomas not associated with HCV, HBV-associated HCC, and HCC of nonviral origin, did not show such amplification of somatic mutations. Thus, the ability of HCV to induce the mutator phenotype is unique and likely plays a critical role in HCV oncogenesis. It is conceivable that the long latency period of HCV-associated malignancies is due to the need for the induction of multiple mutations by HCV.

The HCV-induced mutator phenotype can be explained by the ability of HCV to cause double-strand DNA breaks (DSBs) and induce error-prone DNA polymerase ζ, polymerase ι, and activation-induced cytidine deaminase (AID) (Machida *et al.*, 2004b). Repair of DSBs by homologous recombination can result in a ~100-fold increase in the rate of point mutations in the vicinity of the breaks in *Saccharomyces cerevisiae* (Strathern *et al.*, 1995). These mutations are dependent on the error-prone polymerase ζ, which has the DNA damage bypass activity (Holbeck & Strathern, 1997). Polymerase ι behaves as a dA•dT mutator in the middle of DNA templates but as a dG•dC mutator at their ends, when acting on a primer terminus with a long template overhang, with extraordinarily low fidelity

(Frank *et al.*, 2001). Polymerase ι also induces somatic hypermutation in *Ig* genes in the BL2 cell line (Faili *et al.*, 2002). Thus, the enhanced expression of error-prone DNA polymerases ζ and ι may be responsible for the mutation frequency in HCV-infected cells. Both error-prone polymerases ζ and ι could be activated as a result of B-cell receptor (BCR) stimulation (Poltoratsky *et al.*, 2001; Zan *et al.*, 2001). Significantly, the HCV envelope protein E2 binds to CD81, which is expressed on both B cells and hepatocytes (Pileri *et al.*, 1998), and to the BCR of HCV-associated lymphoma (Quinn *et al.*, 2001), thus activating the intracellular signal transduction pathway. Note that HCV-induced DNA breaks may also be caused by reactive oxygen species (ROS), which can be induced by HCV core, NS3, and NS5A proteins (Lai, 2002). The induction of DSBs may explain the occurrence of apoptosis associated with hepatitis and chromosomal instability found in B cells and hepatocytes of HCV-infected individuals. Furthermore, the ability of HCV to induce high mutation frequency of cellular genes indicates that HCV may cause tumor formation by a "hit-and-run" mechanism.

2.2. Chromosome Translocation

Defects in DNA repair genes cause genetic instability, gross chromosomal rearrangements, and accumulation of mutations, leading ultimately to neoplastic transformation. Both homologous recombination and nonhomologous end-joining (NHEJ) play a role in the repair of DSBs in mammalian cells (Hiom, 1999). The interaction of broken DNA with members of the Rad52 epistasis group, including Rad51, a mammalian homolog of bacterial RecA, initiates homologous recombination repair (Hiom, 1999). Following DNA damage, Rad51 is redistributed within the nucleus (Baumann & West, 1998; Haaf *et al.*, 1995) and induces the ATP-dependent homologous strand-pairing reaction that initiates recombination. In contrast, NHEJ works by non-homology-dependent ligation of broken DNA ends. DNA-dependent protein kinase (DNA-PK) and its associated proteins Ku70, Ku80, and Xrcc4 mediate NHEJ (Lieber *et al.*, 2003).

Cellular DNA repair proteins prevent potential DNA mutations caused by oxidative damage, but are themselves vulnerable to nitric oxide (NO)-induced oxidative damage because of sulphenyl, tyrosyl, and/or phenolic side chains in their active sites (Jaiswal *et al.*, 2000, 2001; Starke *et al.*, 1997). Suppression of DNA repair, coupled with the induction of DNA breaks by viral proteins, may increase the mutation frequency and chromosome rearrangements in virus-infected cells.

Chromosomal abnormalities are common in PBMC of HCV patients as in most cancers (Kitay-Cohen *et al.*, 2000). As mentioned above, HCV infection induces a mutator phenotype by causing DSBs (Machida *et al.*, 2004b). We have further discovered that HCV induces iNOS mRNA expression and enhances NO production through the action of its core and NS3 proteins, and that NO is responsible for DSBs in most cellular genes (Machida *et al.*, 2004a). The accumulation of DSBs in HCV-infected cells indicates that an HCV-induced oxidative environment may overwhelm cellular antioxidant and DNA-repair mechanisms, leading to chromosomal abnormalities.

2.3. Reactive Oxygen Species (ROS)

ROS are generated as a consequence of mitochondrial electron transport. They are caused by a small proportion of the electron flow interacting with oxygen molecules before reaching the cytochrome oxidase complex. HCV infection induces ROS (Choi & Ou, 2006), which leads to oxidative DNA damages and lipid peroxidation in HCV-infected cells (Machida *et al.*, 2006). Treatment of HCV-infected cells with ROS inhibitors effectively prevented mitochondrial damages and the production of ROS (Machida *et al.*, 2006).

The biochemical mechanisms behind the HCV-mediated mitochondria damage remain largely unclear. We have found that the HCV core and NS3 proteins, as well as the E1 envelope protein, are responsible for ROS production in HCV-infected cells. Transgenic mice that express the HCV core protein have increased levels of lipid peroxides and 8-hydroxy-2′-deoxyguanosine (8-oxodG), a marker of oxidatively damaged DNA, in the absence of liver inflammation. This observation indicates that the HCV core protein can induce oxidative stress (Moriya *et al.*, 2001a,b). HCV core protein and NS3 can induce NO production (Machida *et al.*, 2004a), which causes mitochondrial membrane damage and decreases mitochondrial membrane potential ($\Delta\Psi_m$) due to the opening of permeability transition (PT) pores followed by the depolarization of the inner mitochondrial membrane and massive ROS production (Hortelano *et al.*, 1997). NO can also be activated through reaction with another free radical, superoxide (O_2^-), to form the strong oxidant peroxynitrite anion ($ONOO^-$), which can irreversibly inhibit multiple respiratory complexes (complexes I, II, and IV) and aconitase, as well as activate proton leak and open PT pores (Brown, 2001). Downregulation of complex IV activity leads to upregulation of peroxynitrite anion that results in increases in O_2^- and H_2O_2, which may contribute to NO-induced cell death (Brown, 2001). We had hypothesized that HCV-induced NO would disrupt mitochondria electron transport, leading to outbursts of ROS. Indeed, core and NS3 could activate the iNOS promoter and enhance its expression (Machida *et al.*, 2004a). However, we also found that NO was not enough to account for the HCV-induced DNA damage, since both NO and ROS inhibitors were required for the complete abolition of HCV-induced DNA damage. Thus, core and NS3 proteins may activate other ROS sources to amplify the ROS generation cycle.

In contrast to core and NS3 proteins, the E1-induced lipid and DNA damage were mediated entirely through ROS production (Machida *et al.*, 2006). The mechanism of E1-induced ROS production is still not clear. One possibility is that E1 induces endoplasmic reticulum (ER) stress, leading to mitochondrial membrane damages. ER stress can cause the release of Ca^{2+} from ER stores and their accumulation in mitochondria (Deniaud *et al.*, 2008).

As mentioned above, the HCV core protein can induce oxidative stress in the absence of inflammation. If inflammation is also induced, the oxidative stress is escalated to an extent that cannot be scavenged by the physiological antagonistic system. This may accelerate DNA damage and hepatocarcinogenesis. HCV-induced ROS can also activate *STAT3*. As *STAT3* has been reported to be as an oncogene, its activation may lead to the downstream proliferative responses (Bromberg *et al.*, 1999; Machida *et al.*, 2006). In addition, *STAT3* is also an acute-phase response factor of liver disease (Wegenka *et al.*, 1994), including acute hepatitis associated with HCV infection. The constitutive activation of *STAT3* has been shown to inhibit apoptosis (Catlett-Falcone *et al.*, 1999), induce transformation (Bromberg *et al.*, 1999), and cause B cell differentiation, particularly in the terminal differentiation of B cells into antibody-secreting plasma cells (Fornek *et al.*, 2006; Hirano *et al.*, 2000). Thus, the *STAT3*-induced dysregulation of cellular responses may also explain the high incidence of HCC and lymphoproliferative diseases in hepatitis C patients.

In summary, ROS, together with NO (Machida *et al.*, 2004a), directly or indirectly play important roles in HCV pathogenesis. ROS can induce steatosis (through lipid peroxides) and oncogenesis (through DNA mutations and *STAT3* activation), and may also contribute to protection of hepatocytes from acute damage (through the production of *STAT3*) (Machida *et al.*, 2006). ROS and/or iNOS inhibitors may provide therapeutic measures for HCV patients for the protection of their liver tissues from oxidative stress.

2.4. Nitric Oxide

HCV infection induces iNOS expression and production of NO, which, in turn, causes DNA damage, resulting in enhanced mutations of cellular genes (Machida *et al.*, 2004a). This pathway can be blocked by treatment of HCV-infected cells with iNOS inhibitors or the introduction of an iNOS-specific siRNA (Machida *et al.*, 2004a). As mentioned above, HCV core or NS3 protein alone can activate these sequential events (Machida *et al.*, 2004a). The HCV core protein can activate the NF-κB pathway (Kato *et al.*, 2000). This explains why it can activate the iNOS promoter, which contains several NF-κB-binding sites. Indeed, the HCV core transgenic mice produce a higher level of NO_X in their serum. In contrast, how NS3 affects the iNOS gene expression is not clear. It is significant that both core and

NS3 proteins have been shown to be capable of transforming cells under *in vitro* conditions. The finding that both core and NS3 can induce the production of NO may have provided a mechanism for these transforming activities. Nevertheless, DNA mutations alone cannot fully account for the tumorigenic activity of the core protein, as both the tumor and non-tumor regions of the liver of core transgenic mice have similar mutation frequencies (Machida *et al.*, 2004a). Thus, additional potentiating events such as the correct combinations of mutations are necessary to trigger tumor formation.

NO has been shown to cause predominantly transitional nucleotide substitutions (i.e. purine to purine, and pyrimidine to pyrimidine) of cellular genes (Nguyen *et al.*, 1992). Interestingly, we have recently shown that HCV infection causes predominantly transition mutations in cellular genes (Machida *et al.*, 2004b). NO and reactive NO species (RNOS), such as the strong oxidant peroxynitrite anion ($ONOO^-$) and dinitrogen trioxide peroxynitrite, may cause DNA damage through three chemical mechanisms (Nguyen *et al.*, 1992). The first is the direct reaction of RNOS with DNA, which induces nitrosative/oxidative deamination of DNA bases, leading to DNA strand breakage under cell-free conditions (Routledge, 2000). Indeed, the addition of NO to TK6 cells produced a 40- to 50-fold increase in hypoxanthine and xanthine in cellular DNA (Nguyen *et al.*, 1992). It has also been shown that gaseous NO• can induce predominantly transitional mutations (Routledge, 2000). Thus, HCV-induced NO has the ability to modify genomic DNA with transitional substitutions. The second is through inhibition of DNA repair processes (Jaiswal *et al.*, 2000). The third is through increased production of genotoxic species such as alkylating agents and hydrogen peroxide. Thus, production of NO may explain most of the mutations of cellular genes, such as the *p53* tumor suppressor gene, associated with HCV infection (Machida *et al.*, 2004b). NO inhibits apoptosis, but at higher concentrations; NO may be pro-apoptotic as a result of activation of caspases (Kim *et al.*, 2001). Although NO has been reported to induce cell death (Kim *et al.*, 2001), a low level of NO does not kill the cells and activate angiogenesis and enhance cell survival (Nathan, 1992). Therefore, HCV-induced NO may either inhibit or promote cell survival. We have previously separated the non-apoptotic from apoptotic using HCV-infected and uninfected B cells by Annexin V staining (Machida *et al.*, 2004b). The HCV-infected non-apoptotic cells had a significantly higher level of DSBs than that of the uninfected counterparts, confirming the occurrence of spontaneous DNA strand breakage even in the absence of apoptosis (Machida *et al.*, 2004b).

HCV-infected patients also have higher hepatic iNOS levels (Schweyer *et al.*, 2000). The mutagenic effects of NO induced by HCV vary according to the genes affected. In contrast to the *p53* gene, the mutations found in the V_H gene were not completely blocked by iNOS inhibitors, indicating that other mechanisms also contributed to DNA damage (Machida *et al.*, 2004a). This may be due to HCV-activated AID (Machida *et al.*, 2004b), which also causes transition mutations in the RGYW (R, purine; Y, pyrimidine; W, A/T) motif of DNA (Petersen-Mahrt *et al.*, 2002). The viral protein responsible for the activation of AID has not been identified.

NO is a potent antimicrobial effector molecule capable of nitrating tyrosine residues of proteins into nitrotyrosine to exhibit antiviral activity against a wide range of viruses in rodents (Nathan, 1992). Conceivably, NO may also have an antiviral activity against HCV. This may be part of the reason why HCV replicates at low levels *in vivo* even in the presence of significant liver damage.

2.5. Inhibition of DNA Damage Repair

As discussed above, it has previously been demonstrated that HCV infection induces a mutator phenotype by giving rise to DSBs (Machida *et al.*, 2004b). We have further reported that HCV induces iNOS mRNA expression and enhances NO production through the action of the viral core protein and the NS3 protein, and that NO is responsible for inducing DSBs in most of cellular genes (Machida *et al.*, 2004a). Accumulation of DSBs in HCV-infected cells suggests that an HCV-induced oxidative environment may overwhelm cellular antioxidant and DNA-repair mechanisms, leading to chromosomal abnormalities.

Some viral transforming proteins, such as the X protein of HBV (Becker *et al.*, 1998), the E6 protein of human papillomavirus (Chen & Defendi, 1992; Steller *et al.*, 1996), the E4orf3 and E4orf6–E1b55K complex of adenovirus (Stracker *et al.*, 2002), and the Tax protein of human T-cell leukemia virus type I (Jeang *et al.*, 1990; Kao & Marriott, 1999), disrupt cellular DNA repair, leading to chromosomal abnormalities. Cellular DNA repair proteins prevent potential DNA mutations caused by oxidative damage, but are themselves vulnerable to NO-induced oxidative damage because of their active site sulphenyl, tyrosine, and/or phenol side chains (Jaiswal *et al.*, 2000, 2001; Starke *et al.*, 1997). Suppression of DNA repair, coupled with the induction of DNA breaks by viral proteins, may enhance the mutation frequency and chromosome rearrangements in virus-infected cells. HCV core protein has been reported to inhibit the expression of retinoblastoma (Rb) mRNA (Hassan *et al.*, 2004), impair cell-cycle regulation in stably transformed Chinese hamster ovary cells (Honda *et al.*, 2000), and induce DSBs (Machida *et al.*, 2004a).

2.6. Oncogenic Activities of the HCV Core Protein

Transgenic mouse lines that carry the core protein gene of HCV genotype 1b virus had been produced and studied. These mice expressed the 21-kD core protein at a level similar to that found in the liver of HCV patients (Moriya *et al.*, 1997, 1998). The core transgenic mice of two independent lineages developed HCC (Moriya *et al.*, 1998). In contrast, the envelope protein transgenic mice did not develop HCC, despite high expression levels of both E1 and E2 envelope proteins (Koike *et al.*, 1997). The transgenic mice carrying all the nonstructural genes also did not develop HCC. The core transgenic mice first developed hepatic steatosis, which is one of the histologic characteristics of chronic hepatitis C, along with bile duct damage (Bach *et al.*, 1992). Significant inflammation was not observed in the liver of this animal model. These transgenic mice then progressed to develop HCC later in life. Most hepatic nodules had a pathology characterized by "nodule in nodule," which is the development of HCC with a low degree of differentiation within adenoma or well-differentiated HCC (Moriya *et al.*, 1998). Although numerous lipid droplets were found in cells forming adenoma as well as in non-tumorous cells, they were rarely observed in HCC cells. These histological features closely resemble those observed in hepatitis C patients, in whom prominent lipid droplets are found in small, well-differentiated HCC and its precursors, and poorly differentiated HCC without lipid droplets are found inside differentiated HCC (Moriya *et al.*, 1998). Notably, the development of steatosis and HCC has been reproduced in other HCV transgenic mouse lines, which harbor the entire HCV genome or structural genes including the core gene (Lerat *et al.*, 2002). These outcomes indicate that the HCV core protein per se has an oncogenic potential when expressed *in vivo*.

HCV core protein has been shown to modify intracellular signaling pathways to inhibit immune-mediated cell killing (Chen *et al.*, 1997; Kittlesen *et al.*, 2000; Matsumoto *et al.*, 1997; Zhu *et al.*, 1998). Interfering with cellular signaling pathways may also contribute to cellular transformation through activation of cellular transcription factors or interaction with cellular proteins involved in cell growth regulation (Shrivastava *et al.*, 1998). The core protein interacts with retinoid X receptor-α (RXRα), a nuclear receptor involved in cell proliferation and metabolism (Tsutsumi *et al.*, 2002b). The mitogen-activated protein kinase (MAPK) cascade is also activated in the liver of the core gene transgenic mice. The MAPK pathway, which consists of three routes, c-Jun N-terminal kinase (JNK), p38, and extracellular signal-regulated kinase (ERK), is involved in numerous cellular events, including cell proliferation. In the liver of the core gene transgenic mice prior to HCC development, only the JNK route is activated. Downstream of the JNK activation, the transcription factor-activating factor (AP)-1 activation is markedly enhanced (Tsutsumi *et al.*, 2002b, 2003). Further downstream, both the mRNA and protein levels of cyclin D1 and CDK4 are increased. The suppression by HCV core protein of the suppressor of cytokine signaling-1 (*SOCS-1*), a tumor suppressor gene, may also contribute to hepatocarcinogenesis. Thus, the HCV core protein modulates the intracellular signaling pathways and confers an advantage to hepatocytes in terms of cell proliferation. Taken together, these pleiotropic effects of the core protein on the multiple signaling pathways, combined with that on oxidative stress, can have a profound impact on the HCC development in chronic HCV patients.

Thus, the HCV core protein can serve as a structural protein to encapsidate newly synthesized viral RNA and can also serve as a regulatory protein to modulate the activity of transcription factors and cytokines to promote cellular transformation. The following summarizes a number of signaling pathways that are affected by the HCV core protein.

2.6.1. *TNF-α*

The HCV core protein inhibits tumor necrosis factor-α (TNF-α)-mediated apoptosis through a mechanism that involves interactions with the TNF-α-receptor (Kittlesen *et al.*, 2000; Tai *et al.*, 2000). TNF-α is a major inflammatory cytokine secreted by activated macrophages and T cells, and plays a central role in resolving acute infections. TNF-α stimulates FAS-mediated apoptosis and facilitates clearance of infected cells. HCV core binds to the cytoplasmic domains of TNF receptor 1 (TNFR1), lymphotoxin-β receptor, and gC1q receptor and blocks FAS/TNF-α receptor signaling (Chen *et al.*, 1997; Kittlesen *et al.*, 2000; Matsumoto *et al.*, 1997; Zhu *et al.*, 1998). Blocking TNF-α-mediated signaling would result in the survival of infected cells.

2.6.2. *MAPK and AP-1*

The MAPK cascade and the transcription factor AP-1 are also activated in the liver of the core gene transgenic mice (Tsutsumi *et al.*, 2002a, 2003). Alteration of intracellular signaling cascade of MAPK and AP-1 can cause dysregulation of cell cycle and provoke the development of HCC (Ito *et al.*, 1998). In the liver of the core gene transgenic mice, the JNK pathway is activated before HCC development. AP-1 is a downstream effector of JNK. It activates the expression of

CDK4 and cyclin D1 and confers a proliferative advantage on hepatocytes (Koike *et al.*, 2002; Tsutsumi *et al.*, 2002a).

2.6.3. *NF-κB*

The HCV core activates NF-κB, a transcription factor that is involved in regulating the immune response (Zhu *et al.*, 2001). Hepatocytes from patients chronically infected with HCV show elevated levels of NF-κB and increased NF-κB DNA binding activity (Tai *et al.*, 2000). In addition, these cells are less responsive to TNF-α (Tai *et al.*, 2000).

2.6.4. *Oxidative stress*

Patients with chronic HCV infection have elevated levels of serum thioredoxin, a marker of acute intracellular oxidative stress (Shimoda *et al.*, 1994). In addition, DNA from patients suffering from chronic hepatitis C have elevated levels of 8-hydroxydeoxyguanosine, a DNA modification that is caused by oxidative stress (Shimoda *et al.*, 1994). The HCV core protein can induce oxidative stress. This induction of oxidative stress is believed to originate from mitochondrial dysfunction. Oxidative stress may also activate stellate cells that regulate hepatocyte growth and differentiation. Stellate cells are a major fibrogenic cell type in the liver that responds to cytokines, growth factors, and chemokines in response to liver injury. Their normal function is to produce an extracellular matrix to provide a scaffold for normal growth and differentiation of hepatocytes in response to liver damage. Chronic stellate cell activation in response to oxidative stress can contribute to fibrogenesis. The increased production of extracellular matrix and hepatocyte turnover coupled with activation of MAPKs, which can also be induced by oxidative stress, may ultimately lead to HCC (Finkel & Holbrook, 2000).

2.6.5. *Insulin resistance*

HCV core transgenic mice had markedly elevated serum levels of insulin although they did not develop overt diabetes (Shintani *et al.*, 2004). Plasma glucose levels were somewhat higher in transgenic mice than in their normal control littermates. HCV infection also induces insulin resistance *in vivo* (Shintani *et al.*, 2004).

2.6.6. *PPARα*

The HCV core protein interacts with RXRα and peroxisome proliferator-activated receptor-α (PPARα) (Tsutsumi *et al.*, 2002a). The core protein binds to RXRα, which plays important roles in cell proliferation and metabolism (Tsutsumi *et al.*, 2002a). PPARα activation is essential for HCV core protein-induced hepatic steatosis and HCC in mice (Tanaka *et al.*, 2008). HCV core protein induces spontaneous, persistent, age-dependent, and heterogeneous activation of PPARα in transgenic mice, which may contribute to the age-dependent and multicentric hepatocarcinogenesis mediated by the core protein (Tanaka *et al.*, 2008).

2.6.7. *Proteasome activator PA28γ*

The HCV core protein interacts with the proteasome activator PA28γ (Moriishi *et al.*, 2003). The HCV core protein suppresses insulin signaling through a PA28 γ-dependent pathway (Miyamoto *et al.*, 2007). HCV core protein enhances the binding of LXRα/RXRα to the LXR-responsive element in the presence but not in the absence of PA28γ. These findings suggest that PA28γ plays a crucial role in the development of liver pathology induced by HCV infection (Moriishi *et al.*, 2007).

2.6.8. *SOCS-1*

HCV core protein inhibits the expression of *SOCS-1* (Miyoshi *et al.*, 2005). *SOCS-1* is a negative regulator of cytokine signal pathway and has a tumor suppressor activity. The suppression of its expression has been implicated in the induction of hepatocarcinogenesis (Yoshikawa *et al.*, 2001).

2.6.9. *p53*

The HCV core protein has been shown to bind to *p53* and perturb its activity. This persistent perturbation of the *p53* activity by HCV during chronic infection likely plays an important role in HCV carcinogenesis (Yin *et al.*, 1999).

2.7. Oncogenic Activities of the HCV NS5A Protein

HCV NS5A is a nonstructural protein with no known enzymatic activities. However, it has been implicated in conferring resistance on interferon and altering cellular signaling pathways. Blocking the interferon action not only promotes persistent infection but may also interfere with normal cellular signaling pathways and ultimately lead to cellular transformation. Sequence analysis of NS5A from interferon nonresponder patients showed a high degree of sequence diversity that localized to a region of the NS5A gene (Gale *et al.*, 1998). This region was termed the interferon sensitivity-determining region (ISDR). Mutational analysis of the ISDR showed that this region was required for NS5A interaction with PKR, a protein kinase induced by interferon that downregulates viral translation and partially mediates the antiviral effects of interferons (Gale *et al.*, 1998). Activated PKR has been shown to be a mediator of apoptosis in response to certain types of cellular stress. Introduction of dsRNA into certain cell types activates PKR and leads to apoptosis (Kumar *et al.*, 1999). Expression of NS5A in NIH 3T3 cells can suppress dsRNA-mediated apoptosis and is dependent upon intact ISDR elements for this effect (Tan & Katze, 2001). In a similar study, NS5A prevented TNF-α-mediated apoptosis. While NS5A can suppress dsRNA-dependent apoptosis of NIH 3T3 cells, NS5A fails to block dsRNA-mediated apoptosis of HeLa cells, indicating that cell-type specific factors may also contribute to the dsRNA-dependent apoptotic phenotype. Suppression of dsRNA-mediated or TNF-α-induced apoptosis can also contribute to the induction of HCC. Consistent with this hypothesis, the constitutive expression of NS5A in NIH 3T3 cells induced cellular transformation and tumor formation after injection of the NS5A-expressing cells into nude mice. While NS5A with ISDR mutations also showed a growth stimulatory phenotype, they did not cause tumors in mice (Gale *et al.*, 1998; Ghosh *et al.*, 2000). Thus, it is unclear what role NS5A-dependent inhibition of PKR plays in causing cellular transformation and HCC.

3. Other Causative Factors in HCV-associated HCC

3.1. Chronic Liver Inflammation

Chronic liver inflammation caused by HCV infection is believed to be an important carcinogenic factor. Hepatocellular death due to chronic inflammation and the ensuing regeneration enhance mutagenesis in host cells, the accumulation of which may lead to HCC. This mechanism also applies to HBV, another hepatotropic virus that can cause chronic liver inflammation. However, it is unclear whether chronic inflammation by itself is sufficient to cause the high incidence of HCC in HCV patients, as HCC is rare in patients with persistent autoimmune hepatitis (Burroughs *et al.*, 1981).

HCV infection can cause either acute infection that is frequently clinically inapparent or chronic infection that is long-lasting (Lok & McMahon, 2001). The symptoms associated with chronic HCV infection may not be apparent for years but eventually fatigue, malaise, and other conditions typical of hepatitis may appear (Lok & McMahon, 2001). HCV-specific $CD8^+$ cytotoxic T-lymphocytes (CTL) are detected in HCV-infected patients early after infection (Lechner *et al.*, 2000). However, these HCV-specific CTLs display a "stunned" or anergic phenotype lacking the ability to secret IFN-γ upon proper stimulation. Additionally, persistent anergy of HCV-specific CTLs is found in patients with chronic HCV infection (Lechner *et al.*, 2000). In contrast, self-limited acute infection is associated with IFN-γ-secreting HCV-specific $CD8^+$ cells (Gruner *et al.*, 2000). It is unclear if persistence of the virus induces the anergy or if the recovery of CTLs is responsible for the clearance of the virus. Besides the $CD8^+$ CTLs, HCV-specific $CD4^+$ T cells have also been identified in HCV-infected individuals and are thought to play a role in clearing the virus (Gruner *et al.*, 2000). The maintenance of these $CD4^+$ T cells is important for the control of the virus, as their loss will result in HCV recurrence (Gerlach *et al.*, 1999). Despite the appearance of anti-HCV immune responses, the majority of HCV patients develop chronic infection with persistent viremia. These observations indicate that HCV can suppress cellular immunity, which in turn leads to persistent HCV infection with high incidence of carcinogenesis.

3.2. Alcohol

Ample epidemiological evidence suggests that there is a strong connection between HCV and alcoholic liver diseases (ALD). First, the prevalence of HCV is significantly higher among alcoholics than in the general population. For example, while the HCV positive rate in the general population of the United States is roughly 1%, it is 16% for alcoholics and nearly 30% for alcoholics with liver diseases (Heintges & Wands, 1997). Second, the presence of HCV infection correlates with the severity of the disease in alcoholic subjects, i.e. HCV-infected patients with ALD develop liver cirrhosis and HCC at a significantly younger age than uninfected ALD patients, suggesting that alcohol and HCV work synergistically to cause liver damage (Brechot *et al.*, 1996). Many studies also support synergistic interactions between HCV and alcoholism in hepatocarcinogenesis (Donato *et al.*, 2006; Hassan *et al.*, 2002; Lai *et al.*, 2006; Peters & Terrault, 2002; Yuan *et al.*, 2004). Heavy alcohol consumption and viral hepatitis synergistically increase the risk for HCC among blacks and whites in the United States (Yuan *et al.*, 2004). HCC odds ratio increases from 8.1 to 48.3 and 8.6 to 47.8 in HBV and HCV infected patients, respectively, if they also have concomitant alcohol abuse (Yuan *et al.*, 2004). Indeed, our recent result indicates that chronic alcohol intake increases the incidence of spontaneous HCC in HCV core transgenic mice 2-fold (unpublished observation).

Several possible mechanisms may explain the high prevalence rate of HCV among alcoholics and the increased severity of liver diseases in these patients. First, alcohol may enhance the replication of HCV and thus increase the expression of viral RNA and proteins, resulting in more severe HCV-induced liver injury, independent of the damage induced by alcohol alone. Indeed, HCV titer has been shown to exhibit a positive correlation with the amount of alcohol consumption (Oshita *et al.*, 1994). This enhanced effect on HCV replication could be caused directly by the metabolites of ethanol, such as acetaldehyde and free radicals, which may stimulate HCV replication and gene expression. It could also be caused indirectly through alcohol-induced inhibition of the antiviral immune response. Indeed, HCV replication is more active in immuno-deficient patients, such as HIV-infected patients (Sherman *et al.*, 1993), and ethanol consumption can cause immunosuppression (Paronetto, 1993).

Another potential mechanism is the involvement of cytokines. Both ALD and HCV cause enhanced secretion of TNF and other cytokines, such as IL-1, IL-6, and IL-8 (McClain & Cohen, 1989). TNF is particularly interesting because there is a tight correlation between the serum TNF concentration and the severity of ALD (Bird *et al.*, 1990; Khoruts *et al.*, 1991), and TNF receptor-1 (TNFR1) deficiency ameliorates experimental ALD (Ji *et al.*, 2004). TNF may cause cell death through the activation of the TRADD/FADD signal transduction pathway. On the other hand, a variety of factors can modulate the effects of TNF. For examples, NF-κB (Beg & Baltimore, 1996; Van Antwerp *et al.*, 1996; Wang *et al.*, 1996), manganous superoxide dismutase (MnSOD) (Wong *et al.*, 1989), and GSH inhibit TNF-induced cytotoxicity (Fernandez-Checa *et al.*, 1991). In experimental ALD, the mitochondrial pool of GSH is depleted, and the hepatocytes become hypersensitive to TNF (Fernandez-Checa *et al.*, 1991). We have shown that the HCV core protein binds to lymphotoxin-β receptor and TNF receptor (Matsumoto *et al.*, 1997) and that the expression of this protein in several cell lines sensitizes cells to TNF-induced cytolysis (Zhu *et al.*, 1998). Therefore, HCV-infected cells are particularly sensitive to TNF. It is interesting to note that HCV core protein also sensitizes cells to apoptosis mediated by Fas (Ruggieri *et al.*, 1997), which shares with TNF receptors signal transduction molecules such as FADD. These observations suggest that HCV-infected hepatocytes are very sensitive to TNF and possibly other cytokines as well. This enhanced sensitivity, coupled with the increased secretion of TNF in ALD, may account for the synergistic effects of ALD on HCV.

Alcoholism is associated with endotoxemia that stimulates the expression of proinflammatory cytokines and induces inflammation in the liver and fat tissues (Ribeiro *et al.*, 2004). Recently, we have shown that HCV infection, through its NS5A protein, upregulates toll-like receptor 4 (TLR4) expression. This provides another potential explanation for increased liver inflammation often observed in HCV patients with alcohol abuse, as endotoxin can bind to TLR4, leading to further accentuation of TLR4 signaling and the enhanced production of inflammatory cytokines.

4. Endoplasmic Reticulum Stress and HCV Pathogenesis

HCV can induce the ER stress and the unfolded protein response (Sir *et al.*, 2008). ER stress is a homeostatic mechanism that regulates cellular metabolism and protein synthesis in response to perturbations in protein folding and biosynthesis. In mild or early stage of ER stress, protein synthesis is inhibited and cell growth is slowed down. However, extreme or prolonged ER stress can lead to apoptosis (Moussalli *et al.*, 1999). The long-term consequence of persistent ER stress induced by HCV is not well understood, but it is likely that this persistent ER stress may cause alterations in cell physiology and predispose hepatocytes to cellular transformation.

ER stress signaling is intimately linked to cellular metabolism through connections involving changes in the intracellular redox state. These connections can lead to downregulation of GSH synthesis and the induction of oxidative stress (McCullough *et al.*, 1999). As discussed above, oxidative stress has profound effects on cellular metabolism, leading to increased mutation rates, changes in cellular proliferation, and, at extreme levels, apoptosis and HCC (Collins *et al.*, 1999; Finkel & Holbrook, 2000).

5. Gene Expression Profile of HCC

Microarray analysis of 102 liver tumors from 82 HBV and HCV patients showed no consistent differences between the gene expression profiles of these two patient groups (Chen *et al.*, 2002), although there were clear differences between tumor and non-tumor tissues in this study and other microarray studies (Xu *et al.*, 2001). HCCs, as analyzed by DNA microarrays, have been shown to have gene expression patterns that reveal individualities of the particular clonal tumor as well as to have a small subset of genes whose expression seemed to be distinctly associated with HCC (Chen *et al.*, 2002; Xu *et al.*, 2001). However, no consistent gene sets have been found that can clearly explain how HBV or HCV induces oncogenesis. Comparative gene expression clustering analysis has identified, for example, upregulated transcripts associated with cell growth in HCC tissue and downregulated transcripts associated with growth inhibition. Some caution must be taken in interpreting differential gene expression data, since different patterns of gene expression may reflect different degrees of de-differentiation of tumor cells.

6. HCV and Lymphomagenesis

6.1. Induction of *Ig* Hypermutation by HCV

The HCV virion consists of the core (~21 kDa) and two heavily N-glycosylated envelope proteins E1 (~31 kDa) and E2 (~70 kDa) (Grakoui *et al.*, 1993). Both E1 and E2 are type I transmembrane proteins, with an N-terminal ectodomain and a C-terminal hydrophobic anchor. HCV infection of its host cells requires the interaction of the E2 envelope protein with the cell surface receptor CD81 (Hsu *et al.*, 2003; McKeating *et al.*, 2004; Pileri *et al.*, 1998; Zhang *et al.*, 2004). CD81 is a member of the tetraspanin family and is a component of the multimeric B-cell antigen receptor complex (Levy *et al.*, 1998). It is associated with other membrane proteins, which vary in different B-cell lineages and include the signaling molecule CD19, complement receptor 2 (CD21), and interferon-inducible Leu-13

(CD225) protein (Levy *et al.*, 1998; Takahashi *et al.*, 1990). Binding of E2 or antibodies to CD81 induces B-cell aggregation, inhibits Daudi cell proliferation (Flint *et al.*, 1999), stimulates T cells (Soldaini *et al.*, 2003), and inhibits natural killer cell functions (Crotta *et al.*, 2002; Tseng & Klimpel, 2002). In addition, triggering of the CD81 signaling pathway in B cells enhances the production of TNF-α (Altomonte *et al.*, 1996). Correspondingly, HCV infection of primary macrophages has been reported to induce TNF-α production (Radkowski *et al.*, 2004). Co-engagement of the CD19–CD21–D81 complex and the B-cell antigen receptor lowers the B-cell activation threshold by antigen-presenting cells or lipopolysaccharide (Carter & Fearon, 1992). Lymphocytes in mice lacking CD81 develop normally but have altered proliferative responses and are deficient in antibody production, suggesting that CD81 is one of the essential receptors for the production of antibodies (Miyazaki *et al.*, 1997). These observations suggest that HCV may modify the BCR-associated signaling pathway by binding to CD81.

The engagement of B cells by purified E2 induced DSBs specifically in the variable region of *Ig* (V_H) gene locus, leading to hypermutation in V_H of B cells and the reduction of the antigen-binding activities of the antibodies they produce (Machida *et al.*, 2005, 2008). Other gene loci were not affected. Pre-incubation with the anti-CD81 monoclonal antibody blocked this effect. E2–CD81 interaction on B cells triggered the enhanced expression of AID and also stimulated the production of TNF-α (Machida *et al.*, 2005). Knockdown of the expression of AID with its specific siRNA blocked the E2-induced DSBs and the hypermutation of the V_H gene (Machida *et al.*, 2005). HCV infection, through E2–CD81 interaction, may suppress the host's adaptive immune response by activation of AID and hypermutation of *Ig* gene in B cells.

As mentioned above, we have reported that HCV infection induces hypermutation of many cellular genes, including *Ig* and *p53* genes in B cells (Machida *et al.*, 2004b). More recent studies showed that the HCV-induced mutations of somatic genes, such as *p53*, are mediated by NO, but the mechanism of HCV-induced mutation of *Ig* gene is still not clear (Machida *et al.*, 2004a). Both the somatic

hypermutation and class-switch recombination of *Ig* gene in normal B-cell development involve AID, which triggers deamination of deoxycytidine to deoxyuracil (dU) in the template DNA strand, with preference for certain hot-spot motifs (Petersen-Mahrt *et al.*, 2002). The resulting dU/dG pairs can be resolved by the mismatch repair system (Papavasiliou & Schatz, 2002), uracil glycosylase endonuclease (Di Noia & Neuberger, 2002) and error-prone DNA polymerases (Radkowski *et al.*, 2004). Pol ι, Pol η, and Pol ζ are involved in these pathways (Faili *et al.*, 2002; Zan *et al.*, 2001; Zeng *et al.*, 2001). Interestingly, AID, Pol ζ, and Pol ι are induced in HCV-infected B cells (Machida *et al.*, 2004b). The exact mechanism by which HCV induces AID and other enzymes, thereby causing hypermutation of *Ig* gene in B cells, are not well understood. It is likely that the binding of HCV to CD81 activates AID and other enzymes through the receptor-mediated signal transduction pathway. A model for HCV-induced hypermutation of *Ig* genes is illustrated in Fig. 1.

The E2–CD81 interaction induces AID and DSBs, leading to hypermutation of V_H in B cells. Furthermore, this interaction induces TNF-α production by B cells. These effects were confirmed in the natural HCV infection of B cell (Machida *et al.*, 2005). These findings indicate that, even in the absence of virus replication, the very act of virus binding to B cells can contribute to the pathogenesis of HCV. AID has been shown to promote illegitimate DNA recombination

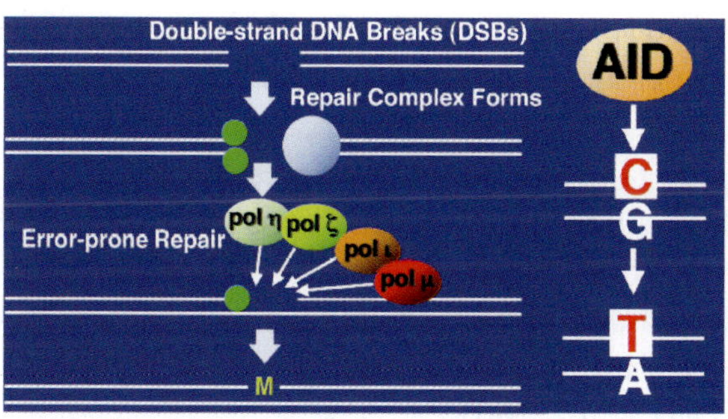

Fig. 1. Possible mechanisms of *Ig* hypermutation.

and somatic mutations of *Ig* as well as non-*Ig* genes. Thus, aberrant expression of AID is potentially oncogenic (Okazaki *et al.*, 2003). Indeed, aberrant expression of AID has been associated with chromosomal aberrations in patients with lymphocytic leukemia and non-Hodgkin's B-cell lymphomas (Heintel *et al.*, 2004), although the functional significance of this association has not been established (Albesiano *et al.*, 2003). In addition, transgenic mice with ectopic and dysregulated AID expression die early because of the development of epithelial and lymphoreticular neoplasm harboring hypermutated *Ig* and non-*Ig* genes (Okazaki *et al.*, 2003). AID may initiate DNA breaks, which are mediated by uracil–DNA glycosylase and apyrimidinic endonuclease (APE) (Di Noia & Neuberger, 2002), and recruit Rad52/Rad51 during somatic hypermutation (Zan *et al.*, 2003). DSB formation is required for the AID-induced mutations (Papavasiliou & Schatz, 2000). However, DSBs in the V_H locus could also occur even in the absence of AID, and could occur in gene segments that did not undergo somatic mutation (Bross *et al.*, 2002; Papavasiliou & Schatz, 2002). Furthermore, in the Burkitt's lymphoma cell line BL2, mutations occurred before DSBs were detected (Faili *et al.*, 2002). Thus, whether AID induction is sufficient to account for the DSBs and mutations induced by E2–CD81 interaction remains to be investigated. It is possible that additional proteins are involved, as the DNA cleavage in V_H is dependent on *de novo* protein synthesis (Nagaoka *et al.*, 2005). Surprisingly, an error-prone DNA polymerase, polymerase ζ, is induced by E2 binding, but it is not involved in the E2-induced DSBs or mutations of V_H gene. Another error-prone DNA polymerase, polymerase ι, which has previously been shown to be stimulated by HCV infection (Machida *et al.*, 2004b), is not induced by E2 binding. Thus, the functional roles of error-prone DNA polymerases in HCV-induced DNA mutations need further investigation. It has been reported that inactivation of polymerase ζ in a Burkitt's cell line (Zan *et al.*, 2001), or expression of polymerase ζ-specific antisense RNA in mice resulted in the reduction of mutation frequency (Diaz *et al.*, 2001).

6.2. Induction of DNA Translocation between *Ig* Genes and Proto-Oncogenes by HCV

The progression from MC to lymphoma is probably due to persistent HCV stimulation followed by a secondary transformation event. The exact mechanism for this transformation is still unclear. One possibility is through accumulation of additional genetic events such as *bcl-2* rearrangement. Indeed, the prevalence of *bcl-2* rearrangement in HCV patients with MC is significantly higher than in HCV patients without MC (Zignego *et al.*, 2002). The immunocytochemical analysis of bone marrow biopsies from 34/39 MC patients revealed that B-lymphocytes strongly expressed the *bcl-2* oncogene product (Monteverde *et al.*, 1995). The aberrant expression of *bcl-2* would lead to extended cell survival, which may predispose lymphocytes to further genetic aberration, such as the translocation of the *myc* oncogene. This may induce malignant lymphomas (Strasser *et al.*, 1990).

6.3. Dual Signaling Model for HCV-induced Mutagenesis in B Cells

HCV-induced NO production causes DSBs and *p53* mutations without significant effect on the V_H gene. The E2–CD81 interaction, conversely, enhances mutations in the V_H gene, but not in the *p53* gene. The basis for such differential effects is still not completely understood. As discussed above, the E2–CD81 interaction may trigger a signaling response similar to that triggered by anti-CD40, IL4 and other cytokines in B cells (Chaudhuri *et al.*, 2003; Muramatsu *et al.*, 1999). The normal somatic hypermutation mechanism of the V_H gene in B cells typically affects the genomic sequences within ~2 Kbp downstream from the transcription initiation site of the *Ig* gene (Rada & Milstein, 2001), under the influence of the *Ig* gene enhancer (Goyenechea *et al.*, 1997). This specificity may explain the differential effects of E2–CD81 interactions on V_H and *p53* genes. E2 will likely bind most cell types since CD81 is expressed ubiquitously. These findings suggest that the other components of the CD81

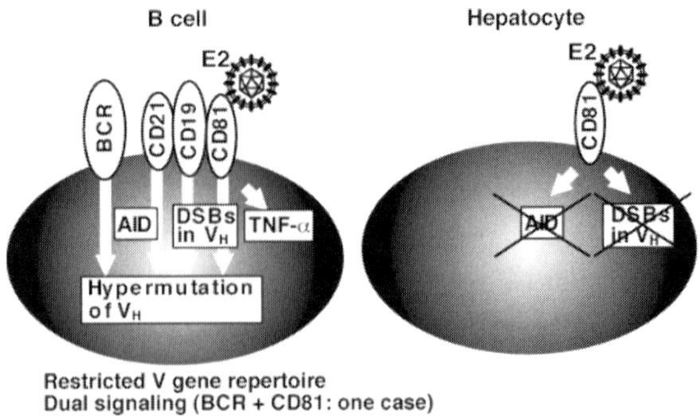

Fig. 2. Dual signaling model for HCV-induced hypermutation of the *Ig* gene in B cells. HCV antigens binding to BCR complex transmit an activation signal (signal 1) that is further amplified by binding of the HCV E2 envelope protein to CD81 (signal 2) to induce DSBs, AID and TNF-α (Weng & Levy, 2003). This leads to the hypermutation of V_H. Such an effect is not observed in hepatocytes, which do not have BCR.

complex, including CD21 and CD19, are also important for the induction of AID. In this regard, it is interesting to note that several protein kinases have been shown to be associated with CD19 and CD21 but not with CD81 (Fearon & Carter, 1995).

The BCR of some HCV-associated NHLs binds the viral E2 envelope protein (Quinn *et al.*, 2001), indicating that HCV can engage both the BCR and CD81 (Fig. 2). Such dual binding and activation of both B-cell signaling complexes would lower their activation threshold. This lower threshold may promote cellular proliferation, resulting initially in a nonmalignant monoclonal or oligoclonal B-cell lymphoproliferative disorder that produces a population of B cells at risk for malignant transformation. This scenario is supported by the observation that monoclonal *IgM* resolved in HCV-infected patients who responded to anti-viral treatment, supporting the linkage between antigen persistence and B-cell proliferation.

6.4. HCV and Non-Hodgkin's B-cell Lymphomas

Most cases of MC are a benign B-cell lymphoproliferative disorder that is associated with HCV infection (Cacoub *et al.*, 2000). However, benign B-cell proliferations may progress to lymphoma, as it has been demonstrated that a pre-malignant B-cell clone could convert to an overt B-cell lymphoma. The B-cell NHL is associated with HCV, but to a lesser degree than HCC. A recent report on regression of splenic marginal zone lymphoma after anti-HCV treatment with interferon and ribavirin has further strengthened the cause–effect relationship between HCV infection and lymphoma (Hermine *et al.*, 2002; Weng & Levy, 2003). In Italy, patients with B-cell NHL have a relative high prevalence rate (9–32%) of HCV infection and B-cell lymphoproliferative disorders (De Rosa *et al.*, 1997; Ferri *et al.*, 1994; Silvestri *et al.*, 1996). In one of these studies, HCV infection was detected in 32% of the NHL cases but in only 3% of patients with Hodgkin's disease and 1.3% of the healthy controls (Ferri *et al.*, 1994). Additional studies from the United States and Japan also showed an increased prevalence of HCV infection in patients with NHL (Zuckerman *et al.*, 1997).

7. Conclusions

Chronic HCV infection results in a high frequency of HCC that displays nonmetastatic and multicentric characteristics, and, to a lesser

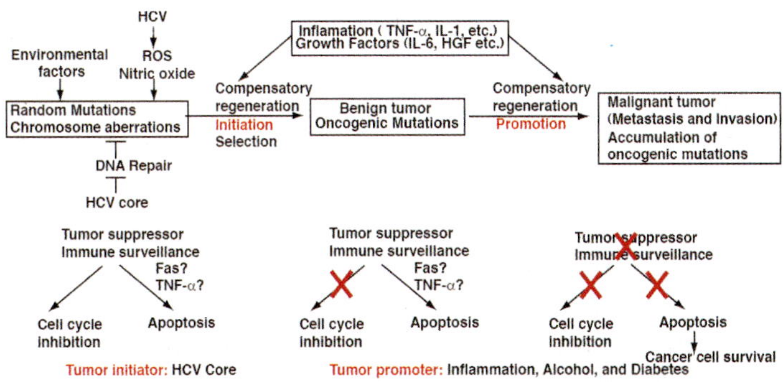

Fig. 3. Mechanisms of HCV carcinogenesis. HCV infection induces random mutations and chromosomal translocations, leading to benign tumor, which is synergized by environmental factors. Additional hits may induce malignant tumor development. Tumor suppressors play a key role in the induction of apoptosis of premalignant cells and the suppression of their malignant transformation, but the inactivation of their activities may cause cancer cell survival, leading to cancer development.

degree, NHL B-cell lymphoma. The molecular pathways of HCV-induced carcinogenesis may involve the indirect, nonvirological factors such as the induction of chronic liver inflammation and regeneration that lead to the emergence of mutated cells with high proliferation rates. In addition, it may also involve virological factors such as viral gene products that stimulate the production of ROS and the expression of error-prone DNA polymerases. These different pathways highlight the complicated interplays between the virus and its host in HCV carcinogenesis. The molecular pathways of HCV carcinogenesis are summarized in Fig. 3.

References

Albesiano E, Messmer BT, Damle RN, Allen SL, Rai KR, Chiorazzi N (2003) Activation-induced cytidine deaminase in chronic lymphocytic leukemia B cells: expression as multiple forms in a dynamic, variably sized fraction of the clone. *Blood* **102**(9): 3333–3339.

Altomonte M, Montagner R, Pucillo C, Maio M (1996) Triggering of target of an antiproliferative antibody-1 (TAPA-1/CD81) up-regulates the release of tumour necrosis factor-alpha by the EBV-B lymphoblastoid cell line JY. *Scand J Immunol* **43**(4): 367–373.

Bach N, Thung SN, Schaffner F (1992) The histological features of chronic hepatitis C and autoimmune chronic hepatitis: a comparative analysis. *Hepatology* **15**(4): 572–577.

Baumann P, West SC (1998) DNA end-joining catalyzed by human cell-free extracts. *Proc Natl Acad Sci USA* **95**(24): 14066–14070.

Becker SA, Lee TH, Butel JS, Slagle BL (1998) Hepatitis B virus X protein interferes with cellular DNA repair. *J Virol* **72**(1): 266–272.

Beg AA, Baltimore D (1996) An essential role for NF-kappaB in preventing TNF-alpha-induced cell death. *Science* **274**(5288): 782–784.

Bird GL, Sheron N, Goka AK, Alexander GJ, Williams RS (1990) Increased plasma tumor necrosis factor in severe alcoholic hepatitis. *Ann Intern Med* **112**(12): 917–920.

Brechot C, Nalpas B, Feitelson MA (1996) Interactions between alcohol and hepatitis viruses in the liver. *Clin Lab Med* **16**(2): 273–287.

Bromberg JF, Wrzeszczynska MH, Devgan G, Zhao Y, Pestell RG, Albanese C, Darnell JE Jr (1999) Stat3 as an oncogene. *Cell* **98**(3): 295–303.

Bross L, Muramatsu M, Kinoshita K, Honjo T, Jacobs H (2002) DNA double-strand breaks: prior to but not sufficient in targeting hypermutation. *J Exp Med* **195**(9): 1187–1192.

Brown GC (2001) Regulation of mitochondrial respiration by nitric oxide inhibition of cytochrome c oxidase. *Biochim Biophys Acta* **1504**(1): 46–57.

Burroughs AK, Bassendine MF, Thomas HC, Sherlock S (1981) Primary liver cell cancer in autoimmune chronic liver disease. *Br Med J (Clin Res Ed)* **282**(6260): 273.

Cacoub P, Hausfater P, Musset L, Piette JC (2000) Mixed cryoglobulinemia in hepatitis C patients. GERMIVIC. *Ann Med Interne (Paris)* **151**(1): 20–29.

Carter RH, Fearon DT (1992) CD19: lowering the threshold for antigen receptor stimulation of B lymphocytes. *Science* **256**(5053): 105–107.

Catlett-Falcone R, Landowski TH, Oshiro MM, Turkson J, Levitzki A, Savino R, Ciliberto G, Moscinski L, Fernandez-Luna JL, Nunez G, Dalton WS, Jove R (1999) Constitutive activation of Stat3 signaling confers resistance to apoptosis in human U266 myeloma cells. *Immunity* **10**(1): 105–115.

Chaudhuri J, Tian M, Khuong C, Chua K, Pinaud E, Alt FW (2003) Transcription-targeted DNA deamination by the AID antibody diversification enzyme. *Nature* **422**(6933): 726–730.

Chen CM, You LR, Hwang LH, Lee YH (1997) Direct interaction of hepatitis C virus core protein with the cellular lymphotoxin-beta receptor modulates the signal pathway of the lymphotoxin-beta receptor. *J Virol* **71**(12): 9417–9426.

Chen TH, Chen CJ, Yen MF, Lu SN, Sun CA, Huang GT, Yang PM, Lee HS, Duffy SW (2002) Ultrasound screening and risk factors for death from hepatocellular carcinoma in a high risk group in Taiwan. *Int J Cancer* **98**(2): 257–261.

Chen TM, Defendi V (1992) Functional interaction of *p53* with HPV18 E6, *c-myc* and H-ras in 3T3 cells. *Oncogene* 7(8): 1541–1547.

Choi J, Ou JH (2006) Mechanisms of liver injury. III. Oxidative stress in the pathogenesis of hepatitis C virus. *Am J Physiol Gastrointest Liver Physiol* **290**(5): G847–851.

Collins CE, Quaggiotto P, Wood L, O'Loughlin EV, Henry RL, Garg ML (1999) Elevated plasma levels of F2 alpha isoprostane in cystic fibrosis. *Lipids* **34**(6): 551–556.

Crotta S, Stilla A, Wack A, D'Andrea A, Nuti S, D'Oro U, Mosca M, Filliponi F, Brunetto RM, Bonino F, Abrignani S, Valiante NM (2002) Inhibition of natural killer cells through engagement of CD81 by the major hepatitis C virus envelope protein. *J Exp Med* **195**(1): 35–41.

De Rosa G, Gobbo ML, De Renzo A, Notaro R, Garofalo S, Grimaldi M, Apuzzo A, Chiurazzi F, Picardi M, Matarazzo M, Rotoli B (1997) High prevalence of hepatitis C virus infection in patients with B-cell lymphoproliferative disorders in Italy. *Am J Hematol* **55**(2): 77–82.

Deniaud A, Sharaf el dein O, Maillier E, Poncet D, Kroemer G, Lemaire C, Brenner C (2008) Endoplasmic reticulum stress induces calcium-dependent permeability transition, mitochondrial outer membrane permeabilization and apoptosis. *Oncogene* **27**(3): 285–299.

Di Bisceglie AM, Lyra AC, Schwartz M, Reddy RK, Martin P, Gores G, Lok AS, Hussain KB, Gish R, Van Thiel DH, Younossi Z, Tong M, Hassanein T, Balart L, Fleckenstein J, Flamm S, Blei A, Befeler AS (2003) Hepatitis C-related hepatocellular carcinoma in the United States: influence of ethnic status. *Am J Gastroenterol* **98**(9): 2060–2063.

Di Noia J, Neuberger MS (2002) Altering the pathway of immunoglobulin hypermutation by inhibiting uracil-DNA glycosylase. *Nature* **419**(6902): 43–48.

Diaz M, Verkoczy LK, Flajnik MF, Klinman NR (2001) Decreased frequency of somatic hypermutation and impaired affinity maturation but intact germinal center formation in mice expressing antisense RNA to DNA polymerase zeta. *J Immunol* **167**(1): 327–335.

Donato F, Gelatti U, Limina RM, Fattovich G (2006) Southern Europe as an example of interaction between various environmental factors: a systematic review of the epidemiologic evidence. *Oncogene* **25**(27): 3756–3770.

El-Serag HB, Mason AC (1999) Rising incidence of hepatocellular carcinoma in the United States. *N Engl J Med* **340**(10): 745–750.

Faili A, Aoufouchi S, Flatter E, Gueranger Q, Reynaud CA, Weill JC (2002) Induction of somatic hypermutation in immunoglobulin genes is dependent on DNA polymerase iota. *Nature* **419**(6910): 944–947.

Fearon DT, Carter RH (1995) The CD19/CR2/TAPA-1 complex of B lymphocytes: linking natural to acquired immunity. *Annu Rev Immunol* **13**: 127–149.

Fernandez-Checa JC, Garcia-Ruiz C, Ookhtens M, Kaplowitz N (1991) Impaired uptake of glutathione by hepatic mitochondria from chronic ethanol-fed rats. Tracer kinetic studies *in vitro* and *in vivo* and susceptibility to oxidant stress. *J Clin Invest* **87**(2): 397–405.

Ferri C, Caracciolo F, Zignego AL, La Civita L, Monti M, Longombardo G, Lombardini F, Greco F, Capochiani E, Mazzoni A *et al.* (1994) Hepatitis C virus infection in patients with non-Hodgkin's lymphoma. *Br J Haematol* **88**(2): 392–394.

Ferri C, La Civita L, Monti M, Longombardo G, Greco F, Pasero G, Zignego AL (1995) Can type C hepatitis infection be complicated by malignant lymphoma? *Lancet* **346**(8987): 1426–1427.

Ferri C, La Civita L, Zignego AL, Pasero G (1997) Viruses and cancers: possible role of hepatitis C virus. *Eur J Clin Invest* **27**(9): 711–718.

Finkel T, Holbrook NJ (2000) Oxidants, oxidative stress and the biology of ageing. *Nature* **408**(6809): 239–247.

Flint M, Maidens C, Loomis-Price LD, Shotton C, Dubuisson J, Monk P, Higginbottom A, Levy S, McKeating JA (1999) Characterization of hepatitis C virus E2 glycoprotein interaction with a putative cellular receptor, CD81. *J Virol* **73**(8): 6235–6244.

Fornek JL, Tygrett LT, Waldschmidt TJ, Poli V, Rickert RC, Kansas GS (2006) Critical role for Stat3 in T-dependent terminal differentiation of IgG B cells. *Blood* **107**(3): 1085–1091.

Frank EG, Tissier A, McDonald JP, Rapic-Otrin V, Zeng X, Gearhart PJ, Woodgate R (2001) Altered nucleotide misinsertion fidelity associated with poliota-dependent replication at the end of a DNA template. *EMBO J* **20**(11): 2914–2922.

Gale M, Jr, Blakely CM, Kwieciszewski B, Tan SL, Dossett M, Tang NM, Korth MJ, Polyak SJ, Gretch DR, Katze MG (1998) Control of PKR protein kinase by hepatitis C virus nonstructural 5A protein: molecular mechanisms of kinase regulation. *Mol Cell Biol* **18**(9): 5208–5218.

Gerlach JT, Diepolder HM, Jung MC, Gruener NH, Schraut WW, Zachoval R, Hoffmann R, Schirren CA, Santantonio T, Pape GR (1999) Recurrence of hepatitis C virus after loss of virus-specific CD4(+) T-cell response in acute hepatitis C. *Gastroenterology* **117**(4): 933–941.

Ghosh AK, Majumder M, Steele R, Meyer K, Ray R, Ray RB (2000) Hepatitis C virus NS5A protein protects against TNF-alpha mediated apoptotic cell death. *Virus Res* **67**(2): 173–178.

Goyenechea B, Klix N, Yelamos J, Williams GT, Riddell A, Neuberger MS, Milstein C (1997) Cells strongly expressing *Ig*(kappa) transgenes show clonal recruitment of hypermutation: a role for both MAR and the enhancers. *Embo J* **16**(13): 3987–3994.

Grakoui A, Wychowski C, Lin C, Feinstone SM, Rice CM (1993) Expression and identification of hepatitis C virus polyprotein cleavage products. *J Virol* **67**(3): 1385–1395.

Gruner NH, Gerlach TJ, Jung MC, Diepolder HM, Schirren CA, Schraut WW, Hoffmann R, Zachoval R, Santantonio T, Cucchiarini M, Cerny A, Pape GR (2000) Association of hepatitis C virus-specific CD8+ T cells with viral clearance in acute hepatitis C. *J Infect Dis* **181**(5): 1528–1536.

Haaf T, Golub EI, Reddy G, Radding CM, Ward DC (1995) Nuclear foci of mammalian Rad51 recombination protein in somatic cells after DNA damage and its localization in synaptonemal complexes. *Proc Natl Acad Sci USA* **92**(6): 2298–2302.

Hassan M, Ghozlan H, Abdel-Kader O (2004) Activation of RB/E2F signaling pathway is required for the modulation of hepatitis C virus core protein-induced cell growth in liver and non-liver cells. *Cell Signal* **16**(12): 1375–1385.

Hassan MM, Hwang LY, Hatten CJ, Swaim M, Li D, Abbruzzese JL, Beasley P, Patt YZ (2002) Risk factors for hepatocellular carcinoma: synergism of alcohol with viral hepatitis and diabetes mellitus. *Hepatology* **36**(5): 1206–1213.

Heintel D, Kroemer E, Kienle D, Schwarzinger I, Gleiss A, Schwarzmeier J, Marculescu R, Le T, Mannhalter C, Gaiger A, Stilgenbauer S, Dohner H, Fonatsch C, Jager U (2004) High expression of activation-induced cytidine deaminase (AID) mRNA is associated with unmutated *IGVH* gene status and unfavourable cytogenetic aberrations in patients with chronic lymphocytic leukaemia. *Leukemia* **18**(4): 756–762.

Heintges T, Wands JR (1997) Hepatitis C virus: epidemiology and transmission. *Hepatology* **26**(3): 521–526.

Hermine O, Lefrere F, Bronowicki JP, Mariette X, Jondeau K, Eclache-Saudreau V, Delmas B, Valensi F, Cacoub P, Brechot C, Varet B, Troussard X (2002) Regression of splenic lymphoma with villous lymphocytes after treatment of hepatitis C virus infection. *N Engl J Med* **347**(2): 89–94.

Hiom K (1999) DNA repair: Rad52 — the means to an end. *Curr Biol* **9**(12): R446–448.

Hirano T, Ishihara K, Hibi M (2000) Roles of *STAT3* in mediating the cell growth, differentiation and survival signals relayed through the IL-6 family of cytokine receptors. *Oncogene* **19**(21): 2548–2556.

Holbeck SL, Strathern JN (1997) A role for REV3 in mutagenesis during double-strand break repair in *Saccharomyces cerevisiae*. *Genetics* **147**(3): 1017–1024.

Honda M, Kaneko S, Shimazaki T, Matsushita E, Kobayashi K, Ping LH, Zhang HC, Lemon SM (2000) Hepatitis C virus core protein induces apoptosis and impairs cell-cycle regulation in stably transformed Chinese hamster ovary cells. *Hepatology* **31**(6): 1351–1359.

Hortelano S, Dallaporta B, Zamzami N, Hirsch T, Susin SA, Marzo I, Bosca L, Kroemer G (1997) Nitric oxide induces apoptosis via triggering mitochondrial permeability transition. *FEBS Lett* **410**(2–3): 373–377.

Hsu M, Zhang J, Flint M, Logvinoff C, Cheng-Mayer C, Rice CM, McKeating JA (2003) Hepatitis C virus glycoproteins mediate pH-dependent cell entry of pseudotyped retroviral particles. *Proc Natl Acad Sci USA* **100**(12): 7271–7276.

Ito Y, Sasaki Y, Horimoto M, Wada S, Tanaka Y, Kasahara A, Ueki T, Hirano T, Yamamoto H, Fujimoto J, Okamoto E, Hayashi N, Hori M (1998) Activation of mitogen-activated protein kinases/extracellular signal-regulated kinases in human hepatocellular carcinoma. *Hepatology* **27**(4): 951–958.

Izumi T, Sasaki R, Miura Y, Okamoto H (1996) Primary hepatosplenic lymphoma: association with hepatitis C virus infection. *Blood* **87**(12): 5380–5381.

Izumi T, Sasaki R, Tsunoda S, Akutsu M, Okamoto H, Miura Y (1997) B cell malignancy and hepatitis C virus infection. *Leukemia* **11**(3): 516–518.

Jaiswal M, LaRusso NF, Burgart LJ, Gores GJ (2000) Inflammatory cytokines induce DNA damage and inhibit DNA repair in cholangiocarcinoma cells by a nitric oxide-dependent mechanism. *Cancer Res* **60**(1): 184–190.

Jaiswal M, LaRusso NF, Shapiro RA, Billiar TR, Gores GJ (2001) Nitric oxide-mediated inhibition of DNA repair potentiates oxidative DNA damage in cholangiocytes. *Gastroenterology* **120**(1): 190–199.

Jeang KT, Widen SG, Semmes OJt, Wilson SH (1990) HTLV-I trans-activator protein, tax, is a trans-repressor of the human beta-polymerase gene. *Science* **247**(4946): 1082–1084.

Ji C, Deng Q, Kaplowitz N (2004) Role of TNF-alpha in ethanol-induced hyperhomocysteinemia and murine alcoholic liver injury. *Hepatology* **40**(2): 442–451.

Kao SY, Marriott SJ (1999) Disruption of nucleotide excision repair by the human T-cell leukemia virus type 1 tax protein. *J Virol* **73**(5): 4299–4304.

Kato N, Yoshida H, Kioko Ono-Nita S, Kato J, Goto T, Otsuka M, Lan K, Matsushima K, Shiratori Y, Omata M (2000) Activation of intracellular signaling by hepatitis B and C viruses: C-viral core is the most potent signal inducer. *Hepatology* **32**(2): 405–412.

Khoruts A, Stahnke L, McClain CJ, Logan G, Allen JI (1991) Circulating tumor necrosis factor, interleukin-1 and interleukin-6 concentrations in chronic alcoholic patients. *Hepatology* **13**(2): 267–276.

Kim WH, Hong F, Jaruga B, Hu Z, Fan S, Liang TJ, Gao B (2001) Additive activation of hepatic NF-kappaB by ethanol and hepatitis B protein X (HBX) or HCV core protein: involvement of TNF-alpha receptor 1-independent and -dependent mechanisms. *Faseb J* **15**(13): 2551–2553.

Kitay-Cohen Y, Amiel A, Hilzenrat N, Buskila D, Ashur Y, Fejgin M, Gaber E, Safadi R, Tur-Kaspa R, Lishner M (2000) *Bcl-2* rearrangement in patients with chronic hepatitis C associated with essential mixed cryoglobulinemia type II. *Blood* **96**(8): 2910–2912.

Kittlesen DJ, Chianese-Bullock KA, Yao ZQ, Braciale TJ, Hahn YS (2000) Interaction between complement receptor gC1qR and hepatitis C virus core protein inhibits T-lymphocyte proliferation. *J Clin Invest* **106**(10): 1239–1249.

Koike K, Moriya K, Ishibashi K, Yotsuyanagi H, Shintani Y, Fujie H, Kurokawa K, Matsuura Y, Miyamura T (1997) Sialadenitis histologically resembling Sjogren syndrome in mice transgenic for hepatitis C virus envelope genes. *Proc Natl Acad Sci USA* **94**(1): 233–236.

Koike K, Tsutsumi T, Fujie H, Shintani Y, Kyoji M (2002) Molecular mechanism of viral hepatocarcinogenesis. *Oncology* **62**(1): 29–37.

Kumar KU, Srivastava SP, Kaufman RJ (1999) Double-stranded RNA-activated protein kinase (PKR) is negatively regulated by 60S ribosomal subunit protein L18. *Mol Cell Biol* **19**(2): 1116–1125.

Lai MM (2002) Hepatitis C virus proteins: direct link to hepatic oxidative stress, steatosis, carcinogenesis and more. *Gastroenterology* **122**(2): 568–571.

Lai MS, Hsieh MS, Chiu YH, Chen TH (2006) Type 2 diabetes and hepatocellular carcinoma: a cohort study in high prevalence area of hepatitis virus infection. *Hepatology* **43**(6): 1295–1302.

Lechner F, Wong DK, Dunbar PR, Chapman R, Chung RT, Dohrenwend P, Robbins G, Phillips R, Klenerman P, Walker BD (2000) Analysis of successful immune responses in persons infected with hepatitis C virus. *J Exp Med* **191**(9): 1499–1512.

Lerat H, Honda M, Beard MR, Loesch K, Sun J, Yang Y, Okuda M, Gosert R, Xiao SY, Weinman SA, Lemon SM (2002) Steatosis and liver cancer in transgenic mice expressing the structural and nonstructural proteins of hepatitis C virus. *Gastroenterology* **122**(2): 352–365.

Levy S, Todd SC, Maecker HT (1998) CD81 (TAPA-1): a molecule involved in signal transduction and cell adhesion in the immune system. *Annu Rev Immunol* **16**: 89–109.

Lieber MR, Ma Y, Pannicke U, Schwarz K (2003) Mechanism and regulation of human non-homologous DNA end-joining. *Nat Rev Mol Cell Biol* **4**(9): 712–720.

Lok AS, McMahon BJ (2001) Chronic hepatitis B. *Hepatology* **34**(6): 1225–1241.

Machida K, Cheng KT, Lai CK, Jeng KS, Sung VM, Lai MM (2006) Hepatitis C virus triggers mitochondrial permeability transition with production of reactive oxygen species, leading to DNA damage and *STAT3* activation. *J Virol* **80**(14): 7199–7207.

Machida K, Cheng KT, Pavio N, Sung VM, Lai MM (2005) Hepatitis C virus E2-CD81 interaction induces hypermutation of the immunoglobulin gene in B cells. *J Virol* **79**(13): 8079–8089.

Machida K, Cheng KT, Sung VM, Lee KJ, Levine AM, Lai MM (2004a) Hepatitis C virus infection activates the immunologic (type II) isoform of nitric oxide synthase and thereby enhances DNA damage and mutations of cellular genes. *J Virol* **78**(16): 8835–8843.

Machida K, Cheng KT, Sung VM, Shimodaira S, Lindsay KL, Levine AM, Lai MY, Lai MM (2004b) Hepatitis C virus induces a mutator phenotype: enhanced mutations of immunoglobulin and protooncogenes. *Proc Natl Acad Sci USA* **101**(12): 4262–4267.

Machida K, Kondo Y, Huang JY, Chen YC, Cheng KT, Keck Z, Foung S, Dubuisson J, Sung VM, Lai MM (2008) Hepatitis C virus (HCV)-induced immunoglobulin hypermutation reduces the affinity and neutralizing activities of antibodies against HCV envelope protein. *J Virol* **82**(13): 6711–6720.

Matsumoto M, Hsieh TY, Zhu N, VanArsdale T, Hwang SB, Jeng KS, Gorbalenya AE, Lo SY, Ou JH, Ware CF, Lai MM (1997) Hepatitis C virus core protein interacts with the cytoplasmic tail of lymphotoxin-beta receptor. *J Virol* **71**(2): 1301–1309.

McClain CJ, Cohen DA (1989) Increased tumor necrosis factor production by monocytes in alcoholic hepatitis. *Hepatology* **9**(3): 349–351.

McCullough AK, Dodson ML, Lloyd RS (1999) Initiation of base excision repair: glycosylase mechanisms and structures. *Annu Rev Biochem* **68**: 255–285.

McKeating JA, Zhang LQ, Logvinoff C, Flint M, Zhang J, Yu J, Butera D, Ho DD, Dustin LB, Rice CM, Balfe P (2004) Diverse hepatitis C virus glycoproteins mediate viral infection in a CD81-dependent manner. *J Virol* **78**(16): 8496–8505.

Miyamoto H, Moriishi K, Moriya K, Murata S, Tanaka K, Suzuki T, Miyamura T, Koike K, Matsuura Y (2007) Involvement of the PA28gamma-dependent pathway in insulin resistance induced by hepatitis C virus core protein. *J Virol* **81**(4): 1727–1735.

Miyazaki T, Muller U, Campbell KS (1997) Normal development but differentially altered proliferative responses of lymphocytes in mice lacking CD81. *Embo J* **16**(14): 4217–4225.

Miyoshi H, Fujie H, Shintani Y, Tsutsumi T, Shinzawa S, Makuuchi M, Kokudo N, Matsuura Y, Suzuki T, Miyamura T, Moriya K, Koike K (2005) Hepatitis C virus core protein exerts an inhibitory effect on suppressor of cytokine signaling (*SOCS*)-*1* gene expression. *J Hepatol* **43**(5): 757–763.

Monteverde A, Sabattini E, Poggi S, Ballare M, Bertoncelli MC, De Vivo A, Briskomatis A, Roncador G, Falini B, Pileri SA (1995) Bone marrow findings further support the hypothesis that essential mixed cryoglobulinemia type II is characterized by a monoclonal B-cell proliferation. *Leuk Lymphoma* **20**(1–2): 119–124.

Moriishi K, Mochizuki R, Moriya K, Miyamoto H, Mori Y, Abe T, Murata S, Tanaka K, Miyamura T, Suzuki T, Koike K, Matsuura Y (2007) Critical role of PA28gamma in hepatitis C virus-associated steatogenesis and hepatocarcinogenesis. *Proc Natl Acad Sci USA* **104**(5): 1661–1666.

Moriishi K, Okabayashi T, Nakai K, Moriya K, Koike K, Murata S, Chiba T, Tanaka K, Suzuki R, Suzuki T, Miyamura T, Matsuura Y (2003) Proteasome activator PA28gamma-dependent nuclear retention and degradation of hepatitis C virus core protein. *J Virol* 77(19): 10237–10249.

Moriya K, Fujie H, Shintani Y, Yotsuyanagi H, Tsutsumi T, Ishibashi K, Matsuura Y, Kimura S, Miyamura T, Koike K (1998) The core protein of hepatitis C virus induces hepatocellular carcinoma in transgenic mice. *Nat Med* **4**(9): 1065–1067.

Moriya K, Fujie H, Yotsuyanagi H, Shintani Y, Tsutsumi T, Matsuura Y, Miyamura T, Kimura S, Koike K (1997) Subcellular localization of hepatitis C virus structural proteins in the liver of transgenic mice. *Jpn J Med Sci Biol* **50**(4–5): 169–177.

Moriya K, Nakagawa K, Santa T, Shintani Y, Fujie H, Miyoshi H, Tsutsumi T, Miyazawa T, Ishibashi K, Horie T, Imai K, Todoroki T, Kimura S, Koike K (2001a) Oxidative stress in the absence of inflammation in a mouse model for hepatitis C virus-associated hepatocarcinogenesis. *Cancer Res* **61**(11): 4365–4370.

Moriya K, Todoroki T, Tsutsumi T, Fujie H, Shintani Y, Miyoshi H, Ishibashi K, Takayama T, Makuuchi M, Watanabe K, Miyamura T, Kimura S, Koike K (2001b) Increase in the concentration of carbon 18 monounsaturated fatty acids in the liver with hepatitis C: analysis in transgenic mice and humans. *Biochem Biophys Res Commun* **281**(5): 1207–1212.

Moussalli M, Pipe SW, Hauri HP, Nichols WC, Ginsburg D, Kaufman RJ (1999) Mannose-dependent endoplasmic reticulum (ER)–Golgi intermediate compartment-53-mediated ER to Golgi trafficking of coagulation factors V and VIII. *J Biol Chem* **274**(46): 32539–32542.

Muramatsu M, Sankaranand VS, Anant S, Sugai M, Kinoshita K, Davidson NO, Honjo T (1999) Specific expression of activation-induced cytidine deaminase (AID), a novel member of the RNA-editing deaminase family in germinal center B cells. *J Biol Chem* **274**(26): 18470–18476.

Nagaoka H, Ito S, Muramatsu M, Nakata M, Honjo T (2005) DNA cleavage in immunoglobulin somatic hypermutation depends on *de novo* protein synthesis but not on uracil DNA glycosylase. *Proc Natl Acad Sci USA* **102**(6): 2022–2027.

Nathan C (1992) Nitric oxide as a secretory product of mammalian cells. *Faseb J* **6**(12): 3051–3064.

Nguyen T, Brunson D, Crespi CL, Penman BW, Wishnok JS, Tannenbaum SR (1992) DNA damage and mutation in human cells exposed to nitric oxide *in vitro*. *Proc Natl Acad Sci USA* **89**(7): 3030–3034.

Okazaki IM, Hiai H, Kakazu N, Yamada S, Muramatsu M, Kinoshita K, Honjo T (2003) Constitutive expression of AID leads to tumorigenesis. *J Exp Med* **197**(9): 1173–1181.

Oshita M, Hayashi N, Kasahara A, Hagiwara H, Mita E, Naito M, Katayama K, Fusamoto H, Kamada T (1994) Increased serum hepatitis C virus RNA levels among alcoholic patients with chronic hepatitis C. *Hepatology* **20**(5): 1115–1120.

Papavasiliou FN, Schatz DG (2000) Cell-cycle-regulated DNA double-stranded breaks in somatic hypermutation of immunoglobulin genes. *Nature* **408**(6809): 216–221.

Papavasiliou FN, Schatz DG (2002) Somatic hypermutation of immunoglobulin genes: merging mechanisms for genetic diversity. *Cell* **109**(Suppl): S35–S44.

Paronetto F (1993) Immunologic reactions in alcoholic liver disease. *Semin Liver Dis* **13**(2): 183–195.

Peters MG, Terrault NA (2002) Alcohol use and hepatitis C. *Hepatology* **36**(5 Suppl 1): S220–S225.

Petersen-Mahrt SK, Harris RS, Neuberger MS (2002) AID mutates *E. coli* suggesting a DNA deamination mechanism for antibody diversification. *Nature* **418**(6893): 99–103.

Pileri P, Uematsu Y, Campagnoli S, Galli G, Falugi F, Petracca R, Weiner AJ, Houghton M, Rosa D, Grandi G, Abrignani S (1998) Binding of hepatitis C virus to CD81. *Science* **282**(5390): 938–941.

Poltoratsky V, Woo CJ, Tippin B, Martin A, Goodman MF, Scharff MD (2001) Expression of error-prone polymerases in BL2 cells activated for *Ig* somatic hypermutation. *Proc Natl Acad Sci USA* **98**(14): 7976–7981.

Quinn ER, Chan CH, Hadlock KG, Foung SK, Flint M, Levy S (2001) The B-cell receptor of a hepatitis C virus (HCV)-associated non-Hodgkin lymphoma binds the viral E2 envelope protein, implicating HCV in lymphomagenesis. *Blood* **98**(13): 3745–3749.

Rada C, Milstein C (2001) The intrinsic hypermutability of antibody heavy and light chain genes decays exponentially. *Embo J* **20**(16): 4570–4576.

Radkowski M, Bednarska A, Horban A, Stanczak J, Wilkinson J, Adair DM, Nowicki M, Rakela J, Laskus T (2004) Infection of primary human macrophages with hepatitis C virus *in vitro*: induction of tumour necrosis factor-alpha and interleukin 8. *J Gen Virol* **85**(Pt 1): 47–59.

Ribeiro PS, Cortez-Pinto H, Sola S, Castro RE, Ramalho RM, Baptista A, Moura MC, Camilo ME, Rodrigues CM (2004) Hepatocyte apoptosis, expression of death receptors, and activation of NF-kappaB in the liver of nonalcoholic and alcoholic steatohepatitis patients. *Am J Gastroenterol* **99**(9): 1708–1717.

Routledge MN (2000) Mutations induced by reactive nitrogen oxide species in the supF forward mutation assay. *Mutat Res* **450**(1–2): 95–105.

Ruggieri A, Harada T, Matsuura Y, Miyamura T (1997) Sensitization to Fas-mediated apoptosis by hepatitis C virus core protein. *Virology* **229**(1): 68–76.

Saito I, Miyamura T, Ohbayashi A, Harada H, Katayama T, Kikuchi S, Watanabe Y, Koi S, Onji M, Ohta Y *et al.* (1990) Hepatitis C virus infection is associated with the development of hepatocellular carcinoma. *Proc Natl Acad Sci USA* **87**(17): 6547–6549.

Schweyer S, Mihm S, Radzun HJ, Hartmann H, Fayyazi A (2000) Liver infiltrating T lymphocytes express interferon gamma and inducible nitric oxide synthase in chronic hepatitis C virus infection. *Gut* **46**(2): 255–259.

Sherman KE, O'Brien J, Gutierrez AG, Harrison S, Urdea M, Neuwald P, Wilber J (1993) Quantitative evaluation of hepatitis C virus RNA in patients with concurrent human immunodeficiency virus infections. *J Clin Microbiol* **31**(10): 2679–2682.

Shimoda R, Nagashima M, Sakamoto M, Yamaguchi N, Hirohashi S, Yokota J, Kasai H (1994) Increased formation of oxidative DNA damage, 8-hydroxydeoxyguanosine, in human livers with chronic hepatitis. *Cancer Res* **54**(12): 3171–3172.

Shintani Y, Fujie H, Miyoshi H, Tsutsumi T, Tsukamoto K, Kimura S, Moriya K, Koike K (2004) Hepatitis C virus infection and diabetes: direct involvement of the virus in the development of insulin resistance. *Gastroenterology* **126**(3): 840–848.

Shrivastava A, Manna SK, Ray R, Aggarwal BB (1998) Ectopic expression of hepatitis C virus core protein differentially regulates nuclear transcription factors. *J Virol* **72**(12): 9722–9728.

Silvestri F, Barillari G, Fanin R, Pipan C, Falasca E, Salmaso F, Zaja F, Infanti L, Patriarca F, Botta GA, Baccarani M (1997) The genotype of the hepatitis C virus in patients with HCV-related B cell non-Hodgkin's lymphoma. *Leukemia* **11**(12): 2157–2161.

Silvestri F, Pipan C, Barillari G, Zaja F, Fanin R, Infanti L, Russo D, Falasca E, Botta GA, Baccarani M (1996) Prevalence of hepatitis C virus infection in patients with lymphoproliferative disorders. *Blood* **87**(10): 4296–4301.

Simonetti RG, Camma C, Fiorello F, Cottone M, Rapicetta M, Marino L, Fiorentino G, Craxi A, Ciccaglione A, Giuseppetti R *et al.* (1992) Hepatitis C virus infection as a risk factor for hepatocellular carcinoma in patients with cirrhosis. A case-control study. *Ann Intern Med* **116**(2): 97–102.

Sir D, Chen WL, Choi J, Wakita T, Yen TS, Ou JH (2008) Induction of incomplete autophagic response by hepatitis C virus via the unfolded protein response. *Hepatology* **48**(4): 1054–1061.

Soldaini E, Wack A, D'Oro U, Nuti S, Ulivieri C, Baldari CT, Abrignani S (2003) T cell costimulation by the hepatitis C virus envelope protein E2 binding to CD81 is mediated by Lck. *Eur J Immunol* **33**(2): 455–464.

Starke DW, Chen Y, Bapna CP, Lesnefsky EJ, Mieyal JJ (1997) Sensitivity of protein sulfhydryl repair enzymes to oxidative stress. *Free Radic Biol Med* **23**(3): 373–384.

Steller MA, Zou Z, Schiller JT, Baserga R (1996) Transformation by human papillomavirus 16 E6 and E7: role of the insulin-like growth factor 1 receptor. *Cancer Res* **56**(21): 5087–5091.

Stracker TH, Carson CT, Weitzman MD (2002) Adenovirus oncoproteins inactivate the Mre11-Rad50-NBS1 DNA repair complex. *Nature* **418**(6895): 348–352.

Strasser A, Harris AW, Bath ML, Cory S (1990) Novel primitive lymphoid tumours induced in transgenic mice by cooperation between *myc* and *bcl-2*. *Nature* **348**(6299): 331–333.

Strathern JN, Shafer BK, McGill CB (1995) DNA synthesis errors associated with double-strand-break repair. *Genetics* **140**(3): 965–972.

Tai DI, Tsai SL, Chen YM, Chuang YL, Peng CY, Sheen IS, Yeh CT, Chang KS, Huang SN, Kuo GC, Liaw YF (2000) Activation of nuclear factor kappaB in hepatitis C virus infection: implications for pathogenesis and hepatocarcinogenesis. *Hepatology* **31**(3): 656–664.

Takahashi S, Doss C, Levy S, Levy R (1990) TAPA-1, the target of an antiproliferative antibody, is associated on the cell surface with the Leu-13 antigen. *J Immunol* **145**(7): 2207–2213.

Takeda S, Shibata M, Morishima T, Harada A, Nakao A, Takagi H, Nagai Y (1992) Hepatitis C virus infection in hepatocellular carcinoma. Detection of plus-strand and minus-strand viral RNA. *Cancer* **70**(9): 2255–2259.

Tan SL, Katze MG (2001) How hepatitis C virus counteracts the interferon response: the jury is still out on NS5A. *Virology* **284**(1): 1–12.

Tanaka N, Moriya K, Kiyosawa K, Koike K, Gonzalez FJ, Aoyama T (2008) PPARalpha activation is essential for HCV core protein-induced hepatic steatosis and hepatocellular carcinoma in mice. *J Clin Invest* **118**(2): 683–694.

Tseng CT, Klimpel GR (2002) Binding of the hepatitis C virus envelope protein E2 to CD81 inhibits natural killer cell functions. *J Exp Med* **195**(1): 43–49.

Tsutsumi T, Suzuki T, Moriya K, Shintani Y, Fujie H, Miyoshi H, Matsuura Y, Koike K, Miyamura T (2003) Hepatitis C virus core protein activates ERK and p38 MAPK in cooperation with ethanol in transgenic mice. *Hepatology* **38**(4): 820–828.

Tsutsumi T, Suzuki T, Moriya K, Yotsuyanagi H, Shintani Y, Fujie H, Matsuura Y, Kimura S, Koike K, Miyamura T (2002a) Alteration of intrahepatic cytokine expression and AP-1 activation in transgenic mice expressing hepatitis C virus core protein. *Virology* **304**(2): 415–424.

Tsutsumi T, Suzuki T, Shimoike T, Suzuki R, Moriya K, Shintani Y, Fujie H, Matsuura Y, Koike K, Miyamura T (2002b) Interaction of hepatitis C virus core protein with retinoid X receptor alpha modulates its transcriptional activity. *Hepatology* **35**(4): 937–946.

Van Antwerp DJ, Martin SJ, Kafri T, Green DR, Verma IM (1996) Suppression of TNF-alpha-induced apoptosis by NF-kappaB. *Science* **274**(5288): 787–789.

Wang CY, Mayo MW, Baldwin AS Jr (1996) TNF- and cancer therapy-induced apoptosis: potentiation by inhibition of NF-kappaB. *Science* **274**(5288): 784–787.

Wegenka UM, Lutticken C, Buschmann J, Yuan J, Lottspeich F, Muller-Esterl W, Schindler C, Roeb E, Heinrich PC, Horn F (1994) The interleukin-6-activated acute-phase response factor is antigenically and functionally related to members of the signal transducer and activator of transcription (STAT) family. *Mol Cell Biol* **14**(5): 3186–3196.

Weng WK, Levy S (2003) Hepatitis C virus (HCV) and lymphomagenesis. *Leuk Lymphoma* **44**(7): 1113–1120.

Wong GH, Elwell JH, Oberley LW, Goeddel DV (1989) Manganous superoxide dismutase is essential for cellular resistance to cytotoxicity of tumor necrosis factor. *Cell* **58**(5): 923–931.

Xu XR, Huang J, Xu ZG, Qian BZ, Zhu ZD, Yan Q, Cai T, Zhang X, Xiao HS, Qu J, Liu F, Huang QH, Cheng ZH, Li NG, Du JJ, Hu W, Shen KT, Lu G, Fu G, Zhong M, Xu SH, Gu WY, Huang W, Zhao XT, Hu GX, Gu JR, Chen Z, Han ZG (2001) Insight into hepatocellular carcinogenesis at transcriptome level by comparing gene expression profiles of hepatocellular carcinoma with those of corresponding noncancerous liver. *Proc Natl Acad Sci USA* **98**(26): 15089–15094.

Yin M, Wheeler MD, Kono H, Bradford BU, Gallucci RM, Luster MI, Thurman RG (1999) Essential role of tumor necrosis factor alpha in alcohol-induced liver injury in mice. *Gastroenterology* **117**(4): 942–952.

Yoshikawa H, Matsubara K, Qian GS, Jackson P, Groopman JD, Manning JE, Harris CC, Herman JG (2001) *SOCS-1*, a negative regulator of the JAK/STAT pathway, is silenced by methylation in human hepatocellular carcinoma and shows growth-suppression activity. *Nat Genet* **28**(1): 29–35.

Yuan JM, Govindarajan S, Arakawa K, Yu MC (2004) Synergism of alcohol, diabetes, and viral hepatitis on the risk of hepatocellular carcinoma in blacks and whites in the U.S. *Cancer* **101**(5): 1009–1017.

Zan H, Komori A, Li Z, Cerutti A, Schaffer A, Flajnik MF, Diaz M, Casali P (2001) The translesion DNA polymerase zeta plays a major role in *Ig* and *bcl-6* somatic hypermutation. *Immunity* **14**(5): 643–653.

Zan H, Wu X, Komori A, Holloman WK, Casali P (2003) AID-dependent generation of resected double-strand DNA breaks and recruitment of Rad52/Rad51 in somatic hypermutation. *Immunity* **18**(6): 727–738.

Zeng X, Winter DB, Kasmer C, Kraemer KH, Lehmann AR, Gearhart PJ (2001) DNA polymerase eta is an A-T mutator in somatic hypermutation of immunoglobulin variable genes. *Nat Immunol* **2**(6): 537–541.

Zhang J, Randall G, Higginbottom A, Monk P, Rice CM, McKeating JA (2004) CD81 is required for hepatitis C virus glycoprotein-mediated viral infection. *J Virol* **78**(3): 1448–1455.

Zhu L, Fukuda S, Cordis G, Das DK, Maulik N (2001) Anti-apoptotic protein survivin plays a significant role in tubular morphogenesis of human coronary arteriolar endothelial cells by hypoxic preconditioning. *FEBS Lett* **508**(3): 369–374.

Zhu N, Khoshnan A, Schneider R, Matsumoto M, Dennert G, Ware C, Lai MM (1998) Hepatitis C virus core protein binds to the cytoplasmic domain of tumor necrosis factor (TNF) receptor 1 and enhances TNF-induced apoptosis. *J Virol* **72**(5): 3691–3697.

Zignego AL, Ferri C, Giannelli F, Giannini C, Caini P, Monti M, Marrocchi ME, Di Pietro E, La Villa G, Laffi G, Gentilini P (2002) Prevalence of *bcl-2* rearrangement in patients with hepatitis C virus-related mixed cryoglobulinemia with or without B-cell lymphomas. *Ann Intern Med* **137**(7): 571–580.

Zuckerman E, Zuckerman T, Levine AM, Douer D, Gutekunst K, Mizokami M, Qian DG, Velankar M, Nathwani BN, Fong TL (1997) Hepatitis C virus infection in patients with B-cell non-Hodgkin lymphoma. *Ann Intern Med* **127**(6): 423–428.

Chapter 4

Human Papillomaviruses and Associated Malignancies

Christine L. Nguyen*,
Margaret E. McLaughlin-Drubin* and Karl Münger*

Abstract: Human papillomaviruses (HPVs) are a DNA virus family of approximately 200 types that specifically infect cutaneous or mucosal epithelia. The most common HPV types are "low-risk" and cause benign epithelial hyperplasias known as warts. However, there is also a group of "high-risk" HPV types that are associated with lesions that can undergo malignant progression. Virtually all cervical carcinoma cases are associated with high-risk HPV infection. Specifically, the two viral proteins, E6 and E7, are required for both the induction and maintenance of the transformed phenotype. E6 and E7 alone contribute to induction and perpetuation of genomic instability, thus generating the host chromosomal abnormalities that are necessary for carcinogenic progression. An understanding of the molecular mechanisms of such an etiologically well-defined model of cancer development can provide invaluable insights into general human cancer development.

1. Introduction

Papillomaviruses (PVs) are a group of small, nonenveloped, double-stranded DNA viruses that comprise the *Papillomaviridae* family.

*The Channing Laboratory, Brigham and Women's Hospital and Department of Medicine, Harvard Medical School, Boston, Massachusetts.

They are found throughout the animal kingdom but are highly species specific (de Villiers, 2001). PVs are nonlytic viruses that infect epithelial cells and cause the formation of papillomas, or warts. Lesions can be cutaneous or can occur on mucosal squamous epithelium. PVs were first identified by Richard Shope in the cottontail rabbit (Shope & Hurst, 1933). However, the discovery of human papillomavirus (HPV) genomes in genital warts was first accomplished in the laboratory of Harald zur Hausen (de Villiers *et al.*, 1981; Gissmann *et al.*, 1982). Using these viral DNAs as hybridization probes under conditions of low stringency, his laboratory succeeded in detecting HPV sequences in cervical cancer tissues (Durst *et al.*, 1983). Since then, great strides have been made to understand and identify HPVs and, to date, more than 200 HPV types have been characterized (de Villiers *et al.*, 2004). New HPV types are defined as sharing less than 90% homology within the L1 open reading frame (ORF) of the closest related type (de Villiers, 2001). Subtypes differ by only 2–10% and variants differ by less than 2% in the L1 ORF. HPV types can also be placed into phylogenetic supergroups depending on their sequence, tropism, and pathogenicity; supergroup A contains genital HPVs, supergroup B contains cutaneous HPVs associated with epidermodysplasia verruciformis (EV), supergroup C contains ungulate fibropapillomaviruses, supergroup D contains cutaneous bovine PVs (BPVs), and supergroup E contains cutaneous PVs (Van Ranst *et al.*, 1992). Furthermore, HPVs have also been classified as either low-risk or high-risk HPVs based on the frequency with which they cause viral-associated malignant tumors. Low-risk HPVs generally cause benign warts, while high-risk HPVs cause lesions that can progress to cervical carcinoma.

2. Viral Life Cycle

The HPV life cycle is closely linked to the differentiation program of the infected epithelial cell. The skin, the largest organ of the human body, is constantly turned over and contains a single layer of dividing cells, the basal cells. Basal cells undergo asymmetric mitosis with one daughter cell remaining a proliferating basal cell while the other daughter cell becomes a suprabasal, differentiating cell. The suprabasal cell withdraws from the cell division cycle and undergoes a program of terminal differentiation, thus ensuring the mechanical stability of the skin and protecting the proliferating basal cells from direct exposure to environmental mutagens. In order to establish a stable infection, PVs need to infect basal cells through mechanisms that remain poorly understood (reviewed in Streeck *et al.*, 2007). Following initial infection, the genomes are maintained at a low copy number in the basal cells and persistent infection is established. The production of infectious virus occurs in the terminally differentiated layers of the epithelium and progeny virions are sloughed off within the terminally differentiated, de-nucleated epithelial squames. The shed virus is stable and retains infectious properties over extended periods (reviewed in Lee & Laimins, 2007).

2.1. Viral Genome

The approximately 8-kb double-stranded circular DNA viral genome is packaged into a 55-nm, icosohedral, nonenveloped virion. Within the virion, the viral DNA is organized into chromatic structures by association with cellular histones. The genome consists of three functional regions: the long control region (LCR), also known as the upstream regulatory region (URR) or the noncoding region (NCR), the early (E) region, and the late (L) region (Seedorf *et al.*, 1985) (Fig. 1). The approximately 1-kb LCR has no coding potentials and contains DNA elements that are responsible for regulating early viral transcription and contribute to both the tissue tropism of HPVs (Sailaja *et al.*, 1999; Sen *et al.*, 2002) and contains the viral origin of replication. Both the early and late ORFs are transcribed from a single DNA strand (Pfister & Fuchs, 1994) and are encoded from each of the three possible reading frames. The early region consists of six to seven ORFs designated E1, E2, E4, E5, E6, E7, and E8. The late region consists of two ORFs designated L1 and L2. During the nonproductive phase of the viral life cycle, E6, E7, E1, and E2 are transcribed from the HPV early promoter (Hummel *et al.*, 1992; Ozbun & Meyers, 1998). During the productive phase of the life cycle, which

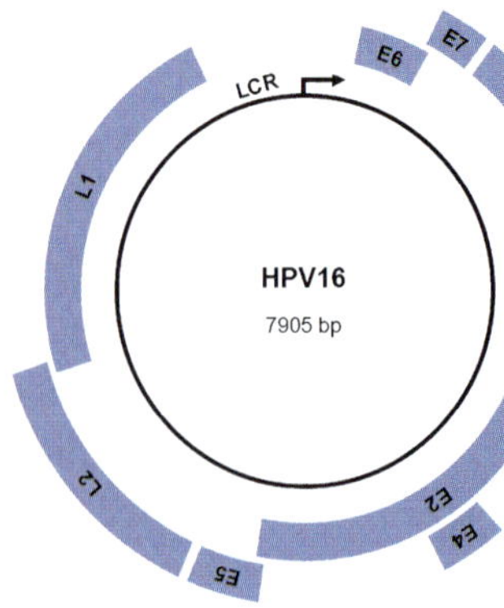

Fig. 1. The HPV16 genome. Schematic representation of the HPV16 double-stranded DNA viral genome. The circular genome (inner circle) is 7905 bp in size and the early (E) and late (L) genes are transcribed from a single strand in each possible reading frame. The arrow indicates the major early promoter, P_{97}.

occurs in the differentiating epithelium (Turek, 1994), the late promoter is active leading to the production of the L1 and L2 capsid proteins (Hummel *et al.*, 1992).

2.2. Infection

HPVs infect epithelial cells; some HPVs display tropism for cutaneous epithelia, while others show preference for mucosal epithelia. Normal squamous epithelia consist of a basal cell layer that is composed of undifferentiated proliferating cells and is protected from the external environment by several layers of differentiated cells that have withdrawn from the cell cycle. Because HPVs depend upon host cell machinery for synthesizing their genomes, the virus must infect the proliferating basal cells in order to establish a persistent infection (reviewed in Munger, 2002). Generally, the virus gains access to basal cells through micro-abrasions in the skin due to physical trauma. Squamocolumnar junctions, such as the transformation zone in the cervix, contain reserve cells that can give rise to squamous or columnar epithelia, and it is thought that the reserve cells are physiologically relevant targets for infection with mucosal HPVs (Martens *et al.*, 2004; Smedts *et al.*, 1992; Tsutsumi *et al.*, 1993).

It remains unclear which receptors are necessary for HPVs to bind and enter cells. Studies suggest that $\alpha6\beta1$ and $\alpha6\beta4$ integrins may serve as receptors (Evander *et al.*, 1997; McMillan *et al.*, 1999), although they are not necessary for infection by all PVs (Sibbet *et al.*, 2000). Additionally, HPV infection requires the presence of heparan sulfate on the cell surface (Giroglou *et al.*, 2001). However, after binding to receptors, the mechanisms through which the virus enters the cell, gains entry to the nucleus, and uncoats its DNA remain enigmatic.

2.3. Productive Viral Infection

The HPV life cycle is closely linked to the differentiation program of infected epithelial cells. A number of promoters are involved in producing the various mRNA species for the genital tract HPVs. In HPV16, the P_{97} promoter is active in non-terminally differentiated cells and, upon differentiation, the P_{670} promoter becomes active and directs the expression of late gene products (reviewed in Howley & Lowy, 2007). Elements in the LCR of the HPV genome also are important in the coordination of viral transcription with the differentiation state of the infected epithelial cell. The LCR contains enhancer elements that are responsive to cellular factors, some of which impart tissue or cell-type specificity (Sailaja *et al.*, 1999). Additionally, the LCR contains a number of transcription factor-binding sites, including sites for AP1, SP1, Oct-1, and YY1 (reviewed in Howley & Lowy, 2007).

In basal cells, the viral genome is maintained episomally and low levels of viral DNA synthesis occur; after initial infection, the viral genome is amplified to 50–100 copies per cell, and then is maintained as a multicopy plasmid in infected cells. This is known as the non-productive phase of the viral life cycle. In this phase, the viral DNA is replicated bi-directionally through theta structure intermediates, but no progeny virus is produced. The replication factors, E1 and E2, are among the first viral proteins to be expressed. E1 and E2 form a complex that binds to the viral origin of replication and recruits the cellular DNA polymerase α/primase and other cellular factors to mediate replication (Conger *et al.*, 1999; Frattini & Laimins, 1994; Mohr *et al.*, 1990). Furthermore, E1 exhibits ATPase and DNA helicase activity (Hughes & Romanos, 1993), and is required for the initiation and elongation of viral DNA synthesis (Liu *et al.*, 1995). E2 also recruits host factors, such as replication protein A (RPA), to the origin to stimulate viral DNA replication (Li & Botchan, 1994), but unlike E1, does not play an enzymatic role in viral DNA replication. E1 associates with a number of host cellular proteins, such as histone H1, SW1/SNF5, cyclin E/CDK2, Hsp40/Hsp70, and Ubc9, although understanding the significances of some of these interactions requires further study (reviewed in Howley & Lowy, 2007).

The E2 protein regulates viral transcription from the early promoter by associating with its cognate sites within the LCR of HPV genomes (Cripe *et al.*, 1987). However, high-risk HPV E2 proteins primarily function as transcriptional repressors of viral early gene expression (Soeda *et al.*, 2006). It was reported that at low concentrations, E2 can activate the early promoter, while at higher levels, E2 acts to repress transcription by preventing the association of cellular transcription factors (Steger & Corbach, 1997). Nevertheless, other factors, such as specific promoters or the cellular environment, may also determine whether E2 functions as an activator or a repressor. E2 is also involved in viral episome maintenance. Since the long-term maintenance of viral episomes requires a *cis* element on the viral plasmid that contains multiple E2-binding sites (Piirsoo *et al.*, 1996), the role of E2 in episome maintenance appears to be due to the ability of E2 to link viral episomes to cellular mitotic chromosomes to ensure the segregation and proper compartmentalization of the viral episome during and following mitosis. It has been shown that E2 associates with mitotic chromosomes (Bastien & McBride, 2000), although the cellular protein(s) that mediates the interaction remains a contentious issue. It was reported that the interaction between E2 and Brd4 was important for the association of E2 with mitotic chromosomes

(You *et al.*, 2004; Baxter *et al.*, 2005), but not all HPVs utilize this mechanism of genome partitioning (McPhillips *et al.*, 2006). However, it was also shown that E2 associates with a DNA helicase, ChlR1, and that this interaction is necessary for loading E2 onto chromosomes and for genome maintenance (Parish *et al.*, 2006). Other mechanisms of genome segregation, such as a direct association between E2 and microtubules, have been proposed for some HPVs (Van Tine *et al.*, 2004). Ultimately, the mechanism by which E2 participates in viral genome segregation requires further study and the possibility exists that this mechanism is just not conserved between HPV types. Regardless of the mechanism of HPV genome maintenance in basal cells, it is thought that PVs infect basal cells that have stem cell-like properties (Martens *et al.*, 2004); alternatively, PVs may reprogram an infected cell to a more stem cell-like state. Recently it was reported that normal diploid cells can be converted to stem cells via the alteration of the expression of genes that are usually epigentically silenced (Takahashi *et al.*, 2007; Yu *et al.*, 2007).

As the infected basal cell divides, the daughter cell moves upwards and begins to differentiate. In order for the virus to continue replicating its genome, however, a DNA replication competent cellular milieu must be preserved despite the differentiation of infected epithelial cells. The E6 and E7 proteins are necessary for abrogating cell-cycle withdrawal in differentiating cells. High-risk E6 associates with the p53 tumor suppressor protein and a cellular ubiquitin ligase, E6AP, leading to the aberrant degradation of p53 (Huibregtse *et al.*, 1991; Scheffner *et al.*, 1994; Werness *et al.*, 1990). E7 associates with the retinoblastoma (pRB) tumor suppressor and the pRB family members, p107 and p130, as well as with other cell-cycle regulators (reviewed in Munger *et al.*, 2007). The biological activities of high-risk HPV E6 and E7, especially those that contribute to immortalization and transformation, are discussed further below. In short, these viral proteins serve to maintain S-phase competence in highly differentiated cells. This process of uncoupling cellular proliferation and differentiation is responsible for the formation of benign hyperproliferative lesions, manifested as warts, which result from productive papillomaviral infection. Furthermore, E6 and E7 appear to be important for the maintenance of viral episomes in the infected basal cells, although the mechanisms remain unclear (McLaughlin-Drubin *et al.*, 2005; Oh *et al.*, 2004; Park & Androphy, 2002; Thomas *et al.*, 1999).

The late stages of the viral life cycle, including capsid protein synthesis and virion assembly, are restricted to the uppermost layers of the differentiated keratinocytes. Although the E4 and E5 proteins are encoded in the early region, their expression patterns are more consistent with those of late genes. The functions of E4 and E5 are still relatively unclear. E4 proteins associate with the keratin cytoskeleton and induce the collapse of the cytokeratin network (Doorbar *et al.*, 1991; Roberts *et al.*, 1993) and therefore may be important for viral egress. The E5 protein has been proposed to play a role in the modification of differentiation-induced cell-cycle exit (Fehrmann *et al.*, 2003). Transforming activities have been detected for E5 proteins of some HPV types and these are discussed further below.

The L1 and L2 proteins are also expressed late in the viral life cycle. Both L1 and L2 contain a nuclear localization signal (NLS) (Zhou *et al.*, 1995) and virion assembly occurs in the nucleus. L2 plays a role in the selective encapsidation of viral DNA into viral capsids and therefore is required for the infectivity of virions (Zhou *et al.*, 1993). L1 and L2 spontaneously form icosahedral capsids, although L1 alone is sufficient for capsid formation, and full virions contain only one copy of the viral genome. Virus particles are detected in the upper granular layer of the epithelium. Since HPVs are not lytic, it is thought that subsequent infections occur when virus-containing squames are sloughed off.

3. Clinical Disease

3.1. Prevalence

HPVs account for the most common sexually transmitted infection worldwide. Modeling studies suggest that up to 80% of women will have acquired a genital HPV infection by the age of 50 (Myers *et al.*, 2000); while comparable numbers for males are not available, they are likely similar. Worldwide, it is estimated that approximately 630 million individuals are infected with HPV, and 30 million cases of genital HPV infection are diagnosed each year (Scheurer *et al.*, 2005). Furthermore, it is estimated that 20 million people are currently infected with HPV in the United States alone, with approximately 6.2 million people becoming infected each year (Cates, 1999; Koutsky, 1997). Almost half of the currently infected individuals are sexually active adolescents and young adults, 15–24 years of age, and the majority of new infections occur among this age group as well (Weinstock *et al.*, 2004). In the United States, the estimated total of HPV-related costs, which includes the costs of screens and treatments, is in excess of $3 billion per year (Chesson *et al.*, 2004); the vast majority of these costs are spent on the clinical management of potentially premalignant lesions.

3.2. Pathology

3.2.1. *Papillomas*

Papillomas, also referred to as "warts" when found on the skin or "condylomas" when found on genitalia, are benign proliferative epithelial lesions that are composed of all the layers of the differentiated epithelium (reviewed in Howley & Lowy, 2007). Usually, warts and condylomas do not display the nuclear atypia that is commonly observed in the basal-like cells in cervical intraepithelial neoplasia (CIN) (Arends *et al.*, 1998). The types of warts (flat, filiform, plantar, palmar, or mosaic) acquired appear to correlate with infection by specific HPV types (reviewed in Howley & Lowy, 2007). The majority of warts or condylomas are associated with low-risk HPVs with types 6 and 11 being responsible for most condylomas (Greer *et al.*, 1995). Due to the location of condylomas, the prevalence of these lesions, not surprisingly, correlates with sexual activity. Although lesions, may remain for months to years, they may also regress spontaneously or persist indefinitely and only very infrequently progress toward carcinogenesis. Regression is thought to be due to an immunologic response (Coleman *et al.*, 1994; Jablonska *et al.*, 1997).

3.2.2. *Cervical cancer*

According to the World Health Organization, cervical cancer is the second most common cancer among women worldwide (Walboomers *et al.*, 1999). Infection with high-risk HPVs is the most significant risk factor for developing cervical cancer (Walboomers *et al.*, 1999). In fact, HPVs are associated with greater than 99% of all cervical cancer cases, with high-risk HPV types 16, 18, 31, 33, and 45 detected in up to 97% of cervical cancer cases worldwide (Clifford *et al.*, 2003; Walboomers *et al.*, 1999). In addition to squamoous cell carcinomas, HPV DNA has also been detected in most cervical adenocarcinomas, adenosquamous carcinomas, and carcinomas with neuroendocrine differentiation (reviewed in Howley & Lowy, 2007). Interestingly, HPV16 is most frequently associated with squamouse cell carcinomas, whereas HPV18 is the predominant type found in adenocarcinomas and neuroendocrine carcinomas, suggesting that infection by different viral types can result in different pathologies.

It is estimated that in 2008 there will be 11,070 new cervical cancer diagnoses and 3,870 cervical cancer-associated deaths in the United States (Jemal *et al.*, 2008). Cervical cancer rates are double among African-American women as compared to Caucasian women in the United States; this discrepancy appears attributable to socioeconomic differences (Schwartz *et al.*, 2003). Worldwide, there is an estimation of 510,000 new diagnoses of cervical cancer and 288,000 associated deaths per year (Saslow *et al.*, 2007); 80% of these cases are reported in developing countries where screening programs have not been established (World Health Organization, 2005). Despite the decrease in cases in developed countries, cervical cancer remains the second leading cause of cancer death in young women worldwide.

Cervical cancer is generally caused by high-risk HPV types, which cause premalignant lesions that have a propensity to progress toward malignancy. Malignant progression is relatively infrequent and usually occurs many years or even decades after the initial infection (Richart & Barron, 1969; Wright *et al.*, 2002b). Invasive cervical cancer is preceded by cervical dysplasia, which is classified by the degree to which basaloid cells replace the squamous epithelium (reviewed in Howley & Lowy, 2007) (Fig. 2). Previously, CINs were categorized into grades,

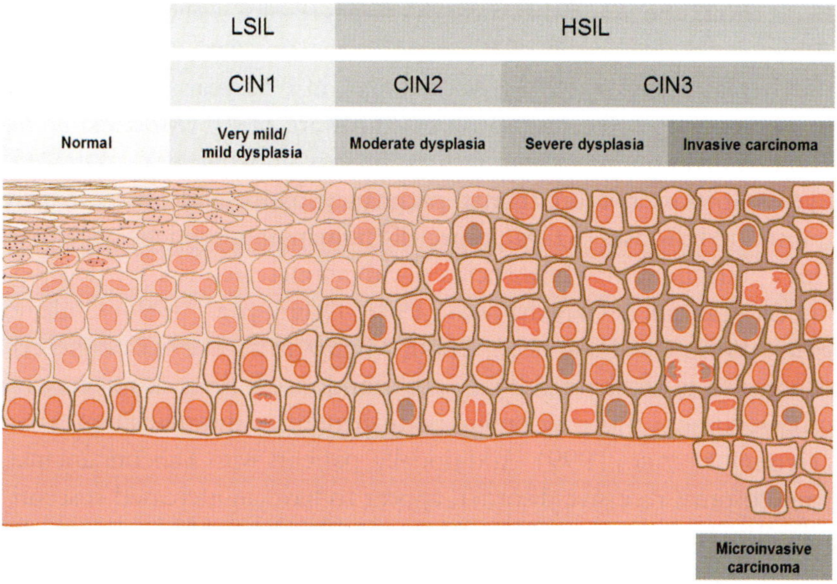

Fig. 2. Degrees of HPV-induced dysplasia. Image shows the progression from normal epithelial tissue to invasive carcinoma. Top row of gray bars (LSIL and HSIL) correspond to the Bethesda System used for classification of cervical cytological screens. The middle gray bars (CIN1-3) refer to histological classifications. See text for details.

where grade I corresponded to mild dysplasia, grade II corresponded to moderate dysplasia, and grade III corresponded to severe dysplasia or carcinoma *in situ*. However, according to the Bethesda System, abnormal cervical cytology results from Pap smears, named after their inventor, Georgios Papanicolaou, are now classified as atypical squamous cells (ASC) or squamous intraepithelial lesions (SIL) (Kurman *et al.*, 1991). ASCs are further designated as ASCs of undetermined significance (ASCUS) or "ASCs, cannot exclude high-grade SILs" (ASC-H) (Solomon *et al.*, 2002). SILs are further categorized as low-grade SILs (LSILs), which correspond to mild dysplasia and CIN grade I, or high-grade SIL (HSIL), which correspond to moderate and severe dysplasia, CIN grade II and III, and carcinoma *in situ* (Solomon *et al.*, 2002). In invasive cervical carcinoma, the dysplastic cells penetrate the basement membrane, invade the stromal tissue, and metastasize to additional sites in the body (Shah *et al.*, 1996).

It should be noted that most dysplasias resolve without treatment, although the likelihood of regression decreases with the severity of the dysplasia (Ostor, 1993). Accordingly, in a 10-year study, only 3% of women with LSIL cases progressed toward HSIL (Moscicki *et al.*, 2004). Furthermore, certain factors, such as smoking, oral contraceptives, nutrition, micronutrients, pregnancy, parity, and other sexually transmitted diseases (STDs), especially human immunodeficiency virus (HIV) infection, may be associated with an increased risk for developing cervical cancer (Batieha *et al.*, 1993; Daling *et al.*, 1996; Giuliano *et al.*, 1997; Kjellberg *et al.*, 2000; Munoz *et al.*, 1994). Some evidence also exists for hereditary contributions to the risk for cervical cancer, though this may be linked to hereditary immunosuppression (Hemminki *et al.*, 1999). Additionally, patients with Fanconi anemia, an autosomal recessive disorder, appear to have an increased susceptibility to HPV-induced carcinogenesis (Kutler *et al.*, 2003), potentially due to an HPV-mediated acceleration of chromosomal instability in cells from these patients (Spardy *et al.*, 2007).

3.2.3. *Other HPV-associated carcinomas*

In addition to cervical carcinomas, HPVs have been associated with other malignancies as well. High-risk HPVs are associated with approximately 40–60% of vaginal carcinomas, vaginal intraepithelial neoplasias, and penile carcinomas, up to 50% of vulvar carcinomas, and approximately 90% of anal carcinomas (reviewed in Parkin & Bray, 2006). Similar to cervical carcinoma, HPV-associated anal carcinomas arise in the transition zone between columnar and squamous epithelia (reviewed in Howley & Lowy, 2007). The risk for developing anal cancer is higher among HIV-infected individuals than in the general population (Frisch *et al.*, 2000).

HPV-associated cancers can also be found in the oral pharynx (tonsils, tonsillar fossa, base of tongue, and soft palate) and, while the most common risk factors for oral cancer are cigarette smoking and alcohol consumption, some oral cancers have been attributed to HPV infection (Gillison *et al.*, 2000; Mellin *et al.*, 2000; Schwartz *et al.*, 1998; Snijders *et al.*, 1996). At least 20% of tumors from the tongue and tonsils contain viral DNA from high-risk HPV types with HPV16 being the most common type isolated from oral cancers (Gillison *et al.*, 2000). The mode of transmission has not yet been fully determined, but oral sex practices have been implicated (Kreimer *et al.*, 2004). Infection with HPV may also contribute to some cases of esophageal cancer (Sur & Cooper, 1998), but the role of the virus is less clear in these cancers. Unlike the case with cervical cancers, there are no standard screening programs available to aid in the early detection of oropharyngeal lesions.

In immunosuppressed individuals, HPVs have also been associated with 90% of nonmelanoma skin cancers (NMSC) (de Villiers *et al.*, 1999; Kiviat, 1999; Pfister & Ter Schegget, 1997), which can affect both basal cells and squamous cells. Nevertheless, the link between NMSC and HPV infection is not as strong as that between squamous cell carcinomas found in individuals with epidermodysplasia verruciformis (EV), a rare autosomal recessive genodermatosis caused by mutations in the *EVER1/TMC6* and *EVER2/TMC8* genes (Ramoz *et al.*, 2002) and viral infection. Individuals with EV have a unique susceptibility to cutaneous HPV infection (Majewski *et al.*, 1997), but the warts do not usually regress and can lead to squamous cell cancers. HPV5 and -8 are associated with approximately 90% of the skin cancers from EV individuals. Malignant tumors in these individuals tend to remain local, but metastases may occur.

Lesions caused by low-risk mucosal HPVs have a low risk for malignant progression; however, in rare cases, low-risk HPV infections can cause serious disease, as in the case of recurrent respiratory papillomatosis (RRP) and giant condylomas of Buschke-Lowenstein. RRP is caused by infection with HPV6 or -11 at birth. While there is presumably a genetic component to disease development, the exact genetic locus remains to be elucidated. Patients with RRP develop rapidly growing wart-like lesions in the larynx and around the vocal cords, which can then spread to the trachea and lung. This disease is associated with considerable morbidity and mortality, as patients require frequent surgeries to keep the airways clear (reviewed in Tasca & Clarke, 2006).

HPV6 and -11 infections can also cause giant condyloma of Buschke-Lowenstein; and, similar to the case with RRP, patients are unable to control or clear the infection. While the tumor is slow growing, it is extremely destructive to adjacent tissue. Unlike RRP, Buschke-Lowenstein condyloma can give rise to local and distant metastases (reviewed in Frega *et al.*, 2002; Rhea *et al.*, 1998).

4. Detection, Treatment, and Prevention

4.1. Screening and Detection

As evidenced in the United States, screening for cervical cancer can dramatically reduce mortality rates. Pap smears or tests were designed to detect premalignant and malignant lesions in the ectocervix and sometimes in the endocervix. The National Cancer Institute currently recommends that women have a Pap test performed at least once every three years and, in 2003, it was estimated that 65.6 million Pap tests were performed (Solomon *et al.*, 2007). The test has changed slightly since its first inception and now involves collecting cells from the outer opening of the cervix and placing the cells on a slide to be checked for the above-mentioned cervical cytological abnormalities (Virtej & Vasiliu, 2003). Liquid-based monolayer cytology is being increasingly used; this method is based on the preservation of cells in a vial of liquid fixative medium after the Pap test. The cells are then processed into a thin layer, stained, and examined for abnormalities (Selvaggi, 2001). The liquid-based monolayer cytology method appears to have a reduced rate of false-positivity since the sample is immediately fixed (Selvaggi, 2001; Uyar *et al.*, 2003). While nuclear features are currently used for diagnoses, attempts are underway to identify new biomarkers for cervical neoplasias.

Because infection with high-risk HPVs is associated with cervical cancer, part of the screening and diagnosis protocol involves testing for the presence of HPV DNA in abnormal samples (Chatterjee *et al.*, 2003; Giovannelli *et al.*, 2004; Nonogaki *et al.*, 2004; Rosenthal, 2004; Sotlar *et al.*, 2004). High-risk HPV DNA is detected through polymerase chain reactions (PCR) or nucleic acid hybridization.

This additional test is recommended by the American Cancer Society (ACS) and the American College of Obstetricians and Gynecologists (ACOG) for women over the age of 30 in order to determine screening intervals (Solomon *et al.*, 2007).

Interestingly, aside from the obvious benefits of screening, it was recently reported that the act of performing a Pap smear may be associated with an inflammatory response that may initiate immunologic clearance of HPV (Passmore *et al.*, 2007). Even a single Pap smear seemed to reduce the risk of cervical cancer, and a significant decline in the detection of HPV was correlated with the lifetime number of Pap smears received (Passmore *et al.*, 2007). Nevertheless, another report suggests that Pap smears could actually increase the likelihood of infection since micro-abrasions could arise from sample collection; mice pretreated with a Cytobrush Plus cell collector (cytobrush) were highly susceptible to infection after inoculation with pseudovirus (Roberts *et al.*, 2007).

4.2. Diagnosis and Treatment

Viral warts are commonly diagnosed based on appearance. Warts tend to regress spontaneously; however, various therapies exist if patients seek treatment for warts. It should be noted that no specific antiviral therapy exists for HPV lesions (Phelps *et al.*, 1998). Therapies to remove or reduce the size of warts include topical application of caustic agents, cryotherapy, inhibitors of DNA synthesis, and surgical therapy or laser treatment; for genital warts, immunomodulating agents appear to be effective (reviewed in Howley & Lowy, 2007).

If a Pap test reveals ASC-H, LSIL, or HSIL cells, a follow-up test called a colposcopy will often be performed where abnormal tissue is detected via a staining solution. If abnormal tissue is indeed found, a biopsy is performed so that the tissue could be further examined under a microscope. If the abnormal tissue appears to be at a high risk for carcinogenic progression, further treatment is required. Treatment options include cryotherapy, laser therapy, or loop electrosurgical excision repair (Wright *et al.*, 2002a).

4.3. Prevention and Vaccines

Since HPV infection can occur in drastically different ways depending on the virus type, controlling infections clearly requires different approaches. For genital HPV infections, the approach to reducing infections would be similar to those for other STDs. The use of condoms has been shown to be effective in reducing the risk of cervical and vulvovaginal infection in newly sexually active women and in reducing the transmission of external genital warts to men (Hippelainen *et al.*, 1994; Winer *et al.*, 2006). Additionally, decreased sexual promiscuity of both partners would clearly reduce the likelihood of infection.

Recently, Gardasil® (quadrivalent HPV [HPV types 6, 11, 16, and 18] recombinant vaccine), a prophylactic vaccine against four types (6, 11, 16, and 18) of HPV, was developed by Merck Pharmaceuticals. Gardasil® is currently approved for use in girls and women of 9 to 26 years of age and is administered as three doses over the course of six months; studies regarding vaccination of women older than 26 years and males are underway. The vaccine is composed of virus-like particles (VLPs) that are made up of self-assembled L1 proteins (Barr & Tamms, 2007). The efficacy of Gardasil® is mediated by the development of humoral immune responses and works against HPV-related CIN or genital warts. Protection remained high for at least five years following vaccination (Barr & Tamms, 2007). Nevertheless, Gardasil® did not protect against HPV types that subjects were PCR-positive and/or seropositive for.

Another pharmaceutical company, GlaxoSmithKline (GSK) has also developed a vaccine for cervical cancer. This vaccine, Cervarix™, is a bivalent L1 VLP vaccine against HPV types 16 and 18, although GSK reports some protection against types 31 and 45 as well (Harper *et al.*, 2004). The vaccine shows sustained efficacy up to 4.5 years after vaccination (Harper *et al.*, 2006).

It is important to note that since the vaccines against HPV are not designed to prevent the development of HPV-associated disease and cancer in individuals that are already infected, there will likely not be a vaccine-attributable decline in HPV-associated cancers for several decades (reviewed in Frazer, 2004). Furthermore, the above-mentioned vaccines do not target every high-risk HPV type. Therefore, recommendations for cervical cytology screening (i.e. Pap smears) remain unchanged and it will continue to be an important tool for the early detection of HPV-associated neoplasias.

5. Carcinogenic Progression and Viral Oncoproteins

5.1. Carcinogenic Progression

During carcinogenic progression, the viral genome often integrates into the host chromosome. This step is considered accidental, as it results in the cessation of the productive viral life cycle. Integration results in the deregulated expression of the viral E6 and E7 proteins because expression of the E2 regulatory protein is usually lost. High-risk HPV E6 and E7 contribute to the initiation and maintenance of the transformed phenotype of HPV-associated cancers. High-risk HPV E6 and E7 perform distinct functions that importantly contribute to carcinogenic progression. Furthermore, in cases where the virus does not integrate and/or where episomes exist or coexist with integrated sequence, the expression of the viral E5 protein may contribute to transformation as well. The transformation capabilities of E5 and high-risk HPV E6 and E7 may reflect a need for the virus to establish persistent infection by creating a proliferative "stem cell-like state," while the low-risk viruses have a life-cycle that is based on rapid production of progeny virus to efficiently transmit virus to new hosts (reviewed in Munger *et al.*, 2004).

5.2. Viral Oncoproteins

5.2.1. *HPV E5*

The E5 proteins of BPV type 1 (BPV1) and HPV16 are small (44 and 83 amino acids, respectively), hydrophobic proteins that localize to membranes of the Golgi apparatus and endoplasmic reticulum (ER) (Burkhardt *et al.*, 1989; Conrad *et al.*, 1993; Disbrow *et al.*, 2003;

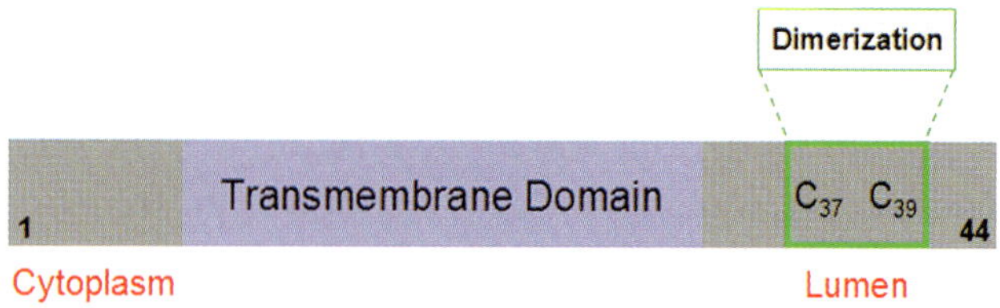

Fig. 3. BPV1 E5. Schematic representation of the 44 amino acid BPV1 E5 protein. The cysteine residues shown are responsible for dimerization and are conserved among the transforming ungulate PV E5 proteins.

Schapiro *et al.*, 2000) (Fig. 3). The oncogenic characteristics of BPV1 E5 have been studied in the greatest detail. Expression of BPV1 E5 is sufficient to transform established rodent cells in culture and is considered to be the major transforming protein of BPV1 (DiMaio *et al.*, 1986; Groff & Lancaster, 1986; Rabson *et al.*, 1986; Schiller *et al.*, 1986; Yang *et al.*, 1985). The protein is associated with intracellular membranes and, in transformed cells, exists as a homodimer that is localized to the ER and the Golgi apparatus; dimerization is necessary for transformation (Burkhardt *et al.*, 1987, 1989; Burnett *et al.*, 1992; Horwitz *et al.*, 1988). The primary transforming mechanism of BPV1 E5 is the aberrant activation of the receptor for the platelet-derived growth factor β (PDGF) (Drummond-Barbosa *et al.*, 1995; Goldstein *et al.*, 1994; Lai *et al.*, 1998; Petti & DiMaio, 1994; Petti *et al.*, 1991). In addition, BPV1 E5 binds to the 16-kDa-pore-forming subunit of the vacuolar H^+-ATPase (16K) and causes Golgi alkalinization by interfering with H^+ transport (Goldstein *et al.*, 1991; Schapiro *et al.*, 2000). The interaction of BPV1 E5 with 16K may play a role in E5-mediated transformation, although the exact role of this function in cellular transformation is not clearly defined.

Similar to BPV E5, the HPV16 E5 protein also localizes to the Golgi apparatus, endosomes, and cellular membranes (Conrad *et al.*, 1993; Disbrow *et al.*, 2003) and can transform fibroblasts to grow in soft agar (Leechanachai *et al.*, 1992; Pim *et al.*, 1992; Straight *et al.*, 1993). Additionally, HPV16 E5 is mitogenic in primary keratinocytes, particularly in cooperation with epidermal growth factor (EGF) and HPV16 E7 (Bouvard *et al.*, 1994; Storey *et al.*, 1992;

Straight *et al.*, 1993; Valle & Banks, 1995; Venuti *et al.*, 1998). HPV16 E5 associates with 16K (Adam *et al.*, 2000; Ashby *et al.*, 2001; Conrad *et al.*, 1993; Rodriguez *et al.*, 2000) and also binds to the EGF receptor (EGFR), PDGFR, and colony stimulating factor-1 receptor (Hwang *et al.*, 1995). Furthermore, the expression of HPV16 E5 in mice alters the growth and differentiation of stratified epithelia and causes epithelial tumors at a high frequency; these properties of E5 require the EGFR (Genther Williams *et al.*, 2005). Using a multi-stage mouse model for skin cancer, it was further shown that HPV16 E5 contributes to the promotion and malignant progression of carcinogenesis (Maufort *et al.*, 2007).

In most HPV-positive cancers, where the viral genome is integrated, E5 is not expressed. Therefore, it is clear that E5 is not necessary for the maintenance of the transformed phenotype. This does not, however, rule out the possibility that E5 contributes to the initiation of the carcinogenic process.

5.2.2. *HPV E6*

The HPV E6 proteins are approximately 150 amino acids in size and contain two zinc-binding domains that consist of a total of four Cys-X-X-Cys motifs (Barbosa *et al.*, 1989; Grossman & Laimins, 1989) (Fig. 4). The high-risk HPV E6 proteins localize to both the nucleus and cytoplasm (Barbosa *et al.*, 1989; Cole & Danos, 1987). The most well-characterized function of high-risk HPV E6 is its ability to interfere

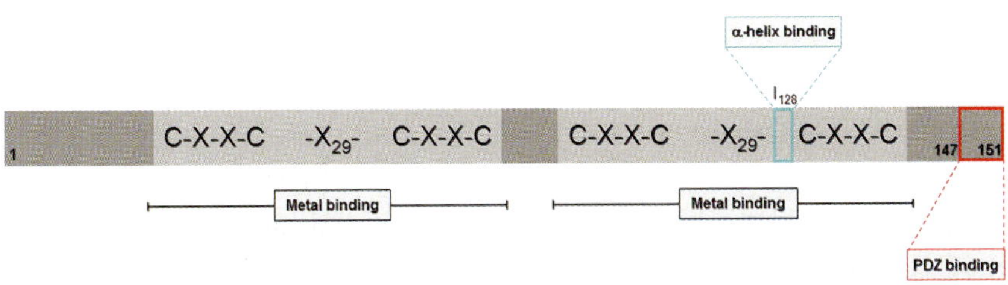

Fig. 4. HPV16 E6. Schematic representation of the HPV16 E6 protein. The 151-amino-acid protein contains two metal-binding motifs as well as α-helix-binding and PDZ-binding motifs, as indicated. The α-helix-binding motif is responsible for the association between HPV16 E6 and E6AP, as well as other cellular targets.

with p53 tumor suppressor activity. The p53 tumor suppressor is involved in various cell-cycle checkpoints and regulates cell-cycle arrest and/or apoptosis in response to DNA damage or other cellular stress; p53 achieves such regulation via activating the transcription of the $p21^{CIP1}$ cyclin-dependent kinase inhibitor (CDKI) gene and other genes such as *Bax*, *GADD45*, *IGF-BP3*, *cyclin G*, and *14-3-3σ* (reviewed in Slee *et al.*, 2004). Since it is beneficial for many viruses to establish persistent infections, mechanisms to block the induction of apoptosis, which may occur during infection, are advantageous to the virus. Accordingly, simian vacuolating virus 40 (SV40) and adenovirus 5 (Ad5) encode proteins, large tumor antigen (T) by the former (Mietz *et al.*, 1992) and E1B and E4orf6 by the latter (Hobom & Dobbelstein, 2004; Yew & Berk, 1992), that also abrogate p53 activity. To overcome proapoptotic activities of p53, high-risk HPV E6 forms a complex with p53 and the cellular ubiquitin ligase E6AP, resulting in the ubiquitination and rapid degradation of p53 (Huibregtse *et al.*, 1991, 1993; Scheffner *et al.*, 1990). Low-risk HPV E6 is unable to bind or promote the degradation of p53 (Scheffner *et al.*, 1990). Accordingly, levels of p53 are low in high-risk HPV E6-immortalized cells or in HPV-associated cancer cells (Scheffner *et al.*, 1991; Werness *et al.*, 1990). Expression of high-risk HPV E6 also prevents a p53-mediated cellular response to DNA damage (Kessis *et al.*, 1993), and eliminates the trophic sentinel response, an apoptotic response to oncogenic insults, induced by high-risk HPV E7 expression (Jones *et al.*, 1997b). Alternative splicing of the E6 transcript results in the production mRNAs that have the potential to encode truncated E6 proteins, which are referred to as E6*. E6* has been reported to interact with E6 and E6AP (Pim *et al.*, 1994) and to inhibit E6-mediated p53 degradation and, therefore, may function in a dominant negative manner (Pim *et al.*, 1997).

High-risk HPV E6 also displays p53-independent activities that may contribute to its transforming activities. It has been suggested that the modulation of E6AP activity by E6 may alter normal E6AP function in such a way that the aberrant and/or decreased ubiquitination of cellular proteins may contribute to high-risk HPV E6-induced transformation (reviewed in Howley & Lowy, 2007). Furthermore, the carboxyl termini of high-risk HPV E6 proteins contain PDZ-binding domains (Kiyono *et al.*, 1997; Lee *et al.*, 1997). PDZ proteins are often localized to areas of cell-to-cell contact and likely play a role in signal transduction and regulation of cell polarity (Craven & Bredt, 1998). High-risk HPV E6 associates with several PDZ proteins including hDLG, MUPP-1, and hSCRIB, leading to their degradation (Kiyono *et al.*, 1997; Lee *et al.*, 1997, 2000; Nakagawa & Huibregtse, 2000). The interaction between high-risk HPV E6 and PDZ proteins is important for E6-mediated transformation, as transgenic mice that express high-risk HPV E6 that lacks a PDZ-binding domain do not develop epidermal hyperplasias as seen with the expression of wild type high-risk HPV E6 (Nguyen *et al.*, 2003). Low-risk HPV E6 proteins lack the ability to associate with PDZ proteins (Kiyono *et al.*, 1997; Lee *et al.*, 1997).

Another important function of high-risk HPV E6 is the ability to activate telomerase. In embryonic cells, telomerase adds hexamer repeats to the telomeres of chromosomes. This activity is absent in somatic cells resulting in the shortening of telomeres after successive cell divisions, ultimately leading to senescence (Liu, 1999). The reactivation of hTERT, the catalytic subunit of telomerase, occurs in most cancer cells (reviewed in Blasco & Hahn, 2003). It has been proposed that high-risk HPV E6 activates the expression of hTERT by associating with both c-Myc and its cofactor Max, leading to the transcriptional activation of the hTERT promoter (Veldman *et al.*, 2001, 2003). However, there is also a report that shows that the induction of hTERT transcription is not dependent upon HPV16 E6-mediated induction of c-Myc, but instead requires an association between E6 and E6AP (Gewin & Galloway, 2001). Moreover, it was shown that the E6–E6AP complex associates with and degrades NFX1-91, a repressor of the hTERT promoter (Gewin *et al.*, 2004). Nevertheless, the interaction between HPV16 E6 and E6AP is not necessary for the activation of hTERT (Sekaric *et al.*, 2008), and E6 can associate with NFX1-91 and NFX1-123, a coactivator of the hTERT promoter, in the absence of E6AP (Katzenellenbogen *et al.*, 2007). Ultimately, induction of hTERT transcription is necessary for high-risk HPV E6-mediated cellular immortalization. Accordingly, low-risk

HPV E6 proteins do not induce telomerase activity (Klingelhutz *et al.*, 1996).

High-risk HPV E6 proteins interact with a number of other cellular proteins as well, including the interferon regulatory factor-3 (IRF-3) (Ronco *et al.*, 1998), the focal adhesion protein paxillin (Tong & Howley, 1997; Vande Pol *et al.*, 1998), and the EF-hand calcium-binding protein E6-BP (Chen *et al.*, 1995). Although the importance of these interactions are being further delineated, the observed interaction between high-risk E6 and the transcriptional coactivator p300/CBP (Patel *et al.*, 1999; Zimmermann *et al.*, 1999) is of notable interest since p300/CBP is also targeted by adenovirus E1A and SV40 large T antigen (Dorsman *et al.*, 1997; Eckner *et al.*, 1996).

5.2.3. *HPV E7*

The HPV E7 proteins are approximately 100 amino acids in size and contain a zinc-binding domain that may also function as a dimerization domain (Barbosa *et al.*, 1989; Clemens *et al.*, 1995; McIntyre *et al.*, 1993) (Fig. 5). E7 proteins are phosphorylated at an amino terminal domain by casein kinase II (CK II) and at a carboxyl terminal

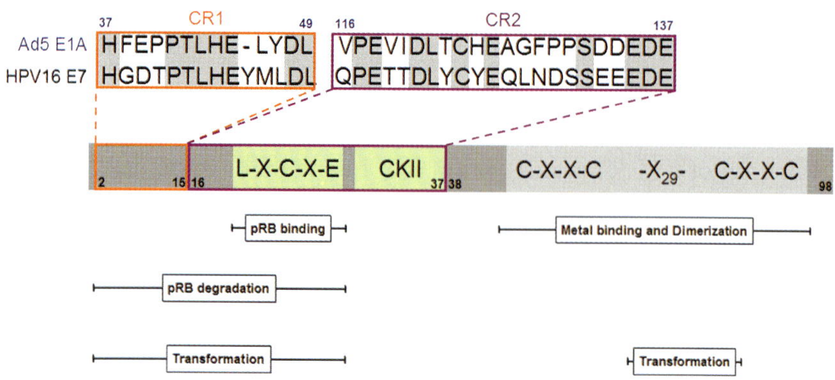

Fig. 5. HPV16 E7. Schematic representation of the HPV16 E7 protein. The 98-amino-acid protein contains one metal-binding motif that is similar to those in E6. The indicated amino-terminal residues have sequence similarity to a portion of CR1 and to CR2 of Ad5 E1A. CR2 includes an LXCXE motif that is necessary for pRB binding and cellular transformation as well as a CKII consensus phosphorylation site.

domain by an unidentified kinase (reviewed in Munger *et al.*, 2004). The localization of E7 is largely cytoplasmic but E7 is also found in the nucleus. HPV E7 proteins have functional similarities with the Ad 12S E1A protein and amino acid sequence similarities with Ad E1A as well as the SV40 large T antigen. The regions of amino acid sequence similarity are designated as conserved region 1 (CR1) and conserved region 2 (CR2) (reviewed in Munger & Howley, 2002) (Fig. 5). The conserved regions are necessary for the transforming activities of all three viral oncoproteins; an LXCXE sequence in CR2 of Ad E1A, HPV E7, and SV40 large T antigen are responsible for complex formation with the retinoblastoma tumor suppressor protein, pRB (DeCaprio *et al.*, 1988; Dyson *et al.*, 1989; Whyte *et al.*, 1988). While the conserved LXCXE pRB-binding motif in CR2 is necessary for pRB association, sequences in the carboxyl terminus of E7 are also involved in the disruption of the pRB–E2F complex, resulting in activated E2F-mediated transcriptional activation (Huang *et al.*, 1993; Wu *et al.*, 1993).

The ability to associate with and promote the degradation of pRB is the most studied function of high-risk HPV E7. pRB is a member of the "pocket protein" family that includes p107 and p130, which also associate with high-risk HPV E7. pRB, p107, and p130 are involved in the regulation of the G1 to S transition (discussed in more detail below). The phosphorylation of pRB by cyclin-dependent kinases (CDKs) in G1 results in the disruption of the pRB–E2F repressor complex and dissociated E2F acts as a transcriptional activator of genes involved in S-phase progression. pRB is dephosphorylated late in mitosis and "active" hypophoshorylated pRB inhibits S-phase entry. High-risk HPV E7 preferentially associates with hypophosphorylated pRB (Dyson *et al.*, 1992) and targets it for proteasomal degradation (Boyer *et al.*, 1996; Jones & Münger, 1997) via a mechanism that relies upon the interaction between HPV16 E7 and the cullin 2 ubiquitin ligase complex (Huh *et al.*, 2007). The high-risk HPV E7-induced aberrant degradation of pRB and the consequential activation of E2F-mediated transcription are thought to be a primary mechanism by which the virus achieves S-phase competence in infected cells. Furthermore, similar to Ad E1A and SV40 large T antigen, this function of high-risk HPV E7 tightly correlates with its ability to transform cells (Jones & Münger, 1997).

The E7 proteins from low-risk HPVs bind pRB with much lower efficiency (approximately 10-fold lower) than the E7 proteins from high-risk viruses (Gage *et al.*, 1990; Münger *et al.*, 1989b). Interestingly, this difference in binding efficiency maps to a single amino acid (Asp 21 in HPV16 E7 versus Gly 22 in HPV6 E7) and substitution experiments revealed that the single amino acid residue was the primary determinant for pRB-binding affinity and transformation capacity of the E7 proteins (Heck *et al.*, 1992; Sang & Barbosa, 1992).

In addition to pRB, high-risk HPV E7 interacts with other cellular proteins that contribute to E7-mediated cellular transformation. In fact, it was shown that complex formation between E7 and the "pocket protein" family is not sufficient to account for its immortalization and transformation functions (Jewers *et al.*, 1992). High-risk HPV E7 has been shown to interact with and abrogate the growth-inhibitory activities of the CDKIs $p21^{CIP1}$ (Funk *et al.*, 1997; Jones *et al.*, 1997a) and $p27^{KIP1}$ (Zerfass-Thome *et al.*, 1996). $p21^{CIP1}$ and $p27^{KIP1}$ are induced by anti-proliferative signals such as growth factor withdrawal (Firpo *et al.*, 1994), activation of p53 (El-Deiry *et al.*, 1993), and loss of cellular adhesion (Assoian, 1997; Fang *et al.*, 1996). Furthermore, $p21^{CIP1}$ has been implicated in coupling cell-cycle arrest and differentiation in keratinocytes (Alani *et al.*, 1998; Di Cunto *et al.*, 1998; Missero *et al.*, 1996). Therefore, inhibition of these CDKIs by high-risk HPV E7 may play an important role in the virus-mediated uncoupling of cellular differentiation and proliferation necessary for viral replication.

As mentioned above, high-risk HPV E7 alters E2F-mediated transcription by disrupting the pRB–E2F complex. It has also been shown that E7 can directly bind the E2F family member E2F1 and promote E2F1-mediated transcription (Hwang *et al.*, 2002). Moreover, E7 interacts with class I histone deacetylases (HDACs) (Brehm *et al.*, 1999; Longworth & Laimins, 2004). HDACs can induce chromatin remodeling through histone modification and thereby can act as transcriptional corepressors. The association between E7 and HDACs increases levels of E2F2-mediated transcription in differentiating cells (Longworth *et al.*, 2005). These additional functions of high-risk HPV E7 likely influence S-phase progression.

High- and low-risk E7s as well as BPV1 E7 also associate with the 600-kDa retinoblastoma protein-associated factor, p600 (DeMasi *et al.*, 2005; Huh *et al.*, 2005). Because p600 is a conserved target between BPV1 and HPV E7s, it appears that the association between E7 and p600 plays an important role in the life cycle of PVs. The biological functions of p600 have not been fully identified in mammalian cells but reports on p600 homologs in *Drosophila* and *Arabidopsis* suggest that p600 may play a role in chromosome segregation (Sekelsky *et al.*, 1999), synaptic transmission at the neuromuscular junction (Richards *et al.*, 1996), calcium influx (Xu *et al.*, 1998), and/or polar auxin transport (Gil *et al.*, 2001). Additionally, p600 family members contain a RING finger domain that is similar to the domain found on N-recognin, a ubiquitin ligase in the N-end rule pathway that is involved in the proteolysis of proteins through an interaction with their N-terminus (Kwon *et al.*, 1998; Madura *et al.*, 1993). Through RNAi knockdown of p600 in mammalian cells, p600 has been implicated in apoptosis induced during anchorage-independent growth, which is known as anoikis (reviewed in Frisch & Screaton, 2001). Therefore, it has been suggested that the interaction between E7 and p600 may deregulate anoikis and protect detached cells from apoptosis, thereby contributing to viral transformation (DeMasi *et al.*, 2007; Huh *et al.*, 2005). Consistent with this hypothesis, HPV16 E7 associates with p600 through the CR1 domain, which, as mentioned above, is necessary for the transformation capability of HPV16 E7 (Gulliver *et al.*, 1997; Phelps *et al.*, 1992). Further studies will be necessary to determine the role of p600 in the viral life cycle and in high-risk HPV E7-mediated cellular transformation.

Similar to E6, high-risk HPV E7 associates with a considerable number of other cellular proteins. The significances of many of these interactions remain unclear and are subjects of continued study.

6. Genomic Instability in HPV-Associated Cancers

Genomic instability refers to the dynamic changes that occur at the genome level over time. The two main types of genomic instability are microsatellite instability, which affects chromatin structure and gene expression, and chromosomal instability, including aneuploidy, which refers to the gains or losses of whole chromosomes (reviewed in Jefford & Irminger-Finger, 2006). Aneuploidy accounts for most of the chromosomal defects in tumor cells (Lengauer *et al.*, 1998) and is consistently observed in almost all cancers (Rajagopalan & Lengauer, 2004). Although genomic instability has often been considered to be a downstream corollary of transformation, evidence mounts for a causal role of aneuploidy in tumorigenic initiation and progression (Lengauer *et al.*, 1998; Nowak *et al.*, 2002; Shih *et al.*, 2001). Aneuploidy can arise through multiple mechanisms that can generally be grouped into one of two mechanistic classes. Cells can acquire genomic instability through mechanisms that decrease the vigilance and/or repair of cellular and chromosomal errors, thereby allowing for the perpetuation of mutations in the genome that could eventually contribute to carcinogenic progression; these include, but are not limited to, defects in the spindle assembly checkpoint and in DNA damage repair pathways (reviewed in Jefford & Irminger-Finger, 2006). Alternatively, genomic instability could be promoted in a cell through mechanisms that actively destabilize the genome, which has been referred to as a "mutator phenotype." Examples of this are the elevation of reactive oxygen species (ROS) levels upon c-Myc overexpression that correlates with the induction of DNA damage (Vafa *et al.*, 2002) or the induction of supernumerary centrosomes (reviewed in Chi & Jeang, 2007; Münger *et al.*, 2006) (see below). "Active" and "passive" mechanisms are not mutually exclusive, however, and, as described below for HPV oncoproteins, it is possible for a cell to acquire defects in cellular checkpoints and repair mechanisms in addition to facing the constant generation of mutagenic events.

It has been shown that the expression of high-risk HPV E6 and E7 dramatically increases genomic instability in cells where spontaneous mutagenesis occurs at an exceedingly low rate (Solinas-Toldo *et al.*, 1997; White *et al.*, 1994). Furthermore, the development of aneuploidy is clearly associated with high-risk HPV infection (Rihet *et al.*, 1996) and can be detected as early as in premalignant lesions (Bibbo *et al.*, 1989; Steinbeck, 1997) and even prior to the integration of HPV genomes into host chromosomes (Bulten *et al.*, 1998; Southern *et al.*, 1997), supporting a causal role for HPV in genomic instability. In agreement, cytogenetic abnormalities were detected in HPV-immortalized keratinocytes (Cottage *et al.*, 2001). Not surprisingly, genomic alterations have been implicated in cervical cancer development. The introduction of chromosome 11 suppresses the malignant phenotype of the HPV-positive HeLa cervical carcinoma cell line (Rösl *et al.*, 1988; Stanbridge *et al.*, 1981). Also, gains of chromosome 3q appear to correlate with the progression of severe dysplasia to invasive carcinoma (Heselmeyer *et al.*, 1996, 1997).

Although the high-risk HPV oncoproteins contribute to cellular transformation and immortalization, further abnormalities in the host genome are required for the malignant progression of HPV-associated neoplasias. Despite acquiring an extended life span and histomorphological hallmarks of HSILs, primary human epithelial cells that express high-risk HPV E6 and E7 remain non-tumorigenic at low passage after immortalization (Hawley-Nelson *et al.*, 1989; McCance *et al.*, 1988; Munger *et al.*, 1989a). Malignant progression of these cells occurs after extended growth in tissue culture or when additional oncogenes such as *ras* and *fos* are expressed (Durst *et al.*, 1989; Pei *et al.*, 1993). Similarly, in transgenic mice where HPV16 E6 and E7 are expressed in basal epithelial cells, the development of cervical cancer is dependent upon long-term exposure to estrogen (Arbeit, 1996).

The necessity for the accumulation of aberrations in the host genome accounts for the extended period between high-risk HPV infection and the emergence of cervical cancer, which is a rare event in itself. Nevertheless, it has been shown that the high-risk oncoproteins can each subvert genomic integrity and likely induce different types of genomic instability (Livingstone *et al.*, 1992; White *et al.*, 1994), highlighting that they are necessary for the initiation as well as the progression of carcinogenesis. Some of the mechanisms by which the viral oncoproteins may destabilize the host genome are discussed in the following sections but are not yet completely delineated.

6.1. Deregulation of the Cell Cycle in HPV-Associated Cancers

6.1.1. *The cell cycle*

The cell cycle is made up of four phases: the gap phase before DNA replication (G1), the DNA synthesis phase (S), the gap between S-phase and the mitotic phase (G2), and mitosis (M). There also exists a G0 phase, which refers to cells that are in a quiescent state. S-phase and M-phase are considered to be the active phases of the cell cycle and entry into, passage through, and exit out of these phases are controlled by checkpoints that ensure the proper progression and outcome of these phases (Hartwell & Weinert, 1989). A checkpoint between G1-phase and S-phase ensures that DNA is not damaged prior to duplication. The S-phase checkpoint monitors the status of DNA replication. A checkpoint between G2-phase and M-phase certifies that chromosomes are fully duplicated and checkpoints during mitosis ensure that chromosomes are properly attached to spindle microtubules. Even with all of these checkpoints, a post-mitotic checkpoint exists to prevent cells that incorrectly complete mitosis from re-entering the cell cycle. Because cyclins and CDKs drive the cell cycle, they are tightly regulated not only by CDK inhibitors but also by a panel of activating and inhibitory kinases and phosphatases.

Clearly, cell-cycle checkpoints are necessary to ensure proper cellular proliferation and disruption of these checkpoints could be detrimental to cells as well as organisms. Interfering with the ability of a cell to detect deficiencies in cellular machinery or to sense DNA damage would result in a cell entering an active phase of the cell cycle without the proper environment to successfully complete that phase. Such events increase the likelihood of acquiring mutations, aneuploidy, and other manifestations of genomic instability. Accordingly, the viral E6 and E7 oncoproteins deregulate the cell cycle to allow for efficient viral replication but in doing so, also contribute to the genomic instability that is key to malignant progression.

6.1.2. *Deregulation of the G1/S transition*

Cyclin D/CDK4 and/or cyclin D/CDK6 are responsible for entry into S-phase; they phosphorylate pRB, which is in a hypophosphorylated state in G1. As mentioned previously, phosphorylation of pRB results in the dissociation of the pRB–E2F complex, allowing E2F to act as a transcriptional activator. This results in the increased expression of enzymes that are critical for DNA synthesis as well as of cyclin E and cyclin A, the regulatory subunits of CDK2. CDK2 activity is required for passage through and completion of S-phase (reviewed in Sherr, 1994). When p53 levels increase in response to conflicting proliferative signals, DNA damage, and failed mitosis, cells undergo a G1/S cell-cycle arrest (reviewed in Lowe *et al.*, 2004). This arrest occurs due to the upregulation of $p21^{CIP1}$, a p53 transcriptional target that inhibits CDK2 activity (reviewed in Vousden & Lu, 2002).

Considering the well-characterized targets of high-risk HPV E6 and E7, p53 and pRB respectively, it is easy to see how these viral proteins disrupt the G1/S transition. Simply stated, E7 targets pRB for degradation resulting in deregulated E2F-mediated transcription and S-phase entry while E6 targets p53 for degradation to prevent cell-cycle arrest and the elimination of infected cells. Interestingly, aberrant S-phase progression induced by high-risk E7 leads to the activation and increased levels of p53 (Demers *et al.*, 1994b; Jones & Münger, 1997). Stabilized p53 in these cells, however, remains transcriptionally inert and, moreover, E7-expressing cells fail to undergo p53-mediated G1/S arrest in response to DNA damage (Demers *et al.*, 1994a; Eichten *et al.*, 2002; Hickman *et al.*, 1994; Slebos *et al.*, 1994; Vousden *et al.*, 1993). Furthermore, the dysregulated cyclin E expression has also been implicated in HPV16 E7-mediated disruption of the G1/S transition (Martin *et al.*, 1998). These, together with the fact that high-risk E6-mediated degradation of p53 also ensures that E7-induced S-phase progression is uninhibited, further highlight the importance of achieving S-phase competence for the virus.

6.1.3. *Deregulation of S-phase*

Because the proper duplication of chromosomal DNA is a critical event, errors in DNA replication are potent inducers of an S-phase arrest. Specifically, DNA double-stranded breaks are recognized quickly and efficiently by serine/threonine kinases that are responsible for activating a complicated cascade of events resulting in DNA break repair and/or the induction of cell-cycle arrest or cell death (reviewed in Wyman & Kanaar, 2006). Mutations in proteins involved in surveying DNA double-stranded breaks are associated with a number of syndromes that include a predisposition to developing tumors (Casper *et al.*, 2002; O'Driscoll *et al.*, 2003; Xu & Baltimore, 1996). The expression of HPV16 E7 induces an increase in nuclei with γH2AX foci, a mark for damaged DNA, and sub-chromosomal DNA fragments were detected in such cells (Duensing & Münger, 2002). These double-stranded breaks may be responsible for the anaphase bridges seen in HPV oncogene-expressing cells (Duensing & Münger, 2002). The anaphase bridges are formed during breakage fusion bridge cycles whereby the aberrant repair of double-stranded DNA breaks results in the formation of a dicentric chromosome (the product of fusing two chromosomes together) that undergoes breakage during the following round of mitosis (McClintock, 1940). Double-stranded DNA breaks detected in HPV oncogene-expressing epithelial cells could be due to the production of ROS, similar to c-myc (Vafa *et al.*, 2002), or via the inhibition of double-stranded DNA break repair. Either way, the heightened presence of double-stranded DNA breaks likely plays a role in increasing the frequency of mutagenesis upon the expression of the HPV oncogenes.

It was also shown that HPV16 E6 expression reduced error-free DNA end-joining activity and increased incorrect DNA end-joining activity in human oral fibroblasts (Shin *et al.*, 2006). This function was in part dependent upon the zinc-binding domains and the PDZ-binding domain of E6. Error-prone DNA end joining may be a mechanism by which high-risk HPV E6 directly contributes to genomic instability in HPV-associated cancer.

6.1.4. *Deregulation of the G2/M transition*

Cyclin A/CDK2 and the M-phase or maturation-promoting factor (MPF) are necessary for entry into and the progression through mitosis. The checkpoints that control M-phase entry monitor cell size and errors in chromosome duplication, such as double-stranded breaks, that would alter the normal segregation of chromosomes. The key component of the MPF is the cyclin B–CDK1 complex. CDK1 is expressed throughout the cell cycle but, prior to entry into mitosis, remains phosphorylated and therefore inactive. At the G2/M transition, the Cdc25 phosphatase removes the inhibitory phosphorylations, inducing MPF activation and M-phase entry. The active cyclin B–CDK1 complex is disrupted at the end of mitosis by the anaphase-promoting complex (APC), which targets cyclin B for ubiquitin-mediated degradation.

Several functions of HPV16 E6 appear to alter the integrity of the checkpoints regulating the G2/M transition. The p53 tumor suppressor contributes to maintaining a G2 cell-cycle arrest when cells enter G2 with damaged DNA or when they arrest in S-phase due to a lack of essential substrates (reviewed in Taylor & Stark, 2001). Because high-risk HPV E6 proteins target p53 for degradation, the G2/M checkpoint is also compromised in HPV16 E6-expressing cells (Thompson *et al.*, 1997) and, in these cells, DNA damage does not elicit a stable G2 arrest (Baus *et al.*, 2003). G2 arrest in response to DNA damage also depends on the transcriptional repression of mitotic genes mediated by the pocket proteins pRb, p107, and p130 (Jackson *et al.*, 2005). In high-risk HPV E7-expressing cells, this pathway is likely thwarted and, in fact, the expression of mitotic genes is deregulated in cells expressing E6 and/or E7 (Garner-Hamrick *et al.*, 2004; Patel *et al.*, 2004; Thierry *et al.*, 2004). Primary cells that contain HPV16 E6/E7 maintain high levels of active mitotic proteins including cyclin A and B (Steinmann *et al.*, 1994).

Furthermore, in normal cells, $p21^{CIP1}$ accumulates in the nucleus at the G2/M transition and inhibits the cyclin A–CDK2 and cyclin B–CDK1 complexes. In cells expressing high-risk E6, the nuclear $p21^{CIP1}$ accumulation does not occur and cells enter mitosis more swiftly than control cells (Dulic *et al.*, 1998). Since high-risk HPV E7 proteins also abrogate the functions of $p21^{CIP1}$, it is likely that E7-expressing cells will exhibit similar abnormalities.

6.2. Centrosomal Defects in HPV-Associated Cancers

6.2.1. *The centrosome and the centrosome duplication cycle*

Centrosomes are cytoplasmic organelles that act as microtubule-organizing centers (MTOCs) and form the mitotic spindle pole bodies in mitosis. They also play roles in controlling cell division and influence cell polarity, shape, and motility (Bornens, 2002; Hinchcliffe *et al.*, 2001; Khodjakov *et al.*, 2000; Niu *et al.*, 1997; Piel *et al.*, 2001). They consist of two centrioles that are surrounded by a pericentriolar matrix (PCM) that consists of a number of different proteins, including pericentrin (Paintrand *et al.*, 1992). Centrosome duplication is a tightly regulated, albeit poorly understood process that proceeds in temporal synchrony with the cell division cycle (Fig. 6; middle panel) (reviewed in Hinchcliffe & Sluder, 2001; Zimmerman *et al.*, 1999). Following cell division, each cell contains a single centrosome that is licensed for duplication through centriole disengagement at the end of M-phase or in early G1. This process is regulated by separase, a protease that is activated by the APC and is also responsible for sister chromatid separation at the metaphase to anaphase transition (Tsou & Stearns, 2006). After the disengagement of centrioles, a single round of duplication occurs during S-phase during which daughter centrioles are synthesized at right angles adjacent to the maternal centrioles. The two centrosomes then form mitotic spindle poles that promote bipolar and symmetric segregation of chromosomes. Nevertheless, it should be noted that centrosomes are not necessarily required for spindle pole formation (Steffen *et al.*, 1986) and, conversely, multiple centrosomes

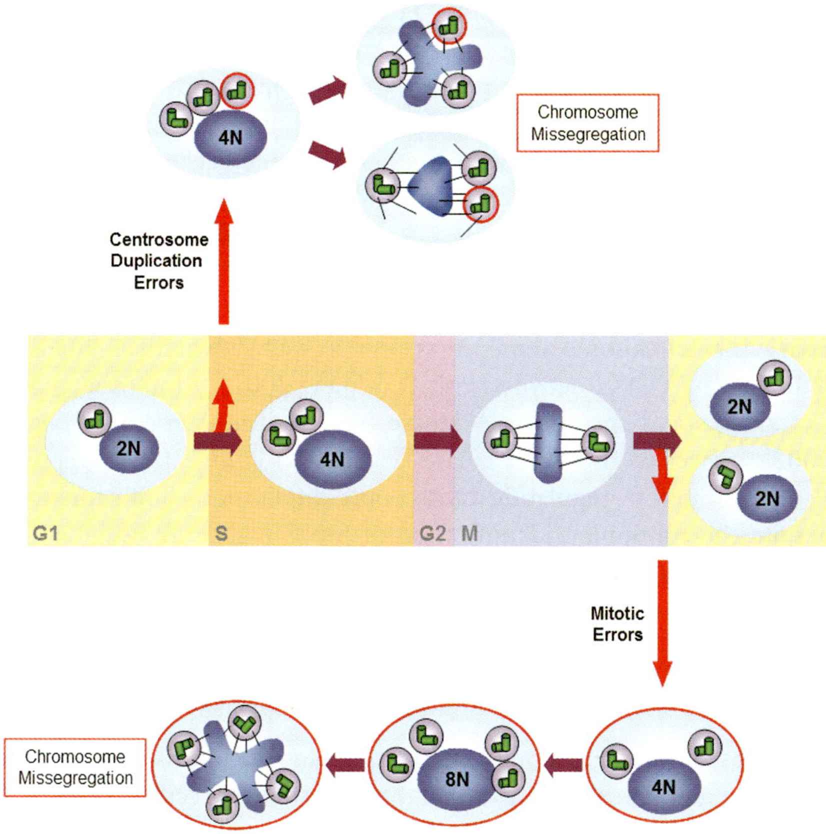

Fig. 6. The centrosome duplication cycle. Normal centrosome duplication is depicted in the middle panel. In G1-phase, cells have only one centrosome. Upon S-phase entry, the two centrioles separate and each serves as a template for synthesis of a daughter. At the end of S-phase, cells contain two centrosomes (each consisting of two centrioles) and 4N DNA content. Please note that cell-cycle designations in the figure are not to scale. In normal cells, bipolar mitosis allows for the symmetric distribution of chromosomes and centrosomes to daughter cells. As described in the text, centrosome abnormalities in cells can arise through two distinct mechanisms. Centrosome overduplication (upper panel) and the accumulation of supernumerary centrosomes as a result of mitotic errors (lower panel) are depicted. In each case, the outline indicates the abnormal feature.

could make up one spindle pole (Fukasawa *et al.*, 1996; Ring *et al.*, 1982). Therefore, alternate mechanisms regulate spindle bipolarization. It is not surprising that a multitude of proteins and/or complexes have been implicated in regulating centrosome duplication since the proper segregation of chromosomes to daughter cells is of utmost importance. Cyclin A/CDK2 and/or cyclin E/CDK2 activity is reportedly necessary for repeated centrosome duplication in arrested cells (Hinchcliffe *et al.*, 1999; Lacey *et al.*, 1999; Matsumoto *et al.*, 1999; Meraldi *et al.*, 1999). The Mps1 kinase also appears to be necessary for centrosome duplication and it was shown that Mps1 is stabilized by CDK2 activity (Fisk & Winey, 2001). Moreover, polo-like kinases and the aurora-A kinase (reviewed in Meraldi & Nigg, 2002), as well as the NDR kinase (Hergovich *et al.*, 2007), were all also implicated in regulating centrosome duplication. Unfortunately, despite the continuing identification of proteins that are essential for the duplication of centrosomes, the actual mechanistic details of centrosome duplication remain enigmatic.

6.2.2. *The establishment of supernumerary centrosomes*

Undoubtedly, deregulation of centrosome duplication could be harmful to the genomic integrity of daughter cells. Excess centrosomes will be acquired if a centrosome is duplicated more than once per cell cycle, through either persistent licensing of newly formed daughter centrioles or via the repeated synthesis of daughter centrioles from the maternal template (Fig. 6; top panel). Supernumerary centrosomes can cause multipolar mitosis leading to asymmetric chromosome segregation and aneuploidy. However, it has been shown that in normal cells multiple centrosomes can coalesce ("cluster") such that only two mitotic spindle poles are formed (Brinkley, 2001; Ring *et al.*, 1982; Sharp *et al.*, 1982). Even under these circumstances, an asymmetric cell division may result from the missegregation of chromosomes due to uneven forces from each pole (Grill *et al.*, 2001). Gains or losses of whole chromosomes as a result of centrosome overduplication could contribute to the carcinogenic potential of a cell.

In addition to hyperamplification of centrosomes, cells can accumulate abnormal centrosome numbers through mitotic errors that result in cytokinesis failure. Cytokinesis failure followed by mitotic slippage causes formation of a 4-N cell in a G1-like state that contains two centrosomes. Therefore, if such a cell were to overcome the post-mitotic checkpoint and re-enter the cell cycle, both centrosomes would be duplicated to yield four centrosomes in mitosis (Fig. 6; bottom panel). One might envision that although a cell contains the "correct" number of centrosomes (4) relative to the amount of DNA (8 N), a tetrapolar mitosis could yield aneuploid progeny. Consistent with this notion, it has been postulated that tetraploidy is a frequent, potentially mandatory, precursor to aneuploidy (Storchova & Pellman, 2004). However, this hypothesis has not been experimentally proven, and in fact, aneuploidy can develop directly from a diploid state (McDermott *et al.*, 2006).

6.2.3. *Centrosomal errors induced by HPV oncoproteins*

Centrosome abnormalities can be detected in numerous cancers; however, whether they are a cause or consequence of mitotic errors and exactly how they contribute to carcinogenic progression has remained a matter of contention. Similar to reports on breast (Lingle *et al.*, 2002) and prostate cancer (Pihan *et al.*, 2003), centrosome abnormalities have been found to arise at early stages of cervical carcinogenesis (Duensing *et al.*, 2000; Skyldberg *et al.*, 2001). High-risk HPV E6 and E7 cooperate to induce supernumerary centrosomes in primary epithelial cells (Duensing *et al.*, 2000). Additionally, centrosomal abnormalities have been detected in cervical and skin lesions that arise in HPV16 E6- and/or E7-expressing transgenic mice (Balsitis *et al.*, 2003; Riley *et al.*, 2003; Schaeffer *et al.*, 2004). It has long been recognized that multipolar mitoses caused by supernumerary centrosomes are histopathological hallmarks of high-risk HPV-associated lesions (Crum *et al.*, 1984; Winkler *et al.*, 1984). The notion that HPV-associated centrosome abnormalities are a primary cause and not merely a consequence of mitotic abnormalities is supported by the fact that the HPV16 E7 oncoprotein induces supernumerary centrosomes in diploid cells.

High-risk HPV E6 and E7 proteins cooperate to induce supernumerary centrosomes in primary human cells, while their low-risk counterparts do not (Duensing *et al.*, 2000). Closer inspection of each oncoprotein elucidated different mechanisms by which they bring about supernumerary centrosomes. Specifically, high-risk HPV E7 is able to rapidly induce centrosome overduplication in primary human cells, and supernumerary centrosomes can be detected in mono-nucleated diploid cells expressing HPV16 E7 (Duensing *et al.*, 2001). Furthermore, multiple daughter centrioles can be detected around a maternal centriole in E7-expressing cells, lending further support to the notion that HPV16 E7 directly causes centrosome duplication errors (Guarguaglini *et al.*, 2005). It is thought that centrosome overduplication is a primary event and not a gradual consequence of the many other functions of E7, as centrosome abnormalities can arise within one or two cell cycles upon HPV16 E7 expression. Since E7-expressing cells display an increase in the incidence of multipolar mitoses (Duensing *et al.*, 2000), it would appear that the effects of E7 on centrosomes greatly contribute to the multipolarity commonly detected in HPV-associated cervical cancers. Although the mechanism by which E7 uncouples centrosome duplication from the cell cycle has not yet been fully delineated, it is known that this function of E7 is not solely dependent upon the inactivation of pRB or the related pocket proteins p107 and p130, as evidenced by the fact that HPV16 E7 can trigger centrosome overduplication in mouse embryo fibroblasts deficient for pRB/p130/p107 (Duensing & Munger, 2003). Interestingly, CDK2 was implicated in E7-mediated centrosome duplication errors. Inhibition of CDK2 activity did not interfere with normal centrosome duplication but impaired the ability of E7 to cause centrosome hyperamplification (Duensing *et al.*, 2004, 2006).

In contrast to the centrosome hyperamplification induced by HPV16 E7, HPV16 E6-expressing cells acquired supernumerary centrosomes through mitotic slippage of cells that encountered cytokinesis failure. Centrosome abnormalities in HPV16 E6-expressing cells occur only in cells that also exhibit nuclear abnormalities; transient HPV16 E6 expression does not result in an increased incidence of supernumerary centrosomes (Duensing *et al.*, 2001). As mentioned below, nuclear abnormalities arise when cells undergo cytokinesis failure and do not complete nuclear and/or cellular division. It is likely that atypical nuclei and the accumulation of centrosomes are a result of tetraploid cells escaping arrest due to E6-mediated p53 abrogation as well as persistent cytokinesis defects (Bunz *et al.*, 1998). Therefore, these cells will likely not give rise to viable daughters or contribute to the genomic instability required for the malignant progression of HPV-associated lesions. Nevertheless, recent reports suggest a role for centrosomally localized p53 in the regulation of centrosome duplication in a manner independent of its transactivation function (Shinmura *et al.*, 2007). It will be interesting to determine whether this pool of p53 is also targeted by E6 and, if so, how this may alter centrosome duplication.

Interestingly, it has been observed that p53 inactivation and cyclin E overexpression result in a synergistic induction of centrosome hyperamplification (Kawamura *et al.*, 2006) and aneuploidy (Karakaidos *et al.*, 2004) in human cells. As such, concomitant occurrence of cyclin E overexpression and p53 mutation strongly correlates with poor prognosis of renal pelvis, ureter, and gastric carcinomas (Furihata *et al.*, 1998; Sakaguchi *et al.*, 1998). Although it has not been documented, it would appear that, through this mechanism, the expression of high-risk HPV E6 and E7 would produce this synergistic effect as well. In fact, high-risk HPV E6 and E7 appear to have a cooperative effect on centrosome overduplication in normal human keratinocytes (Duensing *et al.*, 2000).

6.2.4. *Structural centrosome abnormalities in HPV-associated cancers*

In addition to numerical centrosome abnormalities, high-risk HPV-associated clinical lesions also exhibit structural centrosome abnormalities, including increased size and excess pericentriolar material (Duensing *et al.*, 2000). While the exact mechanism and consequences of HPV-associated structural centrosome abnormalities have not yet been determined, one could envision that irregularity in centrosome structure could contribute to errors in mitosis and/or chromosomal segregation. Excess nucleation of mitotic spindles from a structurally abnormal centrosome may potentially result in asymmetric cell division. Consistent with this idea, it has been shown that uneven net forces that act on spindle poles can alter the symmetry of mitosis (Grill *et al.*, 2001). Additionally, given that the process of centrosome duplication remains enigmatic, structural centrosome abnormalities may alter centrosome duplication in currently unforeseen ways.

6.3. Mitotic Errors in HPV-Associated Cancers

6.3.1. *Mitosis*

Mitosis is the cell division stage of the cell cycle and is divided into six steps. Prophase occurs at the initial transition between G2- and M-phase, where the chromatin condenses into chromosomes, the interphase cytoskeleton disassembles, and the centrosomes begin to move toward the poles. Soon after, when the nuclear envelope breaks down, prometaphase begins. With the dissolution of the nuclear envelope, the spindle microtubules anchored by the centrosomes can now begin attaching to the kinetochores. Metaphase is the stage at which the chromosomes are all captured by a microtubule from each centrosome such that the chromosomes align along a "metaphase plate" that is halfway between the spindle poles. With the appropriate signals, anaphase begins and the sister chromatids are divided and separated toward each pole. At telophase, chromosomes arrive at the poles and nuclear envelopes re-form around the two sets of chromosomes, at which point they begin to decondense. Lastly, the end of mitosis is called cytokinesis, which is the stage where a contractile ring between the soon-to-be daughter cells creates a cleavage furrow that ultimately leads to the daughter cells breaking apart from one another. Predictably, the stages of mitosis, especially those related to the proper attachment of chromosomes, are tightly regulated and monitored.

6.3.2. *Spindle pole formation and chromosome alignment*

Spindle poles consist of an array of microtubules that are anchored at the centrosome by their minus ends and emanate toward to center of the cell. Together with other proteins, such as microtubule motors, they play a pivotal role in aligning chromosomes at the metaphase plate. The nuclear mitotic apparatus protein 1 (NuMA) is necessary for the formation and stabilization of mitotic spindle poles (Merdes *et al.*, 1996) by essentially acting like a microtubule crosslinker; it also regulates the size of mitotic spindles. NuMA localizes to the spindles in both dynein/dynactin (a microtubule motor complex)-dependent and -independent manners (Kisurina-Evgenieva *et al.*, 2004; Merdes *et al.*, 2000). Accordingly, a number of microtubule motor proteins, the kinesins and dyneins, are implicated in regulating various stages of mitosis (Zhu *et al.*, 2005). Alongside the dynamic growth of microtubules, the motor proteins help to provide the forces necessary for chromosome alignment (reviewed in Sharp *et al.*, 2000). Both NuMA and the kinesin Kid were shown to contribute to chromosome alignment in mammalian cells (Levesque *et al.*, 2003).

6.3.3. *Defects in the mitotic spindle assembly checkpoint in HPV-associated cancers*

The mitotic spindle assembly checkpoint regulates metaphase–anaphase progression by monitoring proper attachment of spindle microtubules to centromeres and ensuring that sister chromatid separation only occurs once chromosomes are properly attached to the mitotic spindle poles. This process is regulated by Cdc20-mediated activation of the APC. The mitotic spindle assembly checkpoint is engaged by the recruitment of checkpoint proteins, which include Bub1, Bub3, BubR1, Mad1, Mad2, Mps1, and Cdc20, to unattached kinetochores (reviewed in Yu, 2002). The Bub and Mad proteins directly associate with Cdc20 and thereby inhibit its ability to activate the APC. Several reports suggest that the microtubule motor dynein is also recruited to kinetochores and contributes to the inactivation of the spindle checkpoint (Griffis *et al.*, 2007; Howell *et al.*, 2001; Wojcik *et al.*, 2001). When all kinetochores are properly attached, Cdc20 is able to associate with the APC and the active APC–Cdc20 complex induces the degradation of anaphase inhibitors including securin, which results in the activation of separase. Separase cleaves a subunit of the cohesin protein complex and therefore allows sister chromatid separation (reviewed in Hoffmann, 2006; Malmanche *et al.*, 2006). As discussed earlier, activation of separase also provides the initial licensing event for centrosome duplication.

Mitotic spindle assembly checkpoint errors cause gains and losses of chromosomes during cell division resulting in aneuploid progeny; as discussed, aneuploidy is the most common manifestation of genomic instability in human solid tumors and cervical cancers are frequently aneuploid. Moreover, mutations in mitotic spindle assembly checkpoint genes have been discovered in many chromosomally unstable cancer cell lines (Ohshima *et al.*, 2000; Ru *et al.*, 2002). Additionally, mitotic spindle assembly checkpoint defects may contribute to the genomic instability seen in cervical cancer, as high-risk HPV E6 and E7 oncoproteins have been reported to interfere with multiple mitotic cell-cycle checkpoints, including the mitotic spindle assembly checkpoint (Thomas & Laimins, 1998; Thompson *et al.*, 1997). As mentioned previously, a number of mitotic genes are transcriptional targets of E2F transcriptional regulation (reviewed in Stevaux & Dyson, 2002), including the mitotic spindle assembly checkpoint component Mad2, which is aberrantly expressed in cells with inactivated pRB (Hernando *et al.*, 2004). Accordingly, HPV E7-induced inactivation of pRB may compromise the vigilance of the mitotic spindle assembly checkpoint.

Early studies with mouse cells showed DNA re-replication in the presence of mitotic spindle poisons suggested that p53 may modulate the mitotic spindle assembly checkpoint (Cross *et al.*, 1995; Di Leonardo *et al.*, 1997; Thompson *et al.*, 1997), it is now generally accepted that the integrity of this checkpoint does not depend on p53 function (reviewed in Duensing & Duensing, 2005). Rather, p53 controls a postmitotic checkpoint that thwarts exit from an aberrant G1-like phase, in which cells that do not complete mitosis enter via "mitotic slippage" (reviewed in Margolis *et al.*, 2003).

6.3.4. *Abrogation of the postmitotic checkpoint by HPV oncoproteins — induction of polyploidy*

HPV16 E6- or E7-expressing cells often undergo polyploidization; in fact, high-risk HPV-associated lesions display an increased degree of tetrasomy (Giannoudis *et al.*, 2000; Southern *et al.*, 1997). High-risk HPV E6's ability to induce polyploidy is often linked to its inactivation of the p53 tumor suppressor. If a cell fails to complete cytokinesis, it will not undergo nuclear and/or cellular division and temporarily arrest in anaphase. Such cells de-condense their chromosomes and enter a G1-like state with tetraploid (4-N) DNA content via mitotic slippage; re-entry of these cells into S-phase is restricted by the p53-dependent postmitotic checkpoint (Lanni & Jacks, 1998; Vogel *et al.*, 2004). However, inactivation of p53 by high-risk HPV E6 proteins may allow tetraploid cells to escape arrest and re-enter the cell division cycle. If such tetraploid cells are able to undergo successful cytokinesis, they have the potential to generate aneuploid progeny such as those detected in high-risk HPV-associated lesions. Studies with p53-deficient mouse embryo fibroblasts, however, revealed that loss of p53 (or its transcriptional target $p21^{CIP1}$) causes persistent cytokinesis failure, resulting in apoptosis (Bunz *et al.*, 1998). Consistent with this notion, HPV16 E6-expressing primary human epithelial cells show an increased incidence of binucleation and other nuclear irregularities and frequently undergo senescence (Duensing *et al.*, 2000).

While a p53-dependent mechanism of tetraploidy induction can be easily envisioned for high-risk HPV E6, generation of polyploidy by high-risk HPV E7 is less well defined. However, it is known that the ability of HPV16 E7 to bind and inactivate the retinoblastoma tumor suppressor is not related to development of polyploidy (Southern *et al.*, 2004).

7. Concluding Remarks

Cancer encompasses a set of complex diseases that share at their core a phenotype of unregulated cell growth. Such aberrant growth control can arise through a myriad of pathways, involving numerous defects in the regulation of cell cycle, DNA repair, and differentiation. Many genes involved in these pathways that play critical roles in cancer development have been identified and characterized over the years. In addition, epigenetic events that impart effects on these genes or their function have been demonstrated. Due to the complexity of studying cancers of various etiologies involving an accumulation of both genetic and epigenetic events, the study of cancer development is confounded by the challenge of extracting information on specific abnormalities that drive cancer development.

In contrast, high-risk HPV infection represents a well-defined oncogenic etiology for the study of carcinogenesis. The transformed phenotype is solely predicated on the expression of two viral proteins, E6 and E7. There is no other human solid tumor type that can be modeled with similar accuracy in cell culture or animal models. Thus, further study of the molecular mechanisms of HPV E6 and E7-mediated cancer development will greatly add to our understanding of general human carcinogenesis.

References

Adam JL, Briggs MW, McCance DJ (2000) A mutagenic analysis of the E5 protein of human papillomavirus type 16 reveals that E5 binding to the vacuolar H(+)-ATPase is not sufficient for biological activity, using mammalian and yeast expression systems. *Virology* **272**: 315–325.

Alani RM, Hasskarl J, Münger K (1998) Alterations in cyclin-dependent kinase 2 function during differentiation of primary human keratinocytes. *Mol Carcinog* **23**: 226–233.

Arbeit JM (1996) Transgenic models of epidermal neoplasia and multistage carcinogenesis. *Cancer Surv* **26**: 7–34.

Arends MJ, Buckley CH, Wells M (1998) Aetiology, pathogenesis, and pathology of cervical neoplasia. *J Clin Pathol* **51**: 96–103.

Ashby AD, Meagher L, Campo MS, Finbow ME (2001) E5 transforming proteins of papillomaviruses do not disturb the activity of the vacuolar H(+)-ATPase. *J Gen Virol* **82**: 2353–2362.

Assoian RK (1997) Anchorage-dependent cell cycle progression. *J Cell Biol* **136**: 1–4.

Balsitis SJ, Sage J, Duensing S, Münger K, Jacks T, Lambert PF (2003) Recapitulation of the effects of the human papillomavirus type 16 E7 oncogene on mouse epithelium by somatic Rb deletion and detection of pRb-independent effects of E7 *in vivo*. *Mol Cell Biol* **23**: 9094–9103.

Barbosa MS, Lowy DR, Schiller JT (1989) Papillomavirus polypeptides E6 and E7 are zinc-binding proteins. *J Virol* **63**: 1404–1407.

Barr E, Tamms G (2007) Quadrivalent human papillomavirus vaccine. *Clin Infect Dis* **45**: 609–607.

Bastien N, McBride AA (2000) Interaction of the papillomavirus E2 protein with mitotic chromosomes. *Virology* **270**: 124–134.

Batieha AM, Armenian HK, Norkus EP, Morris JS, Spate VE, Comstock GW (1993) Serum micronutrients and the subsequent risk of cervical cancer in a population-based nested case-control study. *Cancer Epidemiol Biomarkers Prev* **2**: 335–339.

Baus F, Gire V, Fisher D, Piette J, Dulic V (2003) Permanent cell cycle exit in G2 phase after DNA damage in normal human fibroblasts. *Embo J* **22**: 3992–4002.

Baxter MK, McPhillips MG, Ozato K, McBride AA (2005) The mitotic chromosome binding activity of the papillomavirus E2 protein correlates with interaction with the cellular chromosomal protein, Brd4. *J Virol* **79**: 4806–4818.

Bibbo M, Dytch HE, Alenghat E, Bartels PH, Wied GL (1989) DNA ploidy profiles as prognostic indicators in CIN lesions. *Am J Clin Pathol* **92**: 261–265.

Blasco MA, Hahn WC (2003) Evolving views of telomerase and cancer. *Trends Cell Biol* **13**: 289–294.

Bornens M (2002) Centrosome composition and microtubule anchoring mechanisms. *Curr Opin Cell Biol* **14**: 25–34.

Bouvard V, Matlashewski G, Gu ZM, Storey A, Banks L (1994) The human papillomavirus type 16 E5 gene cooperates with the E7 gene to stimulate proliferation of primary cells and increases viral gene expression. *Virology* **203**: 73–80.

Boyer SN, Wazer DE, Band V (1996) E7 protein of human papilloma virus-16 induces degradation of retinoblastoma protein through the ubiquitin-proteasome pathway. *Cancer Res* **56**: 4620–4624.

Brehm A, Nielsen SJ, Miska EA, McCance DJ, Reid JL, Bannister AJ, Kouzarides T (1999) The E7 oncoprotein associates with Mi2 and histone deacetylase activity to promote cell growth. *Embo J* **18**: 2449–2458.

Brinkley BR (2001) Managing the centrosome numbers game: from chaos to stability in cancer cell division. *Trends Cell Biol* **11**: 18–21.

Bulten J, Poddighe PJ, Robben JCM, Gemmink JH, de Wilde PCM, Hanselaar AGJM (1998) Interphase cytogenetic analysis of cervical intraepithelial neoplasia. *Am J Pathol* **152**: 495–503.

Bunz F, Dutriaux A, Lengauer C, Waldman T, Zhou S, Brown JP, Sedivy JM, Kinzler KW, Vogelstein B (1998) Requirement for p53 and p21 to sustain G2 arrest after DNA damage. *Science* **282**: 1497–1501.

Burkhardt A, DiMaio D, Schlegel R (1987) Genetic and biochemical definition of the bovine papillomavirus E5 transforming protein. *Embo J* **6**: 2381–2385.

Burkhardt A, Willingham M, Gay C, Jeang KT, Schlegel R (1989) The E5 oncoprotein of bovine papillomavirus is oriented asymmetrically in Golgi and plasma membranes. *Virology* **170**: 334–339.

Burnett S, Jareborg N, DiMaio D (1992) Localization of bovine papillomavirus type 1 E5 protein to transformed basal keratinocytes and permissive differentiated cells in fibropapilloma tissue. *Proc Natl Acad Sci USA* **89**: 5665–5669.

Casper AM, Nghiem P, Arlt MF, Glover TW (2002) ATR regulates fragile site stability. *Cell* **111**: 779–789.

Cates W Jr (1999) Estimates of the incidence and prevalence of sexually transmitted diseases in the United States. American Social Health Association Panel. *Sex Transm Dis* **26**: S2–S7.

Chatterjee R, Mandal B, Bandyopadhyay S (2003) Detection of HPV DNA in cervical carcinomas by PCR and hybrid capture assay. *Indian J Pathol Microbiol* **46**: 596–599.

Chen JJ, Reid CE, Band V, Androphy EJ (1995) Interaction of papillomavirus E6 oncoproteins with a putative calcium-binding protein. *Science* **269**: 529–531.

Chesson HW, Blandford JM, Gift TL, Tao G, Irwin KL (2004) The estimated direct medical cost of sexually transmitted diseases among American youth, 2000. *Perspect Sex Reprod Health* **36**: 11–19.

Chi YH, Jeang KT (2007) Aneuploidy and cancer. *J Cell Biochem* **102**: 531–538.

Clemens KE, Brent R, Gyuris J, Munger K (1995) Dimerization of the human papillomavirus E7 oncoprotein *in vivo*. *Virology* **214**: 289–293.

Clifford GM, Smith JS, Aguado T, Franceschi S (2003) Comparison of HPV type distribution in high-grade cervical lesions and cervical cancer: a meta-analysis. *Br J Cancer* **89**: 101–105.

Cole ST, Danos O (1987) Nucleotide sequence and comparative analysis of the human papillomavirus type 18 genome. Phylogeny of papillomaviruses and repeated structure of the E6 and E7 gene products. *J Mol Biol* **193**: 599–608.

Coleman N, Birley HD, Renton AM, Hanna NF, Ryait BK, Byrne M, Taylor-Robinson D, Stanley MA (1994) Immunological events in regressing genital warts. *Am J Clin Pathol* **102**: 768–774.

Conger KL, Liu JS, Kuo SR, Chow LT, Wang TS (1999) Human papillomavirus DNA replication. Interactions between the viral E1 protein and two subunits of human DNA polymerase alpha/primase. *J Biol Chem* **274**: 2696–2705.

Conrad M, Bubb VJ, Schlegel R (1993) The human papillomavirus types 6 and 16 E5 proteins are membrane-associated proteins which associate with the 16-kilodalton pore-forming protein. *J Virol* **67**: 6170–6178.

Cottage A, Dowen S, Roberts I, Pett M, Coleman N, Stanley M (2001) Early genetic events in HPV immortalised keratinocytes. *Genes Chromosomes Cancer* **30**: 72–79.

Craven SE, Bredt DS (1998) PDZ proteins organize synaptic signaling pathways. *Cell* **93**: 495–498.

Cripe TP, Haugen TH, Turk JP, Tabatabai F, Schmid PGR, Dürst M, Gissmann L, Roman A, Turek LP (1987) Transcriptional regulation of the human papillomavirus-16 E6–E7 promoter by a keratinocyte-dependent enhancer, and by viral E2 trans-activator and repressor gene products: implications for cervical carcinogenesis. *EMBO J* **6**: 3745–3753.

Cross SM, Sanchez CA, Morgan CA, Schimke MK, Ramel S, Idzerda RL, Raskind WH, Reid BJ (1995) A p53-dependent mouse spindle checkpoint. *Science* **267**: 1353–1356.

Crum CP, Ikenberg H, Richart RM, Gissman L (1984) Human papillomavirus type 16 and early cervical neoplasia. *N Engl J Med* **310**: 880–883.

Daling JR, Madeleine MM, McKnight B, Carter JJ, Wipf GC, Ashley R, Schwartz SM, Beckmann AM, Hagensee ME, Mandelson MT, Galloway DA (1996) The relationship of human papillomavirus-related cervical tumors to cigarette smoking, oral contraceptive use, and prior herpes simplex virus type 2 infection. *Cancer Epidemiol Biomarkers Prev* **5**: 541–548.

de Villiers EM (2001) Taxonmic classification of papillomaviruses. *Papillomavirus Report* **12**: 57–63.

de Villiers EM, Fauquet C, Broker TR, Bernard HU, zur Hausen H (2004) Classification of papillomaviruses. *Virology* **324**: 17–27.

de Villiers EM, Gissmann L, zur Hausen H (1981) Molecular cloning of viral DNA from human genital warts. *J Virol* **40**: 932–935.

de Villiers EM, Ruhland A, Sekaric P (1999) Human papillomaviruses in non-melanoma skin cancer. *Semin Cancer Biol* **9**: 413–422.

DeCaprio JA, Ludlow JW, Figge J, Shew JY, Huang CM, Lee WH, Marsilio E, Paucha E, Livingston DM (1988) SV40 large tumor antigen forms a specific complex with the product of the retinoblastoma susceptibility gene. *Cell* **54**: 275–283.

DeMasi J, Chao MC, Kumar AS, Howley PM (2007) Bovine papillomavirus E7 oncoprotein inhibits anoikis. *J Virol* **81**: 9419–9425.

DeMasi J, Huh KW, Nakatani Y, Munger K, Howley PM (2005) Bovine papillomavirus E7 transformation function correlates with cellular p600 protein binding. *Proc Natl Acad Sci USA* **102**: 11486–11491.

Demers GW, Foster SA, Halbert CL, Galloway DA (1994a) Growth arrest by induction of p53 in DNA damaged keratinocytes is bypassed by human papillomavirus 16 E7. *Proc Natl Acad Sci USA* **91**: 4382–4386.

Demers GW, Halbert CL, Galloway DA (1994b) Elevated wild-type p53 protein levels in human epithelial cell lines immortalized by the human papillomavirus type 16 E7 gene. *Virology* **198**: 169–174.

Di Cunto F, Topley G, Calautti E, Hsiao J, Ong L, Seth PK, Dotto GP (1998) Inhibitory function of p21Cip1/WAF1 in differentiation of primary mouse keratinocytes independent of cell cycle control. *Science* **280**: 1069–1072.

Di Leonardo A, Khan SH, Linke SP, Greco V, Seidita G, Wahl GM (1997) DNA rereplication in the presence of mitotic spindle inhibitors in human and mouse fibroblasts lacking either p53 or pRb function. *Cancer Res* **57**: 1013–1019.

DiMaio D, Guralski D, Schiller JT (1986) Translation of open reading frame E5 of bovine papillomavirus is required for its transforming activity. *Proc Natl Acad Sci USA* **83**: 1797–1801.

Disbrow GL, Sunitha I, Baker CC, Hanover J, Schlegel R (2003) Codon optimization of the HPV-16 E5 gene enhances protein expression. *Virology* **311**: 105–114.

Doorbar J, Ely S, Sterling J, McLean, C, Crawford L (1991) Specific interaction between HPV-16 E1-E4 and cytokeratins results in collapse of the epithelial cell intermediate filament network. *Nature* **352**: 824–827.

Dorsman JC, Teunisse AF, Zantema A, van der Eb AJ (1997) The adenovirus 12 E1A proteins can bind directly to proteins of the p300 transcription co-activator family, including the CREB-binding protein CBP and p300. *J Gen Virol* **78**(Pt 2): 423–426.

Drummond-Barbosa DA, Vaillancourt, RR, Kazlauskas A, DiMaio D (1995) Ligand-independent activation of the platelet-derived growth factor beta receptor: requirements for bovine papillomavirus E5-induced mitogenic signaling. *Mol Cell Biol* **15**: 2570–2581.

Duensing A, Duensing S (2005) Guilt by association? p53 and the development of aneuploidy in cancer. *Biochem Biophys Res Commun* **331**: 694–700.

Duensing A, Liu Y, Tseng M, Malumbres M, Barbacid M, Duensing S (2006) Cyclin-dependent kinase 2 is dispensable for normal centrosome duplication but required for oncogene-induced centrosome overduplication. *Oncogene* **25**: 2943–2949.

Duensing S, Duensing A, Crum CP, Münger K (2001) Human papillomavirus type 16 E7 oncoprotein-induced abnormal centrosome synthesis is an early event in the evolving malignant phenotype. *Cancer Res* **61**: 2356–2360.

Duensing S, Duensing A, Lee DC, Edwards KM, Piboonniyom SO, Manuel E, Skaltsounis L, Meijer L, Munger K (2004) Cyclin-dependent kinase inhibitor indirubin-3′-oxime selectively inhibits human papillomavirus type 16 E7-induced numerical centrosome anomalies. *Oncogene* **23**: 8206–8215.

Duensing S, Lee LY, Duensing A, Basile J, Piboonniyom S, Gonzalez S, Crum CP, Munger K (2000) The human papillomavirus type 16 E6 and E7 oncoproteins cooperate to induce mitotic defects and genomic instability by uncoupling centrosome duplication from the cell division cycle. *Proc Natl Acad Sci USA* **97**: 10002–10007.

Duensing S, Münger K (2003) Human papillomavirus type 16 E7 oncoprotein can induce abnormal centrosome duplication through a mechanism independent of inactivation of retinoblastoma protein family members. *J Virol* **77**: 12331–12335.

Duensing S, Münger K (2002) The human papillomavirus type 16 E6 and E7 oncoproteins independently induce numerical and structural chromosome instability. *Canc Res* **62**: 7075–7082.

Dulic V, Stein GH, Far DF, Reed SI (1998) Nuclear accumulation of p21Cip1 at the onset of mitosis: a role at the G2/M-phase transition. *Mol Cell Biol* **18**: 546–557.

Durst M, Gallahan D, Jay G, Rhim JS (1989) Glucocorticoid-enhanced neoplastic transformation of human keratinocytes by human papillomavirus type 16 and an activated ras oncogene. *Virology* **173**: 767–771.

Durst M, Gissmann L, Ikenberg H, zur Hausen H (1983) A papillomavirus DNA from a cervical carcinoma and its prevalence in cancer biopsy samples from different geographic regions. *Proc Natl Acad Sci USA* **80**: 3812–3815.

Dyson N, Guida P, Münger K, Harlow E (1992) Homologous sequences in adenovirus E1A and human papillomavirus E7 proteins mediate interaction with the same set of cellular proteins. *J Virol* **66**: 6893–6902.

Dyson N, Howley PM, Münger K, Harlow E (1989) The human papillomavirus-16 E7 oncoprotein is able to bind to the retinoblastoma gene product. *Science* **243**: 934–937.

Eckner R, Ludlow JW, Lill NL, Oldread E, Arany Z, Modjtahedi N, Decaprio JA, Livingston DM, Morgan JA (1996) Association of p300 and CBP with simian virus 40 large T antigen. *Mol Cell Biol* **16**: 3454–3464.

Eichten A, Westfall M, Pietenpol JA, Münger K (2002) Stabilization and functional impairment of the tumor suppressor p53 by the human papillomavirus type 16 E7 oncoprotein. *Virology* **295**: 74–95.

El-Deiry WS, Tokino T, Velculescu VE, Levy DB, Parsons R, Trent JM, Lin D, Mercer WE, Kinzler KW, Vogelstein B (1993) WAF1, a potential mediator of p53 tumor suppression. *Cell* **75**: 817–825.

Evander M, Frazer IH, Payne E, Qi YM, Hengst K, McMillan NA (1997) Identification of the alpha6 integrin as a candidate receptor for papillomaviruses. *J Virol* **71**: 2449–2456.

Fang F, Orend G, Watanabe N, Hunter T, Ruoslahti E (1996) Dependence of cyclin E-CDK2 kinase activity on cell anchorage. *Science* **271**: 499–502.

Fehrmann F, Klumpp DJ, Laimins LA (2003) Human papillomavirus type 31 E5 protein supports cell cycle progression and activates late viral functions upon epithelial differentiation. *J Virol* 77: 2819–2831.

Firpo EJ, Koff A, Solomon MJ, Roberts JM (1994) Inactivation of a cdk2 inhibitor during interleukin 2-induced proliferation of human T lymphocytes. *Mol Cell Biol* **14**: 4889–4901.

Fisk HA, Winey M (2001) The mouse Mps1p-like kinase regulates centrosome duplication. *Cell* **106**: 95–104.

Frattini MG, Laimins LA (1994) Binding of the human papillomavirus E1 origin-recognition protein is regulated through complex formation with the E2 enhancer-binding protein. *Proc Natl Acad Sci USA* **91**: 12398–12402.

Frazer IH (2004) Prevention of cervical cancer through papillomavirus vaccination. *Nat Rev Immunol* **4**: 46–54.

Frega A, Stentella P, Tinari A, Vecchione A, Marchionni M (2002) Giant condyloma acuminatum or buschke-Lowenstein tumor: review of the literature and report of three cases treated by CO2 laser surgery. A long-term follow-up. *Anticancer Res* **22**: 1201–1204.

Frisch M, Biggar RJ, Goedert JJ (2000) Human papillomavirus-associated cancers in patients with human immunodeficiency virus infection and acquired immunodeficiency syndrome. *J Natl Cancer Inst* **92**: 1500–1510.

Frisch SM, Screaton RA (2001) Anoikis mechanisms. *Curr Opin Cell Biol* **13**: 555–562.

Fukasawa K, Choi T, Kuriyama R, Rulong S, Vande Woude GF (1996) Abnormal centrosome amplification in the absence of p53. *Science* **271**: 1744–1747.

Funk JO, Waga S, Harry JB, Espling E, Stillman B, Galloway DA (1997) Inhibition of CDK activity and PCNA-dependent DNA replication by p21 is blocked by interaction with the HPV-16 E7 oncoprotein. *Genes Dev* **11**: 2090–2100.

Furihata M, Ohtsuki Y, Sonobe H, Shuin T, Yamamoto A, Terao N, Kuwahara M (1998) Prognostic significance of cyclin E and p53 protein overexpression in carcinoma of the renal pelvis and ureter. *Br J Cancer* **77**: 783–788.

Gage JR, Meyers C, Wettstein FO (1990) The E7 proteins of the nononcogenic human papillomavirus type 6b (HPV-6b) and of the oncogenic HPV-16 differ in retinoblastoma protein binding and other properties. *J Virol* **64**: 723–730.

Garner-Hamrick PA, Fostel JM, Chien WM, Banerjee NS, Chow LT, Broker TR, Fisher C (2004) Global effects of human papillomavirus type 18 E6/E7 in an organotypic keratinocyte culture system. *J Virol* **78**: 9041–9050.

Genther Williams SM, Disbrow GL, Schlegel R, Lee D, Threadgill DW, Lambert PF (2005) Requirement of epidermal growth factor receptor for hyperplasia induced by E5, a high-risk human papillomavirus oncogene. *Cancer Res* **65**: 6534–6542.

Gewin L, Galloway DA (2001) E box-dependent activation of telomerase by human papillomavirus type 16 E6 does not require induction of c-myc. *J Virol* **75**: 7198–7201.

Gewin L, Myers H, Kiyono T, Galloway DA (2004) Identification of a novel telomerase repressor that interacts with the human papillomavirus type-16 E6/E6-AP complex. *Genes Dev* **18**: 2269–2282.

Giannoudis A, Evans MF, Southern SA, Herrington CS (2000) Basal keratinocyte tetrasomy in low-grade squamous intra-epithelial lesions of the cervix is restricted to high and intermediate risk HPV infection but is not type-specific. *Br J Cancer* **82**: 424–428.

Gil P, Dewey E, Friml J, Zhao Y, Snowden KC, Putterill J, Palme K, Estelle M, Chory J (2001) BIG: a calossin-like protein required for polar auxin transport in *Arabidopsis*. *Genes Dev* **15**: 1985–1997.

Gillison ML, Koch WM, Capone RB, Spafford M, Westra WH, Wu L, Zahurak ML, Daniel RW, Viglione M, Symer DE *et al.* (2000) Evidence for a causal association between human papillomavirus and a subset of head and neck cancers. *J Natl Cancer Inst* **92**: 709–720.

Giovannelli L, Lama A, Capra G, Giordano V, Arico P, Ammatuna P (2004) Detection of human papillomavirus DNA in cervical samples: analysis of the new PGMY-PCR compared to the hybrid capture II and MY-PCR assays and a two-step nested PCR assay. *J Clin Microbiol* **42**: 3861–3864.

Giroglou T, Florin L, Schafer F, Streeck RE, Sapp M (2001) Human papillomavirus infection requires cell surface heparan sulfate. *J Virol* **75**: 1565–1570.

Gissmann L, Diehl V, Schultz-Coulon HJ, zur Hausen H (1982) Molecular cloning and characterization of human papilloma virus DNA derived from a laryngeal papilloma. *J Virol* **44**: 393–400.

Giuliano AR, Papenfuss M, Nour M, Canfield LM, Schneider A, Hatch K (1997) Antioxidant nutrients: associations with persistent human papillomavirus infection. *Cancer Epidemiol Biomarkers Prev* **6**: 917–923.

Goldstein DJ, Finbow ME, Andresson T, McLean P, Smith K, Bubb V, Schlegel R (1991) Bovine papillomavirus E5 oncoprotein binds to the 16K component of vacuolar H(+)-ATPases. *Nature* **352**: 347–349.

Goldstein DJ, Li W, Wang LM, Heidaran MA, Aaronson S, Shinn R, Schlegel R, Pierce JH (1994) The bovine papillomavirus type 1 E5 transforming protein specifically binds and activates the beta-type receptor for the platelet-derived growth factor but not other related tyrosine kinase-containing receptors to induce cellular transformation. *J Virol* **68**: 4432–4441.

Greer CE, Wheeler CM, Ladner MB, Beutner K, Coyne MY, Liang H, Langenberg A, Yen TS, Ralston R (1995) Human papillomavirus (HPV) type distribution and serological response to HPV type 6 virus-like particles in patients with genital warts. *J Clin Microbiol* **33**: 2058–2063.

Griffis ER, Stuurman N, Vale RD (2007) Spindly, a novel protein essential for silencing the spindle assembly checkpoint, recruits dynein to the kinetochore. *J Cell Biol* **177**: 1005–1015.

Grill SW, Gonczy P, Stelzer EH, Hyman AA (2001) Polarity controls forces governing asymmetric spindle positioning in the *Caenorhabditis elegans* embryo. *Nature* **409**: 630–633.

Groff DE, Lancaster WD (1986) Genetic analysis of the 3′ early region transformation and replication functions of bovine papillomavirus type 1. *Virology* **150**: 221–230.

Grossman SR, Laimins LA (1989) E6 protein of human papillomavirus type 18 binds zinc. *Oncogene* **4**: 1089–1093.

Guarguaglini G, Duncan PI, Stierhof YD, Holmstrom T, Duensing S, Nigg EA (2005) The forkhead-associated domain protein Cep170 interacts with Polo-like kinase 1 and serves as a marker for mature centrioles. *Mol Biol Cell* **16**: 1095–1107.

Gulliver GA, Herber RL, Liem A, Lambert PF (1997) Both conserved region 1 (CR1) and CR2 of the human papillomavirus type 16 E7 oncogene are required for induction of epidermal hyperplasia and tumor formation in transgenic mice. *J Virol* **71**: 5905–5914.

Harper DM, Franco EL, Wheeler C, Ferris DG, Jenkins D, Schuind A, Zahaf T, Innis B, Naud P, De Carvalho NS, *et al.* (2004) Efficacy of a bivalent L1 virus-like particle vaccine in prevention of infection with human papillomavirus types 16 and 18 in young women: a randomised controlled trial. *Lancet* **364**: 1757–1765.

Harper DM, Franco EL, Wheeler CM, Moscicki AB, Romanowski B, Roteli-Martins CM, Jenkins D, Schuind A, Costa Clemens SA, Dubin G (2006) Sustained efficacy up to 4.5 years of a bivalent L1 virus-like particle vaccine against human papillomavirus types 16 and 18: follow-up from a randomised control trial. *Lancet* **367**: 1247–1255.

Hartwell LH, Weinert TA (1989) Checkpoints: controls that ensure the order of cell cycle events. *Science* **246**: 629–634.

Hawley-Nelson P, Vousden KH, Hubbert NL, Lowy DR, Schiller JT (1989) HPV16 E6 and E7 proteins cooperate to immortalize human foreskin keratinocytes. *EMBO J* **8**: 3905–3910.

Heck DV, Yee CL, Howley PM, Münger K (1992) Efficiency of binding to the retinoblastoma protein correlates with the transforming capacity of the E7 oncoproteins of the human papillomaviruses. *Proc Natl Acad Sci USA* **89**: 4442–4446.

Hemminki K, Dong C, Vaittinen P (1999) Familial risks in cervical cancer: is there a hereditary component? *Int J Cancer* **82**: 775–781.

Hergovich A, Lamla S, Nigg EA, Hemmings BA (2007) Centrosome-associated NDR kinase regulates centrosome duplication. *Mol Cell* **25**: 625–634.

Hernando E, Nahle Z, Juan G, Diaz-Rodriguez E, Alaminos M, Hemann M, Michel L, Mittal V, Gerald W, Benezra R *et al.* (2004) Rb inactivation promotes genomic instability by uncoupling cell cycle progression from mitotic control. *Nature* **430**: 797–802.

Heselmeyer K, Macville M, Schrock E, Blegen H, Hellstrom AC, Shah K, Auer G, Ried T (1997) Advanced-stage cervical carcinomas are defined by a recurrent pattern of chromosomal aberrations revealing high genetic instability and a consistent gain of chromosome arm 3q. *Genes Chromosomes Cancer* **19**: 233–240.

Heselmeyer K, Schrock E, du Manoir S, Blegen H, Shah K, Steinbeck R, Auer G, Ried T (1996) Gain of chromosome 3q defines the transition from severe dysplasia to invasive carcinoma of the uterine cervix. *Proc Natl Acad Sci USA* **93**: 479–484.

Hickman ES, Picksley SM, Vousden KH (1994) Cells expressing HPV16 E7 continue cell cycle progression following DNA damage induced p53 activation. *Oncogene* **9**: 2177–2181.

Hinchcliffe EH, Li C, Thompson EA, Maller JL, Sluder G (1999) Requirement of Cdk2-cyclin E activity for repeated centrosome reproduction in *Xenopus* egg extracts. *Science* **283**: 851–854.

Hinchcliffe EH, Miller FJ, Cham M, Khodjakov A, Sluder G (2001) Requirement of a centrosomal activity for cell cycle progression through G1 into S phase. *Science* **291**: 1547–1550.

Hinchcliffe EH, Sluder G (2001) "It Takes Two to Tango": understanding how centrosome duplication is regulated throughout the cell cycle. *Genes Dev* **15**: 1167–1181.

Hippelainen MI, Hippelainen M, Saarikoski S, Syrjanen K (1994) Clinical course and prognostic factors of human papillomavirus infections in men. *Sex Transm Dis* **21**: 272–279.

Hobom U, Dobbelstein M (2004) E1B-55-kilodalton protein is not required to block p53-induced transcription during adenovirus infection. *J Virol* **78**: 7685–7697.

Hoffmann I (2006) Protein kinases involved in mitotic spindle checkpoint regulation. *Results Probl Cell Differ* **42**: 93–109.

Horwitz BH, Burkhardt AL, Schlegel R, DiMaio D (1988) 44-amino-acid E5 transforming protein of bovine papillomavirus requires a hydrophobic core and specific carboxyl-terminal amino acids. *Mol Cell Biol* **8**: 4071–4078.

Howell BJ, McEwen BF, Canman JC, Hoffman DB, Farrar EM, Rieder C L, Salmon ED (2001) Cytoplasmic dynein/dynactin drives kinetochore protein transport to the spindle poles and has a role in mitotic spindle checkpoint inactivation. *J Cell Biol* **155**: 1159–1172.

Howley PM, Lowy DR (2007) Papillomaviruses. In: Knipe DM, Howley PM (eds.), *Fields Virology*. Philadelphia: Lippincott Williams & Wilkins, pp. 2299–2354.

Huang PS, Patrick DR, Edwards G, Goodhart PJ, Huber HE, Miles L, Garsky VM, Oliff A, Heimbrook DC (1993) Protein domains governing interactions between E2F, the retinoblastoma gene product, and human papillomavirus type 16 E7 protein. *Mol Cell Biol* **13**: 953–960.

Hughes FJ, Romanos MA (1993) E1 protein of human papillomavirus is a DNA Helicase/ATPase. *Nucleic Acids Res* **21**: 5817–5823.

Huh K, Zhou X, Hayakawa H, Cho JY, Libermann TA, Jin J, Harper JW, Münger K (2007) Human papillomavirus type 16 E7 oncoprotein associates with the cullin 2 ubiquitin ligase complex, which contributes to degradation of the retinoblastoma tumor suppressor. *J Virol* **81**: 9737–9747.

Huh KW, DeMasi J, Ogawa H, Nakatani Y, Howley PM, Münger K (2005) Association of the human papillomavirus type 16 E7 oncoprotein with the 600-kDa retinoblastoma protein-associated factor, p600. *Proc Natl Acad Sci USA* **102**: 11492–11497.

Huibregtse JM, Scheffner M, Howley PM (1991) A cellular protein mediates association of p53 with the E6 oncoprotein of human papillomavirus types 16 or 18. *EMBO J* **10**: 4129–4135.

Huibregtse JM, Scheffner M, Howley PM (1993) Localization of the E6-AP regions that direct human papillomavirus E6 binding, association with p53, and ubiquitination of associated proteins. *Mol Cell Biol* **13**: 4918–4927.

Hummel M, Hudson JB, Laimins LA (1992) Differentiation-induced and constitutive transcription of human papillomavirus type 31b in cell lines containing viral episomes. *J Virol* **66**: 6070–6080.

Hwang ES, Nottoli T, Di Maio D (1995) The HPV16 E5 protein: expression, detection, and stable complex formation with transmembrane proteins in COS cells. *Virology* **211**: 227–233.

Hwang SG, Lee D, Kim J, Seo T, Choe J (2002) Human papillomavirus type 16 E7 binds to E2F1 and activates E2F1-driven transcription in a retinoblastoma protein-independent manner. *J Biol Chem* **277**: 2923–2930.

Jablonska S, Majewski S, Obalek S, Orth G (1997) Cutaneous warts. *Clin Dermatol* **15**: 309–319.

Jackson MW, Agarwal MK, Yang J, Bruss P, Uchiumi T, Agarwal ML, Stark GR, Taylor WR (2005) p130/p107/p105Rb-dependent transcriptional repression during DNA-damage-induced cell-cycle exit at G2. *J Cell Sci* **118**: 1821–1832.

Jefford CE, Irminger-Finger I (2006) Mechanisms of chromosome instability in cancers. *Crit Rev Oncol Hematol* **59**: 1–14.

Jemal A, Siegel R, Ward E, Hao Y, Xu J, Murray T, Thun MJ (2008) Cancer statistics, 2008. *CA Cancer J Clin* **58**: 71–96.

Jewers RJ, Hildebrandt P, Ludlow JW, Kell B, McCance DJ (1992) Regions of human papillomavirus type 16 E7 oncoprotein required for immortalization of human keratinocytes. *J Virol* **66**: 1329–1335.

Jones DL, Alani RM, Münger K (1997a) The human papillomavirus E7 oncoprotein can uncouple cellular differentiation and proliferation in human keratinocytes by abrogating $p21^{Cip1}$-mediated inhibition of cdk2. *Genes Dev* **11**: 2101–2111.

Jones DL, Münger K (1997) Analysis of the p53-mediated G1 growth arrest pathway in cells expressing the human papillomavirus type 16 E7 oncoprotein. *J Virol* **71**: 2905–2912.

Jones DL, Thompson DA, Münger K (1997b) Destabilization of the RB tumor suppressor and stabilization of p53 contribute to HPV type 16 E7-induced apoptosis. *Virology* **239**: 97–107.

Karakaidos P, Taraviras S, Vassiliou LV, Zacharatos P, Kastrinakis NG, Kougiou D, Kouloukoussa M, Nishitani H, Papavassiliou AG, Lygerou Z, Gorgoulis VG (2004) Overexpression of the replication licensing regulators hCdt1 and hCdc6 characterizes a subset of non-small-cell lung carcinomas: synergistic effect with mutant p53 on tumor growth and chromosomal instability — evidence of E2F-1 transcriptional control over hCdt1. *Am J Pathol* **165**: 1351–1365.

Katzenellenbogen RA, Egelkrout EM, Vliet-Gregg P, Gewin LC, Gafken PR, Galloway DA (2007) NFX1-123 and poly(A) binding proteins synergistically augment activation of telomerase in human papillomavirus type 16 E6-expressing cells. *J Virol* **81**: 3786–3796.

Kawamura K, Morita N, Domiki C, Fujikawa-Yamamoto K, Hashimoto M, Iwabuchi K, Suzuki K (2006) Induction of centrosome amplification in p53 siRNA-treated human fibroblast cells by radiation exposure. *Cancer Sci* **97**: 252–258.

Kessis TD, Slebos RJ, Nelson WG, Kastan MB, Plunkett BS, Han SM, Lorincz AT, Hedrick L, Cho KR (1993) Human papillomavirus 16 E6 expression disrupts the p53-mediated cellular response to DNA damage. *Proc Natl Acad Sci USA* **90**: 3988–3992.

Khodjakov A, Cole RW, Oakley BR, Rieder CL (2000) Centrosome-independent mitotic spindle formation in vertebrates. *Curr Biol* **10**: 59–67.

Kisurina-Evgenieva O, Mack G, Du Q, Macara I, Khodjakov A, Compton DA (2004) Multiple mechanisms regulate NuMA dynamics at spindle poles. *J Cell Sci* **117**: 6391–6400.

Kiviat NB (1999) Papillomaviruses in non-melanoma skin cancer: epidemiological aspects. *Semin Cancer Biol* **9**: 397–403.

Kiyono T, Hiraiwa A, Fujita M, Hayashi Y, Akiyama T, Ishibashi M (1997) Binding of high-risk human papillomavirus E6 oncoproteins to the human homologue of the *Drosophila* discs large tumor suppressor protein. *Proc Natl Acad Sci USA* **94**: 11612–11616.

Kjellberg L, Hallmans G, Ahren AM, Johansson R, Bergman F, Wadell G, Angstrom T, Dillner J (2000) Smoking, diet, pregnancy and oral contraceptive use as risk factors for cervical intra-epithelial neoplasia in relation to human papillomavirus infection. *Br J Cancer* **82**: 1332–1338.

Klingelhutz AJ, Foster SA, McDougall JK (1996) Telomerase activation by the E6 gene product of human papillomavirus type 16. *Nature* **380**: 79–82.

Koutsky L (1997) Epidemiology of genital human papillomavirus infection. *Am J Med* **102**: 3–8.

Kreimer AR, Alberg AJ, Daniel R, Gravitt PE, Viscidi R, Garrett ES, Shah KV, Gillison ML (2004) Oral human papillomavirus infection in adults is associated with sexual behavior and HIV serostatus. *J Infect Dis* **189**: 686–698.

Kurman RJ, Malkasian GD Jr, Sedlis A, Solomon D (1991) From Papanicolaou to Bethesda: the rationale for a new cervical cytologic classification. *Obstet Gynecol* 77: 779–782.

Kutler DI, Wreesmann VB, Goberdhan A, Ben-Porat L, Satagopan J, Ngai I, Huvos AG, Giampietro P, Levran O, Pujara K, *et al.* (2003). Human papillomavirus DNA and p53 polymorphisms in squamous cell carcinomas from Fanconi anemia patients. *J Natl Cancer Inst* **95**: 1718–1721.

Kwon YT, Reiss Y, Fried VA, Hershko A, Yoon JK, Gonda DK, Sangan P, Copeland NG, Jenkins NA, Varshavsky A (1998) The mouse and human genes encoding the recognition component of the N-end rule pathway. *Proc Natl Acad Sci USA* **95**: 7898–7903.

Lacey KR, Jackson PK, Stearns T (1999) Cyclin-dependent kinase control of centrosome duplication. *Proc Natl Acad Sci USA* **96**: 2817–2822.

Lai CC, Henningson C, DiMaio D (1998) Bovine papillomavirus E5 protein induces oligomerization and *trans*-phosphorylation of the platelet-derived growth factor beta receptor. *Proc Natl Acad Sci USA* **95**: 15241–15246.

Lanni JS, Jacks T (1998) Characterization of the p53-dependent postmitotic checkpoint following spindle disruption. *Mol Cell Biol* **18**: 1055–1064.

Lee C, Laimins LA (2007) The differentiation-dependent life cycle of human papillomaviruses in keratinocytes. In: Garcea RL, DiMaio D (eds.), *The Papillomaviruses*, pp. 45–68. New York: Springer.

Lee SS, Glaunsinger B, Mantovani F, Banks L, Javier RT (2000) Multi-PDZ domain protein MUPP1 is a cellular target for both adenovirus E4-ORF1 and high-risk papillomavirus type 18 E6 oncoproteins. *J Virol* **74**: 9680–9693.

Lee SS, Weiss RS, Javier RT (1997) Binding of human virus oncoproteins to hDlg/SAP97, a mammalian homolog of the *Drosophila* discs large tumor suppressor protein. *Proc Natl Acad Sci USA* **94**: 6670–6675.

Leechanachai P, Banks L, Moreau F, Matlashewski G (1992) The E5 gene from human papillomavirus type 16 is an oncogene which enhances growth factor-mediated signal transduction to the nucleus. *Oncogene* 7: 19–25.

Lengauer C, Kinzler KW, Vogelstein B (1998) Genetic instabilities in human cancers. *Nature* **396**: 643–649.

Levesque AA, Howard L, Gordon MB, Compton DA (2003) A functional relationship between NuMA and kid is involved in both spindle organization and chromosome alignment in vertebrate cells. *Mol Biol Cell* **14**: 3541–3552.

Li R, Botchan MR (1994) Acidic transcription factors alleviate nucleosome-mediated repression of DNA replication of bovine papillomavirus type 1. *Proc Natl Acad Sci USA* **91**: 7051–7055.

Lingle WL, Barrett SL, Negron VC, D'Assoro AB, Boeneman K, Liu W, Whitehead CM, Reynolds C, Salisbury JL (2002) Centrosome amplification drives chromosomal instability in breast tumor development. *Proc Natl Acad Sci USA* **99**: 1978–1983.

Liu JP (1999) Studies of the molecular mechanisms in the regulation of telomerase activity. *Faseb J* **13**: 2091–2104.

Liu JS, Kuo SR, Broker TR, Chow, LT (1995) The functions of human papillomavirus type 11 El, E2, and E2C proteins in cell-free DNA replication. *J Biol Chem* **270**: 27283–27291.

Livingstone LR, White A, Sprouse J, Livanos E, Jacks T, Tlsty TD (1992) Altered cell cycle arrest and gene amplification potential accompany loss of wild-type p53. *Cell* **70**: 923–935.

Longworth MS, Laimins LA (2004) The binding of histone deacetylases and the integrity of zinc finger-like motifs of the E7 protein are essential for the life cycle of human papillomavirus type 31. *J Virol* **78**: 3533–3541.

Longworth MS, Wilson R, Laimins LA (2005) HPV31 E7 facilitates replication by activating E2F2 transcription through its interaction with HDACs. *Embo J* **24**: 1821–1830.

Lowe SW, Cepero E, Evan G (2004) Intrinsic tumour suppression. *Nature* **432**: 307–315.

Madura K, Dohmen RJ, Varshavsky A (1993) N-recognin/Ubc2 interactions in the N-end rule pathway. *J Bio Chem* **268**: 12046–12054.

Majewski S, Jablonska S, Orth G (1997) Epidermodysplasia verruciformis. Immunological and nonimmunological surveillance mechanisms: role in tumor progression. *Clin Dermatol* **15**: 321–334.

Malmanche N, Maia A, Sunkel CE (2006) The spindle assembly checkpoint: preventing chromosome mis-segregation during mitosis and meiosis. *FEBS Lett* **580**: 2888–2895.

Margolis RL, Lohez OD, Andreassen PR (2003) G1 tetraploidy checkpoint and the suppression of tumorigenesis. *J Cell Biochem* **88**: 673–683.

Martens JE, Arends J, Van der Linden PJ, De Boer BA, Helmerhorst TJ (2004) Cytokeratin 17 and p63 are markers of the HPV target cell, the cervical stem cell. *Anticancer Res* **24**: 771–775.

Martin LG, Demers GW, Galloway DA (1998) Disruption of the G1/S transition in human papillomavirus type 16 E7-expressing human cells is associated with altered regulation of cyclin E. *J Virol* **72**: 975–985.

Matsumoto Y, Hayashi K, Nishida E (1999) Cyclin-dependent kinase 2 (Cdk2) is required for centrosome duplication in mammalian cells. *Curr Biol* **9**: 429–432.

Maufort JP, Williams SM, Pitot HC, Lambert PF (2007) Human papillomavirus 16 E5 oncogene contributes to two stages of skin carcinogenesis. *Cancer Res* **67**: 6106–6112.

McCance DJ, Kopan R, Fuchs E, Laimins LA (1988) Human papillomavirus type 16 alters human epithelial cell differentiation *in vitro*. *Proc Natl Acad Sci USA* **85**: 7169–7173.

McClintock B (1940) The stability of broken ends of chromosomes in *Zea mays*. *Genetics* **26**: 234–282.

McDermott KM, Zhang J, Holst CR, Kozakiewicz BK, Singla V, Tlsty TD (2006) p16(INK4a) prevents centrosome dysfunction and genomic instability in primary cells. *PLoS Biol* **4**: e51.

McIntyre MC, Frattini MG, Grossman SR, Laimins LA (1993) Human papillomavirus type 18 E7 protein requires intact Cys-X-X-Cys motifs for zinc binding, dimerization, and transformation but not for Rb binding. *J Virol* **67**: 3142–3150.

McLaughlin-Drubin ME, Bromberg-White JL, Meyers C (2005) The role of the human papillomavirus type 18 E7 oncoprotein during the complete viral life cycle. *Virology* **338**: 61–68.

McMillan NA, Payne E, Frazer IH, Evander M (1999) Expression of the alpha6 integrin confers papillomavirus binding upon receptor-negative B-cells. *Virology* **261**: 271–279.

McPhillips MG, Oliveira JG, Spindler JE, Mitra R, McBride AA (2006) Brd4 is required for E2-mediated transcriptional activation but not genome partitioning of all papillomaviruses. *J Virol* **80**: 9530–9543.

Mellin H, Friesland S, Lewensohn R, Dalianis T, Munck-Wikland E (2000) Human papillomavirus (HPV) DNA in tonsillar cancer: clinical correlates, risk of relapse, and survival. *Int J Cancer* **89**: 300–304.

Meraldi P, Lukas J, Fry AM, Bartek J, Nigg EA (1999) Centrosome duplication in mammalian somatic cells requires E2F and Cdk2-cyclin A. *Nat Cell Biol* **1**: 88–93.

Meraldi P, Nigg EA (2002) The centrosome cycle. *FEBS Lett* **521**: 9–13.

Merdes A, Heald R, Samejima K, Earnshaw WC, Cleveland DW (2000) Formation of spindle poles by dynein/dynactin-dependent transport of NuMA. *J Cell Biol* **149**: 851–862.

Merdes A, Ramyar K, Vechio JD, Cleveland DW (1996) A complex of NuMA and cytoplasmic dynein is essential for mitotic spindle assembly. *Cell* **87**: 447–458.

Mietz JA, Unger T, Huibregtse JM, Howley PM (1992) The transcriptional transactivation function of wild-type p53 is inhibited by SV40 large T-antigen and by HPV-16 E6 oncoprotein. *EMBO J* **11**: 5013–5020.

Missero C, Di Cunto F, Kiyokawa H, Koff A, Dotto GP (1996) The absence of p21Cip1/WAF1 alters keratinocyte growth and differentiation and promotes ras-tumor progression. *Genes Dev* **10**: 3065–3075.

Mohr IJ, Clark R, Sun S, Androphy EJ, MacPherson P, Botchan MR (1990) Targeting the E1 replication protein to the papillomavirus origin of replication by complex formation with the E2 transactivator. *Science* **250**: 1694–1699.

Moscicki AB, Shiboski S, Hills NK, Powell KJ, Jay N, Hanson EN, Miller S, Canjura-Clayton KL, Farhat S, Broering JM, Darragh TM (2004) Regression of low-grade squamous intra-epithelial lesions in young women. *Lancet* **364**: 1678–1683.

Münger K (2002) The role of human papillomaviruses in human cancers. *Front Biosci* 7: d641–649.

Münger K, Baldwin A, Edwards KM, Hayakawa H, Nguyen CL, Owens M, Grace M, Huh K (2004) Mechanisms of human papillomavirus-induced oncogenesis. *J Virol* **78**: 11451–11460.

Münger K, Hayakawa H, Nguyen CL, Melquiot NV, Duensing A, Duensing S (2006) Viral carcinogenesis and genomic instability. *Exs* (96): 179–199.

Münger K, Howley PM (2002) Human papillomavirus immortalization and transformation functions. *Virus Res* **89**: 213–228.

Münger K, Howley PM, DiMaio D (2007) Human papillomavirus E6 and E7 oncogenes. In: Garcea R, DiMaio D (eds.), *The Papillomaviruses.* New York: Springer Verlag.

Münger K, Phelps WC, Bubb V, Howley PM, Schlegel R (1989a) The E6 and E7 genes of the human papillomavirus type 16 together are necessary and sufficient for transformation of primary human keratinocytes. *J Virol* **63**: 4417–4421.

Münger K, Werness BA, Dyson N, Phelps WC, Harlow E, Howley PM (1989b) Complex formation of human papillomavirus E7 proteins with the retinoblastoma tumor suppressor gene product. *Embo J* **8**: 4099–4105.

Munoz N, Bosch FX, de Sanjose S, Shah KV (1994) The role of HPV in the etiology of cervical cancer. *Mutat Res* **305**: 293–301.

Myers ER, McCrory DC, Nanda K, Bastian L, Matchar DB (2000). Mathematical model for the natural history of human papillomavirus infection and cervical carcinogenesis. *Am J Epidemiol* **151**: 1158–1171.

Nakagawa S, Huibregtse JM (2000) Human scribble (Vartul) is targeted for ubiquitin-mediated degradation by the high-risk papillomavirus E6 proteins and the E6AP ubiquitin-protein ligase. *Mol Cell Biol* **20**: 8244–8253.

Nguyen ML, Nguyen MM, Lee D, Griep AE, Lambert PF (2003) The PDZ ligand domain of the human papillomavirus type 16 E6 protein is required for E6's induction of epithelial hyperplasia *in vivo*. *J Virol* 77: 6957–6964.

Niu MY, Mills JC, Nachmias VT (1997) Development of polarity in human erythroleukemia cells: roles of membrane ruffling and the centrosome. *Cell Motil Cytoskeleton* **36**: 203–215.

Nonogaki S, Wakamatsu A, Longatto Filho A, Pereira SM, Utagawa ML, Ferreira Alves VA, Di Loreto C, Sakamoto Maeda MY, Lima TP, Roteli-Martins C, Syrjanen K (2004) Hybrid capture II and polymerase chain reaction for identifying HPV infections in samples collected in a new collection medium: a comparison. *Acta Cytol* **48**: 514–520.

Nowak MA, Komarova NL, Sengupta A, Jallepalli PV, Shih Ie M, Vogelstein B, Lengauer C (2002) The role of chromosomal instability in tumor initiation. *Proc Natl Acad Sci USA* **99**: 16226–16231.

O'Driscoll M, Ruiz-Perez VL, Woods CG, Jeggo PA, Goodship JA (2003) A splicing mutation affecting expression of ataxia-telangiectasia and Rad3-related protein (ATR) results in Seckel syndrome. *Nat Genet* **33**: 497–501.

Oh ST, Longworth MS, Laimins LA (2004) Roles of the E6 and E7 proteins in the life cycle of low-risk human papillomavirus type 11. *J Virol* **78**: 2620–2626.

Ohshima K, Haraoka S, Yoshioka S, Hamasaki M, Fujiki T, Suzumiya J, Kawasaki C, Kanda M, Kikuchi M (2000). Mutation analysis of mitotic checkpoint genes (hBUB1 and hBUBR1) and microsatellite instability in adult T-cell leukemia/lymphoma. *Cancer Lett* **158**: 141–150.

Ostor AG (1993) Natural history of cervical intraepithelial neoplasia: a critical review. *Int J Gynecol Pathol* **12**: 186–192.

Ozbun MA, Meyers C (1998) Human papillomavirus type 31b E1 and E2 transcript expression correlates with vegetative viral genome amplification. *Virology* **248**: 218–230.

Paintrand M, Moudjou M, Delacroix H, Bornens M (1992) Centrosome organization and centriole architecture: their sensitivity to divalent cations. *J Struct Biol* **108**: 107–128.

Parish JL, Bean AM, Park RB, Androphy EJ (2006) ChlR1 is required for loading papillomavirus E2 onto mitotic chromosomes and viral genome maintenance. *Mol Cell* **24**: 867–876.

Park RB, Androphy EJ (2002) Genetic analysis of high-risk e6 in episomal maintenance of human papillomavirus genomes in primary human keratinocytes. *J Virol* **76**: 11359–11364.

Parkin DM, Bray F (2006) Chapter 2: The burden of HPV-related cancers. *Vaccine* **24**(3): S11–S25.

Passmore JA, Morroni C, Shapiro S, Williamson AL, Hoffman M (2007) Papanicolaou smears and cervical inflammatory cytokine responses. *J Inflamm* (London) **4**: 8.

Patel D, Huang SM, Baglia LA, McCance DJ (1999) The E6 protein of human papillomavirus type 16 binds to and inhibits co-activation by CBP and p300. *Embo J* **18**: 5061–5072.

Patel D, Incassati A, Wang N, McCance DJ (2004) Human papillomavirus type 16 E6 and E7 cause polyploidy in human keratinocytes and up-regulation of G2-M-phase proteins. *Cancer Res* **64**: 1299–1306.

Pei XF, Meck JM, Greenhalgh D, Schlegel R (1993) Cotransfection of HPV-18 and v-fos DNA induces tumorigenicity of primary human keratinocytes. *Virology* **196**: 855–860.

Petti L, DiMaio D (1994) Specific interaction between the bovine papillomavirus E5 transforming protein and the beta receptor for platelet-derived growth factor in stably transformed and acutely transfected cells. *J Virol* **68**: 3582–3592.

Petti L, Nilson LA, DiMaio D (1991) Activation of the platelet-derived growth factor receptor by the bovine papillomavirus E5 transforming protein. *Embo J* **10**: 845–855.

Pfister H, Fuchs PG (1994) Anatomy, taxonomy and evolution of papillomaviruses. *Intervirology* **37**: 143–149.

Pfister H, Ter Schegget J (1997) Role of HPV in cutaneous premalignant and malignant tumors. *Clin Dermatol* **15**: 335–347.

Phelps WC, Barnes JA, Lobe DC (1998) Molecular targets for human papillomaviruses: prospects for antiviral therapy. *Antivir Chem Chemother* **9**: 359–377.

Phelps WC, Münger K, Yee CL, Barnes JA, Howley PM (1992) Structure-function analysis of the human papillomavirus E7 oncoprotein. *J Virol* **66**: 2418–2427.

Piel M, Nordberg J, Euteneuer U, Bornens M (2001) Centrosome-dependent exit of cytokinesis in animal cells. *Science* **291**: 1550–1553.

Pihan GA, Wallace J, Zhou Y, Doxsey SJ (2003) Centrosome abnormalities and chromosome instability occur together in pre-invasive carcinomas. *Cancer Res* **63**: 1398–1404.

Piirsoo M, Ustav E, Mandel T, Stenlund A, Ustav M (1996) *Cis* and *trans* requirements for stable episomal maintenance of the BPV-1 replicator. *Embo J* **15**: 1–11.

Pim D, Collins M, Banks L (1992) Human papillomavirus type 16 E5 gene stimulates the transforming activity of the epidermal growth factor receptor. *Oncogene* 7: 27–32.

Pim D, Massimi P, Banks L (1997) Alternatively spliced HPV-18 E6* protein inhibits E6 mediated degradation of p53 and suppresses transformed cell growth. *Oncogene* **15**: 257–264.

Pim D, Storey A, Thomas M, Massimi P, Banks L (1994) Mutational analysis of HPV-18 E6 identifies domains required for p53 degradation *in vitro*, abolition of p53 transactivation *in vivo* and immortalisation of primary BMK cells. *Oncogene* **9**: 1869–1876.

Rabson MS, Yee C, Yang YC, Howley PM (1986) Bovine papillomavirus type 1 3′ early region transformation and plasmid maintenance functions. *J Virol* **60**: 626–634.

Rajagopalan H, Lengauer C (2004) Aneuploidy and cancer. *Nature* **432**: 338–341.

Ramoz N, Rueda LA, Bouadjar B, Montoya LS, Orth G, Favre M (2002) Mutations in two adjacent novel genes are associated with epidermodysplasia verruciformis. *Nat Genet* **32**: 579–581.

Rhea WG, Jr, Bourgeois BM, Sewell DR (1998) Condyloma acuminata: a fatal disease? *Am Surg* **64**: 1082–1087.

Richards S, Hillman T, Stern M (1996) Mutations in the *Drosophila* pushover gene confer increased neuronal excitability and spontaneous synaptic vesicle fusion. *Genetics* **142**: 1215–1223.

Richart RM, Barron BA (1969) A follow-up study of patients with cervical dysplasia. *Am J Obstet Gynecol* **105**: 386–393.

Rihet S, Lorenzato M, Clavel C (1996) Oncogenic human papillomaviruses and ploidy in cervical lesions. *J Clin Pathol* **49**: 892–896.

Riley RR, Duensing, S, Brake T, Münger K, Lambert PF, Arbeit JM (2003) Dissection of human papillomavirus E6 and E7 function in transgenic mouse models of cervical carcinogenesis. *Cancer Res* **63**: 4862–4871.

Ring D, Hubble R, Kirschner M (1982) Mitosis in a cell with multiple centrioles. *J Cell Biol* **94**: 549–556.

Roberts JN, Buck CB, Thompson CD, Kines R, Bernardo M, Choyke PL, Lowy DR, Schiller JT (2007) Genital transmission of HPV in a mouse model is potentiated by nonoxynol-9 and inhibited by carrageenan. *Nat Med* **13**: 857–861.

Roberts S, Ashmole I, Johnson GD, Kreider JW, Gallimore PH (1993) Cutaneous and mucosal human papillomavirus E4 proteins form intermediate filament-like structures in epithelial cells. *Virology* **197**: 176–187.

Rodriguez MI, Finbow ME, Alonso A (2000) Binding of human papillomavirus 16 E5 to the 16 kDa subunit c (proteolipid) of the vacuolar H(+)-ATPase can be dissociated from the E5-mediated epidermal growth factor receptor overactivation. *Oncogene* **19**: 3727–3732.

Ronco LV, Karpova AY, Vidal M, Howley PM (1998) Human papillomavirus 16 E6 oncoprotein binds to interferon regulatory factor-3 and inhibits its transcriptional activity. *Genes Dev* **12**: 2061–2072.

Rosenthal DL (2004) Cervical disease screening and detection: emerging techniques in molecular diagnostic assays. *Med Lab Obs* **36**: 10–11, 14–16; quiz 18–19.

Rösl F, Dürst M, zur Hausen H (1988) Selective suppression of human papillomavirus transcription in non-tumorigenic cells by 5-azacytidine. *EMBO J* **7**: 1321–1327.

Ru HY, Chen RL, Lu WC, Chen JH (2002) hBUB1 defects in leukemia and lymphoma cells. *Oncogene* **21**: 4673–4679.

Sailaja G, Watts RM, Bernard HU (1999) Many different papillomaviruses have low transcriptional activity in spite of strong epithelial specific enhancers. *J Gen Virol* **80**: 1715–1724.

Sakaguchi T, Watanabe A, Sawada H, Yamada Y, Yamashita J, Matsuda M, Nakajima M, Miwa T, Hirao T, Nakano H (1998) Prognostic value of cyclin E and p53 expression in gastric carcinoma. *Cancer* **82**: 1238–1243.

Sang BC, Barbosa MS (1992) Single amino acid substitutions in "low-risk" human papillomavirus (HPV) type 6 E7 protein enhance features characteristic of the "high risk" HPV E7 oncoproteins. *Proc Natl Acad Sci USA* **89**: 8063–8067.

Saslow D, Castle PE, Cox JT, Davey DD, Einstein MH, Ferris DG, Goldie SJ, Harper DM, Kinney W, Moscicki AB, *et al.* (2007). American Cancer Society guideline for human papillomavirus (HPV) vaccine use to prevent cervical cancer and its precursors. *CA Cancer J Clin* **57**: 7–28.

Schaeffer AJ, Nguyen M, Liem A, Lee D, Montagna C, Lambert PF, Ried T, Difilippantonio MJ (2004) E6 and E7 oncoproteins induce distinct patterns of chromosomal aneuploidy in skin tumors from transgenic mice. *Cancer Res* **64**: 538–546.

Schapiro F, Sparkowski J, Adduci A, Suprynowicz F, Schlegel R, Grinstein S (2000) Golgi alkalinization by the papillomavirus E5 oncoprotein. *J Cell Biol* **148**: 305–315.

Scheffner M, Huibregtse JM, Howley PM (1994) Identification of a human ubiquitin-conjugating enzyme that mediates the E6-AP-dependent ubiquitination of p53. *Proc Natl Acad Sci USA* **91**: 8797–8801.

Scheffner M, Münger K, Byrne JC, Howley PM (1991) The state of the p53 and retinoblastoma genes in human cervical carcinoma cell lines. *Proc Natl Acad Sci USA* **88**: 5523–5527.

Scheffner M, Werness BA, Huibregtse JM, Levine AJ, Howley PM (1990) The E6 oncoprotein encoded by human papillomavirus types 16 and 18 promotes the degradation of p53. *Cell* **63**: 1129–1136.

Scheurer ME, Tortolero-Luna G, Adler-Storthz K (2005) Human papillomavirus infection: biology, epidemiology, and prevention. *Int J Gynecol Cancer* **15**: 727–746.

Schiller JT, Vass WC, Vousden KH, Lowy DR (1986) E5 open reading frame of bovine papillomavirus type 1 encodes a transforming gene. *J Virol* **57**: 1–6.

Schwartz KL, Crossley-May H, Vigneau FD, Brown K, Banerjee M (2003) Race, socioeconomic status and stage at diagnosis for five common malignancies. *Cancer Causes Control* **14**: 761–766.

Schwartz SM, Daling JR, Doody DR, Wipf GC, Carter JJ, Madeleine MM, Mao EJ, Fitzgibbons ED, Huang S, Beckmann AM, *et al.* (1998) Oral cancer risk in relation to sexual history and evidence of human papillomavirus infection. *J Natl Cancer Inst* **90**: 1626–1636.

Schweiger MR, You J, Howley PM (2006) Bromodomain protein 4 mediates the papillomavirus E2 transcriptional activation function. *J Virol* **80**: 4276–4285.

Seedorf K, Krammer G, Durst M, Suhai S, Rowekamp WG (1985) Human papillomavirus type 16 DNA sequence. *Virology* **145**: 181–185.

Sekaric P, Cherry JJ, Androphy EJ (2008) Binding of human papillomavirus type 16 E6 to E6AP is not required for activation of hTERT. *J Virol* **82**: 71–76.

Sekelsky JJ, McKim KS, Messina L, French RL, Hurley WD, Arbel T, Chin GM, Deneen B, Force SJ, Hari KL, *et al.* (1999) Identification of novel *Drosophila* meiotic genes recovered in a P-element screen. *Genetics* **152**: 529–542.

Selvaggi SM (2001) Implications of low diagnostic reproducibility of cervical cytologic and histologic diagnoses. *JAMA* **285**: 1506–1508.

Sen E, Bromberg-White JL, Meyers C (2002) Genetic analysis of *cis* regulatory elements within the 5′ region of the human papillomavirus type 31 upstream regulatory region during different stages of the viral life cycle. *J Virol* **76**: 4798–4809.

Shah KV, Kessis TD, Shah F, Gupta JW, Shibata D, Jones RW (1996) Human papillomavirus investigation of patients with cervical intraepithelial neoplasia 3, some of whom progressed to invasive cancer. *Int J Gynecol Pathol* **15**: 127–130.

Sharp DJ, Rogers GC, Scholey JM (2000) Microtubule motors in mitosis. *Nature* **407**: 41–47.

Sharp GA, Weber K, Osborn M (1982) Centriole number and process formation in established neuroblastoma cells and primary dorsal root ganglion neurones. *Eur J Cell Biol* **29**: 97–103.

Sherr CJ (1994) G1 phase progression: cycling on cue. *Cell* **79**: 551–555.

Shih IM, Zhou W, Goodman SN, Lengauer C, Kinzler KW, Vogelstein B (2001) Evidence that genetic instability occurs at an early stage of colorectal tumorigenesis. *Cancer Res* **61**: 818–822.

Shin KH, Ahn JH, Kang MK, Lim PK, Yip FK, Baluda MA, Park NH (2006) HPV-16 E6 oncoprotein impairs the fidelity of DNA end-joining via p53-dependent and -independent pathways. *Int J Oncol* **28**: 209–215.

Shinmura K, Bennett RA, Tarapore P, Fukasawa K (2007) Direct evidence for the role of centrosomally localized p53 in the regulation of centrosome duplication. *Oncogene* **26**: 2939–2944.

Shope RE, Hurst EW (1933) Infectious papillomatosis of rabbits; with a note on the histopathology. *J Exp Med* **58**: 607–624.

Sibbet G, Romero-Graillet C, Meneguzzi G, Saveria Campo M (2000) alpha6 integrin is not the obligatory cell receptor for bovine papillomavirus type 4. *J Gen Virol* **81**(Pt 6): 1629.

Skyldberg B, Fujioka K, Hellstrom AC, Sylven L, Moberger B, Auer G (2001) Human papillomavirus infection, centrosome aberration, and genetic stability in cervical lesions. *Mod Pathol* **14**: 279–284.

Slebos RJ, Lee MH, Plunkett BS, Kessis TD, Williams BO, Jacks T, Hedrick L, Kastan MB, Cho KR (1994) p53-dependent G1 arrest involves pRB-related proteins and is disrupted by the human papillomavirus 16 E7 oncoprotein. *Proc Natl Acad Sci USA* **91**: 5320–5324.

Slee EA, O'Connor DJ, Lu X (2004) To die or not to die: how does p53 decide? *Oncogene* **23**: 2809–2818.

Smedts F, Ramaekers F, Troyanovsky S, Pruszczynski M, Robben H, Lane B, Leigh I, Plantema F, Vooijs P (1992) Basal-cell keratins in cervical reserve cells and a comparison to their expression in cervical intraepithelial neoplasia. *Am J Pathol* **140**: 601–612.

Snijders PJF, Scholes AGM, Hart CA, Jones AS, Vaughan ED, Woolgar JA, Mejer C, Walboomers JMM, Field JK (1996) Prevalence of mucosotropic human papillomaviruses in squamous-cell carcinomas of the head and neck. *Int J Cancer* **66**: 464–469.

Soeda E, Ferran MC, Baker CC, McBride AA (2006) Repression of HPV16 early region transcription by the E2 protein. *Virology* **351**: 29–41.

Solinas-Toldo S, Durst M, Lichter P (1997) Specific chromosomal imbalances in human papillomavirus-transfected cells during progression toward immortality. *Proc Natl Acad Sci USA* **94**: 3854–3859.

Solomon D, Breen N, McNeel T (2007) Cervical cancer screening rates in the United States and the potential impact of implementation of screening guidelines. *CA Cancer J Clin* **57**: 105–111.

Solomon D, Davey D, Kurman R, Moriarty A, O'Connor D, Prey M, Raab S, Sherman M, Wilbur D, Wright T Jr, Young N (2002) The 2001 Bethesda System: terminology for reporting results of cervical cytology. *JAMA* **287**: 2114–2119.

Sotlar K, Diemer D, Dethleffs A, Hack Y, Stubner A, Vollmer N, Menton S, Menton M, Dietz K, Wallwiener D, *et al.* (2004) Detection and typing of human papillomavirus by e6 nested multiplex PCR. *J Clin Microbiol* **42**: 3176–3184.

Southern SA, Evans MF, Herrington CS (1997) Basal cell tetrasomy in low-grade cervical squamous intraepithelial lesions infected with high-risk human papillomaviruses. *Cancer Res* **57**: 4210–4213.

Southern SA, Lewis MH, Herrington CS (2004) Induction of tetrasomy by human papillomavirus type 16 E7 protein is independent of pRb binding and disruption of differentiation. *Br J Cancer* **90**: 1949–1954.

Spardy N, Duensing A, Charles D, Haines N, Nakahara T, Lambert PF, Duensing S (2007) The human papillomavirus type 16 E7 oncoprotein activates the Fanconi anemia (FA) pathway and causes accelerated chromosomal instability in FA cells. *J Virol* **81**: 13265–13270.

Stanbridge EJ, Flandermeyer RR, Daniels DW, Nelson-Rees WA (1981) Specific chromosome loss associated with the expression of tumorigenicity in human cell hybrids. *Somatic Cell Genet* 7: 699–712.

Steffen W, Fuge H, Dietz R, Bastmeyer M, Muller G (1986) Aster-free spindle poles in insect spermatocytes: evidence for chromosome-induced spindle formation? *J Cell Biol* **102**: 1679–1687.

Steger G, Corbach S (1997) Dose-dependent regulation of the early promoter of human papillomavirus type 18 by the viral E2 protein. *J Virol* **71**: 50–58.

Steinbeck RG (1997) Proliferation and DNA aneuploidy in mild dysplasia imply early steps of cervical carcinogenesis. *Acta Oncol* **36**: 3–12.

Steinmann KE, Pei XF, Stoppler H, Schlegel R, Schlegel R (1994) Elevated expression and activity of mitotic regulatory proteins in human papillomavirus immortalized keratinocytes. *Oncogene* **9**: 387–394.

Stevaux O, Dyson NJ (2002) A revised picture of the E2F transcriptional network and RB function. *Curr Opin Cell Biol* **14**: 684–691.

Storchova Z, Pellman D (2004) From polyploidy to aneuploidy, genome instability and cancer. *Nat Rev Mol Cell Biol* **5**: 45–54.

Storey A, Greenfield I, Banks L, Pim D, Crook T, Crawford L, Stanley M (1992) Lack of immortalizing activity of a human papillomavirus type 16 variant DNA with a mutation in the E2 gene isolated from normal human cervical keratinocytes. *Oncogene* 7: 459–465.

Straight SW, Hinkle PM, Jewers RJ, Mccance DJ (1993) The E5 oncoprotein of human papillomavirus type-16 transforms fibroblasts and effects the downregulation of the epidermal growth factor receptor in keratinocytes. *J Virol* **67**: 4521–4532.

Streeck RE, Selinka HC, Sapp M (2007) Viral entry and receptors. In: Garcea RL, DiMaio D (eds.), *The Papillomaviruses*, pp. 89–108. New York: Springer.

Sur M, Cooper K (1998) The role of the human papilloma virus in esophageal cancer. *Pathology* **30**: 348–354.

Takahashi K, Tanabe K, Ohnuki M, Narita M, Ichisaka T, Tomoda K, Yamanaka S (2007) Induction of pluripotent stem cells from adult human fibroblasts by defined factors. *Cell* **131**: 861–872.

Tasca RA, Clarke RW (2006) Recurrent respiratory papillomatosis. *Arch Dis Child* **91**: 689–691.

Taylor WR, Stark GR (2001) Regulation of the G2/M transition by p53. *Oncogene* **20**: 1803–1815.
Thierry F, Benotmane MA, Demeret C, Mori M, Teissier S, Desaintes C (2004) A genomic approach reveals a novel mitotic pathway in papillomavirus carcinogenesis. *Cancer Res* **64**: 895–903.
Thomas JT, Hubert WG, Ruesch MN, Laimins LA (1999) Human papillomavirus type 31 oncoproteins E6 and E7 are required for the maintenance of episomes during the viral life cycle in normal human keratinocytes. *Proc Natl Acad Sci USA* **96**: 8449–8454.
Thomas JT, Laimins LA (1998) Human papillomavirus oncoproteins E6 and E7 independently abrogate the mitotic spindle checkpoint. *J Virol* **72**: 1131–1137.
Thompson DA, Belinsky G, Chang TH, Jones DL, Schlegel R, Münger K (1997) The human papillomavirus-16 E6 oncoprotein decreases the vigilance of mitotic checkpoints. *Oncogene* **15**: 3025–3035.
Tong X, Howley PM (1997) The bovine papillomavirus E6 oncoprotein interacts with paxillin and disrupts the actin cytoskeleton. *Proc Nat Acad Sci USA* **94**: 4412–4417.
Tsou MF, Stearns T (2006) Mechanism limiting centrosome duplication to once per cell cycle. *Nature* **442**: 947–951.
Tsutsumi K, Sun Q, Yasumoto S, Kikuchi K, Ohta Y, Pater A, Pater MM (1993) *In vitro* and *in vivo* analysis of cellular origin of cervical squamous metaplasia. *Am J Pathol* **143**: 1150–1158.
Turek LP (1994) The structure, function, and regulation of papillomaviral genes in infection and cervical cancer. *Adv Virus Res* **44**: 305–356.
Uyar DS, Eltabbakh GH, Mount SL (2003) Positive predictive value of liquid-based and conventional cervical Papanicolaou smears reported as malignant. *Gynecol Oncol* **89**: 227–232.
Vafa O, Wade M, Kern S, Beeche M, Pandita TK, Hampton GM, Wahl GM (2002) c-Myc can induce DNA damage, increase reactive oxygen species, and mitigate p53 function: a mechanism for oncogene-induced genetic instability. *Mol Cell* **9**: 1031–1044.
Valle GF, Banks L (1995) The human papillomavirus (HPV)-6 and HPV-16 E5 proteins co-operate with HPV-16 E7 in the transformation of primary rodent cells. *J Gen Virol* **76**: 1239–1245.
Van Ranst M, Kaplan JB, Burk RD (1992) Phylogenetic classification of human papillomaviruses: correlation with clinical manifestations. *J Gen Virol* **73**(Pt 10): 2653–2660.

Van Tine BA, Dao LD, Wu SY, Sonbuchner TM, Lin BY, Zou N, Chiang CM, Broker TR, Chow LT (2004) Human papillomavirus (HPV) origin-binding protein associates with mitotic spindles to enable viral DNA partitioning. *Proc Natl Acad Sci USA* **101**: 4030–4035.

Vande Pol SB, Brown MC, Turner CE (1998) Association of bovine papillomavirus type 1 E6 oncoprotein with the focal adhesion protein paxillin through a conserved protein interaction motif. *Oncogene* **16**: 43–52.

Veldman T, Horikawa I, Barrett JC, Schlegel R (2001) Transcriptional activation of the telomerase hTERT gene by human papillomavirus type 16 E6 oncoprotein. *J Virol* **75**: 4467–4472.

Veldman T, Liu X, Yuan H, Schlegel R (2003) Human papillomavirus E6 and Myc proteins associate *in vivo* and bind to and cooperatively activate the telomerase reverse transcriptase promoter. *Proc Natl Acad Sci USA* **100**: 8211–8216.

Venuti A, Salani D, Poggiali F, Manni V, Bagnato A (1998) The E5 oncoprotein of human papillomavirus type 16 enhances endothelin-1-induced keratinocyte growth. *Virology* **248**: 1–5.

Virtej P, Vasiliu C (2003) Cytodiagnosis in cervical neoplasia: from the Babes/Papanicolaou smear to the actual Bethesda System. *Clin Exp Obstet Gynecol* **30**: 173–177.

Vogel C, Kienitz A, Hofmann I, Muller R, Bastians H (2004) Crosstalk of the mitotic spindle assembly checkpoint with p53 to prevent polyploidy. *Oncogene* **23**: 6845–6853.

Vousden KH, Lu X (2002) Live or let die: the cell's response to p53. *Nat Rev Cancer* **2**: 594–604.

Vousden KH, Vojtesek B, Fisher C, Lane D (1993) HPV-16 E7 or adenovirus E1A can overcome the growth arrest of cells immortalized with a temperature-sensitive p53. *Oncogene* **8**: 1697–1702.

Walboomers JM, Jacobs MV, Manos MM, Bosch FX, Kummer JA, Shah KV, Snijders PJ, Peto J, Meijer CJ, Munoz N (1999) Human papillomavirus is a necessary cause of invasive cervical cancer worldwide [see comments]. *J Pathol* **189**: 12–19.

Weinstock H, Berman S, Cates W Jr (2004) Sexually transmitted diseases among American youth: incidence and prevalence estimates, 2000. *Perspect Sex Reprod Health* **36**: 6–10.

Werness BA, Levine AJ, Howley PM (1990) Association of human papillomavirus types 16 and 18 E6 proteins with p53. *Science* **248**: 76–79.

White AE, Livanos EM, Tlsty TD (1994) Differential disruption of genomic integrity and cell cycle regulation in normal human fibroblasts by the HPV oncoproteins. *Genes Dev* **8**: 666–677.

Whyte P, Buchkovich KJ, Horowitz JM, Friend SH, Raybuck M, Weinberg RA, Harlow E (1988) Association between an oncogene and an antioncogene: the adenovirus E1a proteins bind to the retinoblastoma gene product. *Nature* **334**: 124–129.

Winer RL, Hughes JP, Feng Q, O'Reilly S, Kiviat NB, Holmes KK, Koutsky LA (2006) Condom use and the risk of genital human papillomavirus infection in young women. *N Engl J Med* **354**: 2645–2654.

Winkler B, Crum CP, Fujii T, Ferenczy A, Boon M, Braun L, Lancaster WD, Richart RM (1984) Koilocytotic lesions of the cervix. The relationship of mitotic abnormalities to the presence of papillomavirus antigens and nuclear DNA content. *Cancer* **53**: 1081–1087.

Wojcik E, Basto R, Serr M, Scaerou F, Karess R, Hays T (2001) Kinetochore dynein: its dynamics and role in the transport of the Rough deal checkpoint protein. *Nat Cell Biol* **3**: 1001–1007.

World Health Organization (2005) Viral cancers. In: *State of the Art of Vaccine Research and Development: Initiative for Vaccine Research*, pp. 92–99 Geneva, Switzerland: World Health Organization.

Wright TC Jr, Cox JT, Massad LS, Twiggs LB, Wilkinson EJ (2002a) 2001 consensus guidelines for the management of women with cervical cytological abnormalities. *J Low Genit Tract Dis* **6**: 127–143.

Wright TC Jr, Kurman R, Ferenczy A (2002b) Precancerous lesions of the cervix. In: Blaustein A, Kurman RJ (eds.), *Blaustein's Pathology of the Female Genital Tract* (5th edn.), pp. 253–324. New York: Springer.

Wu EW, Clemens KE, Heck DV, Münger K (1993) The human papillomavirus E7 oncoprotein and the cellular transcription factor E2F bind to separate sites on the retinoblastoma tumor suppressor protein. *J Virol* **67**: 2402–2407.

Wyman C, Kanaar R (2006) DNA double-strand break repair: all's well that ends well. *Annu Rev Genet* **40**: 363–383.

Xu XZ, Wes PD, Chen H, Li HS, Yu M, Morgan S, Liu Y, Montell C (1998) Retinal targets for calmodulin include proteins implicated in synaptic transmission. *J Biol Chem* **273**: 31297–31307.

Xu Y, Baltimore D (1996) Dual roles of ATM in the cellular response to radiation and in cell growth control. *Genes Dev* **10**: 2401–2410.

Yang YC, Spalholz BA, Rabson MS, Howley PM (1985) Dissociation of transforming and *trans*-activation functions for bovine papillomavirus type 1. *Nature* **318**: 575–577.

Yew PR, Berk AJ (1992) Inhibition of p53 transactivation required for transformation by adenovirus early 1B protein. *Nature* **357**: 82–85.

You J, Croyle JL, Nishimura A, Ozato K, Howley PM (2004) Interaction of the bovine papillomavirus E2 protein with Brd4 tethers the viral DNA to host mitotic chromosomes. *Cell* **117**: 349–360.

Yu H (2002) Regulation of APC-Cdc20 by the spindle checkpoint. *Curr Opin Cell Biol* **14**: 706–714.

Yu J, Vodyanik MA, Smuga-Otto K, Antosiewicz-Bourget J, Frane JL, Tian S, Nie J, Jonsdottir GA, Ruotti V, Stewart R *et al.* (2007) Induced pluripotent stem cell lines derived from human somatic cells. *Science* **318**: 1917–1920.

Zerfass-Thome K, Zwerschke W, Mannhardt B, Tindle R, Botz JW, Jansen-Durr P (1996) Inactivation of the cdk inhibitor p27KIP1 by the human papillomavirus type 16 E7 oncoprotein. *Oncogene* **13**: 2323–2330.

Zhou J, Gissmann L, Zentgraf H, Muller H, Picken M, Muller M (1995) Early phase in the infection of cultured cells with papillomavirus virions. *Virology* **214**: 167–176.

Zhou J, Stenzel DJ, Sun XY, Frazer IH (1993) Synthesis and assembly of infectious bovine papillomavirus particles *in vitro*. *J Gen Virol* **74**: 763–768.

Zhu C, Zhao J, Bibikova M, Leverson JD, Bossy-Wetzel E, Fan JB, Abraham RT, Jiang W (2005) Functional analysis of human microtubule-based motor proteins, the kinesins and dyneins, in mitosis/cytokinesis using RNA interference. *Mol Biol Cell* **16**: 3187–3199.

Zimmerman W, Sparks CA, Doxsey SJ (1999) Amorphous no longer: the centrosome comes into focus. *Curr Opin Cell Biol* **11**: 122–128.

Zimmermann H, Degenkolbe R, Bernard HU, O'Connor, MJ (1999) The human papillomavirus type 16 E6 oncoprotein can down-regulate p53 activity by targeting the transcriptional coactivator CBP/p300. *J Virol* **73**: 6209–6219.

Chapter 5

Epstein-Barr Virus and Its Oncogenesis

Hsin-Pai Li[†], Mei Chao[†], Shu-Jen Chen[‡] and Yu-Sun Chang[*,†,§]

Abstract: Epstein-Barr virus (EBV), a γ-herpesvirus, has been studied for over 40 years, since its first discovery which dates back to 1964. Although more than 90% of the human population have been infected with EBV at early childhood, the majority remain asymptomatic. EBV has been proven to be the etiological agent associated with various human cancers, such as Burkitt's lymphoma (BL), Hodgkin's disease (HD), T-cell lymphoma, nasopharyngeal carcinoma (NPC), and a subset of gastric carcinoma. In this chapter, we specifically discuss the oncogenic properties of EBV latent genes, small RNAs, and microRNAs (miRNAs) that are expressed in EBV-associated cancers.

1. Introduction

Epstein-Barr virus (EBV) was first discovered in Burkitt's lymphoma (BL)-derived cell lines by M.-A. Epstein and Y.-M. Barr (Epstein *et al.*, 1964; Epstein & Barr, 1964). The viruses present in BL cell lines, which are biologically and antigenically distinct from other

*Corresponding author.
[†]Department of Microbiology and Immunology, Chang Gung University, Taoyuan, Taiwan.
[‡]Chang Gung Molecular Medicine Research Center, Chang Gung University, Taoyuan, Taiwan.
[§]Chang Gung Molecular Medicine Research Center and Institute of Biomedical Sciences, Chang Gung University, Taoyuan, Taiwan.
Email: ysc@mail.cgu.edu.tw

members of the herpesvirus family (Epstein *et al.*, 1965; Henle & Henle, 1966), were designated EBV or human herpesvirus 4 (HHV4), as they represented the fourth human herpesvirus discovered. EBV was the first virus to be recognized as a human tumor virus candidate; it now forms the oncogenic γ-herpesvirus subfamily together with human herpesvirus 8 (HHV8), which is also called Kaposi's sarcoma-associated herpesvirus (KSHV). Similar to other herpesviruses, EBV has a DNA-wrapped, toroid-shaped protein core, a nucleocapsid comprising 162 capsomeres, a protein tegument between the nucleocapsid and the envelope, and an outer envelope with external glycoprotein spikes (Dolyniuk *et al.*, 1976a,b).

The EBV genome contains a linear double-stranded DNA molecule that is ~172 kb in length and potentially encodes ~100 genes (Kieff & Rickinson, 2007). The *Bam*HI restriction enzyme map of the EBV genome and the location of known genes expressed in malignant tumors are shown in Fig. 1A. The DNA genome of EBV is

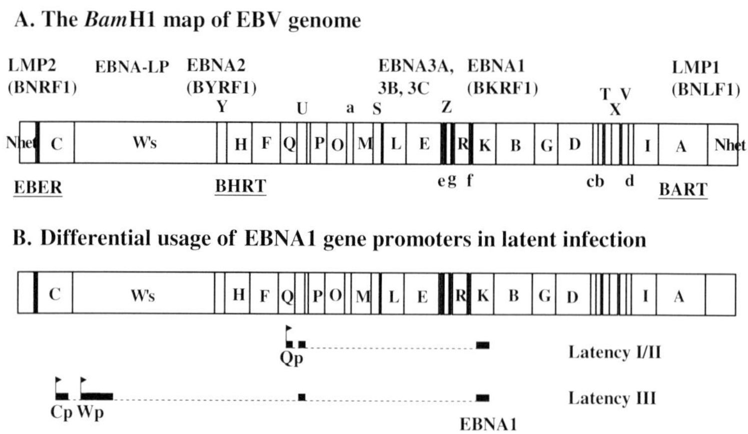

Fig. 1. Schematic diagram of EBV genome. (A) EBV *Bam*HI genomic map. Restriction enzyme digested fragments A–Z, named according to the fragment size in decreasing order, are indicated. The upper panel indicates the relative positions of latent genes that are discussed in this chapter and the lower panel indicates the viral non-coding RNAs, EBERs and miRNA clusters (BHRF and BART). (B) Schematic diagram of differential usage of EBNA1 promoter in latent infection. Qp is used in LatI/II while Cp and Wp are used in LatIII to express EBNA1.

separated into short and long unique sections by a variable number of internal repeats (IRs), and is flanked at both ends by multiple tandem repeats (TRs) (Given & Kieff, 1979; Hayward & Kieff, 1977). EBV infection has both latent and lytic stages. During latent infection, viral gene expression is restricted and no new virions are produced. In contrast, during the lytic cycle, most of the viral genes are expressed and mature virions are produced, which often lead to cell lysis or cell death. Therefore, it is conceivable that latent infection has a greater impact on the cause or pathogenesis of EBV-related cancers than that of the lytic infection. EBV preferentially infects both lymphocytes and epithelial cells. Human peripheral B cells are susceptible to latent EBV infection, which results in transformation of B cells to lymphoblastoid cell lines (LCLs). In B cells, the EBV genome is circularized and maintained in the nuclei of infected cells in an episomal form. Human epithelial cells, in contrast, are fully permissive for lytic EBV infection *in vivo* (Niedobitek *et al.*, 1991), although this infection is inefficient *in vitro*.

EBV is the causative agent of infectious mononucleosis, an acute self-limited disease, and more importantly, it is closely associated with human malignancies, including BL (Neri *et al.*, 1991), Hodgkin's disease (HD) (Ambinder *et al.*, 1993; Peh *et al.*, 1997), T-cell lymphoma (Jones *et al.*, 1988), nasopharyngeal carcinoma (NPC) (Klein, 1976; Brooks *et al.*, 1992; Chen *et al.*, 1992), a subset of gastric carcinoma (Shibata & Weiss, 1992) and lung carcinoma with lymphoepithelioma-like histology (Gal *et al.*, 1991). In these EBV-infected cancers, EBV is predominantly present in its latent forms (Table 1). Therefore, it is important to understand how EBV induces the proliferation of infected cells and contributes to the formation of these tumors. Three major forms of EBV latent gene expression have been described and designated as latency I, II, and III (Kerr *et al.*, 1992; Rowe *et al.*, 1992). Latency III is represented by latently infected LCLs expressing six nuclear antigens (EBNA1, EBNA2, EBNA3A, -3B, -3C, and leader protein), three latent membrane proteins (LMP1, -2A, and -2B), and two highly abundant EBV-encoded small RNAs (EBER1 and EBER2). Latency I is represented by BL cells expressing only EBNA1 and small RNAs (Rowe *et al.*, 1987).

Table 1. EBV-encoded Genes in EBV Associated Malignancies

		EBV Gene Expression[a]					
	Latency	EBNA1	EBNA2, 3A, 3B, 3C, LP	LMP1	LMP2	EBERs	miRNAs
Burkitt's lymphoma	I	+	–	–	–	+	?
Nasopharyngeal carcinoma	I/II	+	–	+	+	+	+[b]
Gastric carcinoma	II	+	–	–	+	+	+
T/NK cell lymphoma	I/II	+	–	+	+	+	?
Hodgkin's lymphoma	II	+	–	+	+	+	?
Post-transplant lymphoma	III	+	+	+	+	+	?
AIDS-associated lymphoma	III	+	+	+	+	+	?

[a]EBV gene expression is identified by gene-specific antibodies and gene transcripts. "+" reported in majority of tumor cells; "–" not reported in most tumor cells; and "?"not been reported.
[b]Unpublished data.

Finally, latency II is represented by NPC and T-cell lymphoma cells expressing EBNA1, LMP1, LMP2A, LMP2B, and the two EBERs (Brooks *et al.*, 1992). Recently, there have been several comprehensive EBV review articles that discussed EBV-associated diseases in detail (Young & Rickinson, 2004; Kieff & Rickinson, 2007; Klein *et al.*, 2007; Rezk & Weiss, 2007). This chapter deals with the oncogenic aspects of EBV by focusing on the functional role of viral latent genes: *EBNA1*, *EBNA2*, *EBNA3s*, *LMP1*, *LMP2*, and viral small RNAs: EBERs and EBV microRNAs (miRNAs) predominantly expressed in EBV-associated cancers.

2. EBNA1

Among the EBV latent proteins, EBNA1 is the only viral protein expressed in all EBV-associated tumors. Its expression is indispensable due to its role in the maintenance and replication of the episomal EBV genome through its DNA-binding activity to the origin of latent replication, *oriP* (Yates *et al.*, 1985; Reisman *et al.*, 1985; Harrison *et al.*, 1994). EBNA1 binds directly to two regions within *oriP*: the family of repeats (FR), as transcription enhancer, and the dyad-symmetry (DS), as initiation site for latent EBV DNA. EBNA1 also associates with the host cell chromosome, which ensures proper partition and retention of EBV genome during mitosis (Marechal *et al.*, 1999). EBNA1 can function both as a transcription activator by activating the expression of other EBV latency genes (Reisman & Sugden, 1986) and a negative regulator by repressing its own transcription (Sample *et al.*, 1992). A more direct involvement of EBNA1 in the oncogenesis of EBV-associated tumors has been demonstrated by introducing EBNA1 antisense DNA oligomer that inhibited proliferation of EBV-immortalized cells and generating EBNA1 transgenic mice that induced lymphoma (Wilson *et al.*, 1996). However, another research group reported their EBNA1 transgenic mice did not suffer from lymphoma (Kang *et al.*, 2005). Therefore, it is still controversial whether the oncogenic potential of EBNA1 can be modeled in transgenic mice. Nevertheless, investigations of EBNA1-interacting cellular proteins and the transcriptional profiling analysis of EBNA1-expressing cells have supported the oncogenic roles of EBNA1 at the cellular level and will be discussed further.

2.1. Differential Promoter Selection of EBNA1 Transcripts

Although the EBNA1 ORF contains a single exon located in the *Bam*HI K fragment, its spliced mRNAs can be transcribed from three different upstream promoters namely, Cp, Wp, and Qp (Fig. 1B). The selective usage of these promoters depends on different EBV latencies. In cases of latency I or II (represented by BL and NPC cells, respectively), the EBNA1-specific 2.4-kb transcript has a unique *Bam*HI Q/U/K spliced form which is initiated at a TATA-less promoter, Qp, in the *Bam*HI Q fragment (Sample *et al.*, 1991; Tsai *et al.*, 1995). In latency III (such as in LCLs), a 3.5-kb EBNA1 transcript is spliced from an approximately 100-kb primary transcript, which is initiated at Cp or Wp (in the *Bam*HI C/W boundary) of the EBV genome (Tierney *et al.*, 1994; Chang *et al.*, 1998). This differential usage of promoters for EBNA1 gene expression is not only important for regulation of EBV genes in infected cells but also useful for distinguishing the latent stages in EBV-infected cells or biopsy tissues.

2.2. EBNA1 Protein Domains and Related Functions

The EBNA1 protein from the prototype B95-8 EBV strain is comprised of 641 amino acids (aa) and has unique N- and C-terminal domains separated by an internal irregular glycine/alanine repeat domain (Fig. 2A) (Dillner *et al.*, 1984). The length of the glycine/alanine repeat determines the size of the EBNA1 protein found in EBV-positive cell lines, which ranges between 69 and 97 kDa (Hennessy *et al.*, 1983). The repeat region also prevents antigen processing and recognition by cytotoxic T-lymphocytes, by inhibiting proteasomal degradation of the mature protein (Levitskaya *et al.*, 1995, 1997). The overall length of the repeat and the presence of

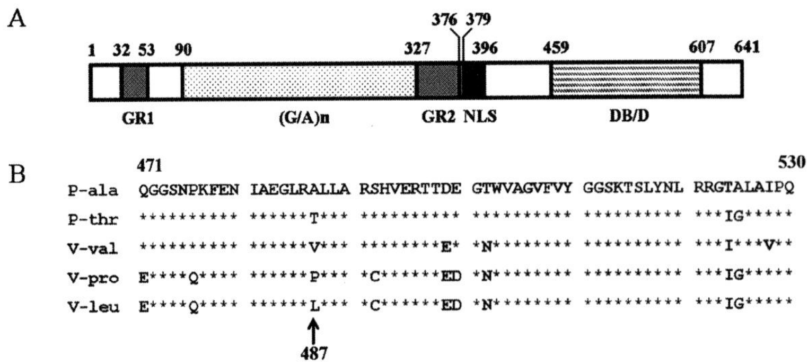

Fig. 2. Schematic diagram of EBNA1. (A) Functional domains of EBNA1. EBNA1 is composed of a gly/arg-rich motif (GR1, aa 32–53) and a second GR2 (aa 328–376); an internal gly/ala repeat [(G/A)n, aa 90–327]; a nuclear localization signal (NLS, aa 379–396); and a DNA-binding or dimmerization (DB/D; aa 459–607) domain. (B) EBNA1 subtypes. The sequence variations between aa 471 and 530 of EBNA1 subtypes (aa 487), P-ala, P-thr, V-val, V-pro, and V-leu, are indicated.

regularly interspersed Ala residues appears to be critical for this effect (Sharipo *et al.*, 1998, 2001). Among the other protein domains, the N-terminal 89 aa of EBNA1 include a glycine/arginine-rich motif (aa 32–53; GR1), while the C-terminus (aa 328–641) contains a nuclear localization signal (aa 379–396; NLS) and a second glycine/arginine-rich region (aa 328–376; GR2). The GR2 region mediates the association of *oriP*-bound EBNA1 molecules, which results in the looping and linking of *oriP* DNA. This interaction stabilizes EBNA1, contributes to DNA replication (Su *et al.*, 1991; Goldsmith *et al.*, 1993; Mackey *et al.*, 1995), and assists in the functions of segregation and transactivation (Wu *et al.*, 2002; Kennedy *et al.*, 2003). Within the C-terminus of EBNA1, the major DNA-binding and dimerization region (DB/D; aa 459–607) is essential for the replication, segregation, and transcriptional regulation functions, as shown by EBNA1-cognate DNA co-crystallization studies (Bochkarev *et al.*, 1995, 1998). Within this region, aa 459–500, particularly aa 462–477, are the core residues for DNA interaction, whereas aa 501–532 and aa 554–598 are the core residues for dimerization (Rawlins *et al.*, 1985; Milman & Hwang, 1987; Ambinder *et al.*, 1991). Thus, all regions of the EBNA1 protein are essential for EBNA1-mediated functions.

2.3. EBNA1 Subtypes

EBV is widespread in human populations and its infection is associated with a variety of lymphoid and epithelial neoplasms; both EBV infection and EBV-associated cancer distribution can show considerable geographic variation. This raises an important question as to whether particular oncogenic EBV strains are linked to specific diseases in genetically susceptible populations, possibly through a change in cell tropism or through the acquisition of mutations in viral latent genes. Indeed, the particular aa sequence alterations of the EBNA1 have been observed more frequently in EBV-associated tumors than in the blood and throat washings of asymptomatic carriers (Snudden *et al.*, 1995; Wrightham *et al.*, 1995; Bhatia *et al.*, 1996; Gutierrez *et al.*, 1998; Habeshaw *et al.*, 1999). Sequence analysis of the C-terminal region of EBNA1 allowed classification of five distinct EBNA1 subtypes; these have been named according to the signature change at residue 487, and include the prototype B95-8 strain sequence, P-ala, a closely related subtype, P-thr, and three more distinct variants, V-leu, V-pro, and V-val (Fig. 2B) (Bhatia *et al.*, 1996; Gutierrez *et al.*, 1997). These EBNA1 subtypes may be associated with BL cases from different geographic areas, but it should be noted that the same subtypes are also prevalent in the general population of those regions (Habeshaw *et al.*, 1999). In the BL endemic area of East Africa, the V-leu subtype of EBNA1 was detected in more than 50% of the analyzed samples, whereas this subtype is rarely found in Southeast Asia (Habeshaw *et al.*, 1999). In contrast, the V-val subtype has been identified in most, if not all, NPC cases occurring in Southeast Asia, especially in southern China. Notably, the V-val subtype is also prevalent in the general population in this region, while being only rarely detected in other parts of the world (Snudden *et al.*, 1995; Chen *et al.*, 1999; Wang *et al.*, 2002, 2003).

The biological functions of the various EBNA1 subtypes have not been well established to date. The first report describing sequence alterations in the V-val subtype of EBNA1 in NPC demonstrated that these variations did not affect the *in vitro* DNA-binding ability of EBNA1 (Snudden *et al.*, 1995). Furthermore, expression of the P-ala, P-thr, and V-val subtypes in cultured human embryonic kidney cells had no apparent effect on cell growth (Mai *et al.*, 2007). However, a recent study, using a luciferase reporter system containing transcriptional enhancer FR, indicated that V-val EBNA1 has higher transcriptional activity than that of P-ala subtype (B95-8 strain EBNA1) (Do *et al.*, 2008). Again, whether this higher transcriptional activity EBNA1 subtype correlates with higher oncogenic activity is not known. At present, the sequences of EBNA1 clearly show geographical polymorphisms; however, it is difficult to conclude thus far the possible presence of tumor-specific EBNA1 subtype(s).

2.4. Posttranslational Modifications of EBNA1

EBNA1 undergoes several posttranslational modifications, such as phosphorylation, ribosylation, and methylation, which are important for its biological functions. For example, EBNA1 is phosphorylated at serine residues (Hearing & Levine, 1985); mutational analyses have indicated that phosphorylation of the serines in the GR2 region of EBNA1 increases its binding to hEBP2, thereby contributing to the segregation function of EBNA1 (Shire *et al.*, 2006). Furthermore, a recent study suggested that phosphorylation at Ser385 of the EBNA1 NLS regulates nuclear transport efficiency by affecting the binding affinity between EBNA1 and NPI1 (importin $\alpha5$) (Kitamura *et al.*, 2006). Studies have shown that poly-ADP ribose polymerase and a protein arginine methyltransferase (PRMT) could bind and modify EBNA1, thereby negatively regulating *oriP*-dependent DNA replication and affecting EBNA1 localization, respectively (Holowaty *et al.*, 2003b; Deng *et al.*, 2005; Shire *et al.*, 2006).

2.5. EBNA1-Interacting Cellular Proteins

EBNA1 not only acts in the maintenance and transcriptional activation of the EBV genome, it also appears to have a direct role in contributing to the oncogenic potential of EBV. Mechanistically, this multifunctional nature seems to arise from the ability of EBNA1 to interact with a spectrum of cellular proteins, in particular, the chromosomal replication-related proteins, such as replication protein A (RPA) (Zhang *et al.*, 1998) and origin recognition complex (ORC) (Dhar *et al.*, 2001). Chromatin-immunoprecipitation (ChIP) and co-immunoprecipitation (co-IP) assays have further indicated that EBNA1 interacts with the human ORC (Schepers *et al.*, 2001). Telomeric repeat binding factor 2 (TRF2), the TRF2-interacting protein, hRap1, and the telomere-associated poly-(ADP-ribose) polymerase have all been shown to bind *oriP* in an EBNA1-dependent fashion (Deng *et al.*, 2002). EBNA1 has also been shown to interact with metastasis inhibition factor Nm23-H1, thereby suppressing the ability of Nm23-H1 to inhibit cell migration (Murakami *et al.*, 2005). These data are consistent with a recent report indicating that EBNA1 can promote metastasis and overcome the metastatic suppressor effects of Nm23-H1 in a nude mouse model (Kaul *et al.*, 2007).

Many other EBNA1-interacting proteins have been obtained through yeast one-hybrid and two-hybrid approaches, including hEBP2, Rch1/importin-α, NPI1, and p32/TAP (Wang *et al.*, 1997; Kim *et al.*, 1997; Fischer *et al.*, 1997; Aiyar *et al.*, 1998; Shire *et al.*, 1999; Ito *et al.*, 2000). It has been suggested that attachment of EBNA1 to mitotic chromosomes occurs through an interaction with cellular hEBP2 proteins present on the mitotic chromosomes (Wu *et al.*, 2000; Kapoor *et al.*, 2005). Since importin-α and NPI1 are nuclear transport factors, their interaction with EBNA1 might be important for the nuclear localization of EBNA1.

EBNA1-interacting cellular proteins have also been profiled using EBNA1 affinity chromatography and tandem affinity purification-tagging approaches; the identified proteins include several important cellular regulatory proteins, such as PRMT5 and HAUSP/USP7 (Holowaty *et al.*, 2003b). As mentioned above, EBNA1 could be methylated by PRMTs, specifically PRMT1 and -5, thereby affecting the localization of EBNA1 (Shire *et al.*, 2006). HAUSP/USP7 is a ubiquitin-specific protease that interacts with and deubiquitinates p53 (Li *et al.*, 2002). EBNA1 and p53 bind the same domain of HAUSP/USP7, with EBNA1 showing higher affinity, suggesting that EBNA1 could sequester HAUSP/USP7, thereby destabilizing p53 and protecting cells from apoptosis (Holowaty *et al.*, 2003a; Saridakis *et al.*, 2005). This is consistent with a report indicating that EBNA1 is required for survival of EBV-positive BL cells, and expression of EBNA1 in uninfected cells can inhibit p53-dependent apoptosis (Kennedy *et al.*, 2003).

3. EBNA2, EBNA3A, EBNA3B, EBNA3C, and EBNA-LP

EBNA2, the three EBNA3s, and EBNA-LP are mainly expressed in EBV-infected cells at latency III, which may be represented by *in vitro* transformed LCLs (Allday *et al.*, 1989). The role played by this set of proteins in oncogenesis *in vivo* still remains to be established.

3.1. EBNA2

EBV can transform primary B lymphocytes efficiently to LCLs *in vitro*, and EBNA2 is one of the key virally encoded proteins involved in this process. This has been established by two main lines of evidence: (1) In the BL cell line, P3HR1, the EBV genome has a deletion in the region containing the EBNA2 coding sequence. This mutant EBV failed to convert primary B lymphocytes to LCLs, but transformation could be restored by reintroduction of the deleted DNA fragment (Cohen *et al.*, 1989; Hammerschmidt & Sugden, 1989). (2) The sequence of EBNA2 differs between two EBV subtypes, with viruses carrying type 1 EBNA2 showing higher efficiency in causing LCL outgrowth than those carrying type 2 EBNA2 (Rickinson *et al.*, 1987; Cohen *et al.*, 1989).

EBNA2 is a transcriptional activator of both viral and cellular genes. In contrast to most transcription factors, EBNA2 does not bind directly to its responsive DNA element but transactivates its target genes through association with the cellular transcription factor recombination signal-binding protein Jk (RBP-Jk) (also called EBV C promoter binding factor 1 [CBF1]/Suppressor of Hairless [Su (H)]) (Henkel *et al.*, 1994; Laux *et al.*, 1994; Waltzer *et al.*, 1994), which recognizes the RBP-JK sites on the viral promoter regions of Cp (Jin & Speck, 1992), LMP1 (Zimber-Strobl *et al.*, 1993; Sjoblom *et al.*, 1995), LMP2A (Johannsen *et al.*, 1995), cellular gene promoters of CD21 (EBV receptor/CR2) (Cordier *et al.*, 1990), and CD23 (Cordier *et al.*, 1990; Henkel *et al.*, 1994). Since RBP-JK associates with the WFP sequence in a key protein–protein interaction domain in the Notch receptor intracellular domain (Tamura *et al.*, 1995) and EBNA2 contains a similar WWP sequence (Yalamanchili *et al.*, 1994), it seems reasonable to suppose that EBNA2 mimics the constitutively active Notch receptor, which has been linked to human T-cell lymphoma in a mouse model (Pear *et al.*, 1996).

3.2. EBNA3A, EBNA3B, and EBNA3C

The three EBNA3 genes are transcribed from Cp or Wp, which are ~100 kb upstream from the coding sequences. EBNA3A, -3B, and -3C belong to a gene family by virtue of having the same gene structure and sharing limited but significant amino-acid sequence homology. Among the three EBNA3 proteins, EBNA3A and -3C are essential for the efficient *in vitro* transformation of B lymphocytes (Tomkinson *et al.*, 1993), and were shown to cooperate with activated Ras in an *in vitro* transformation study of primary rat embryo fibroblasts (Parker *et al.*, 2000). Biochemically, EBNA3A and -3B repress expression of the proapoptotic tumor-suppressor, Bim (Anderton *et al.*, 2008).

The EBNA3s act as transcription repressors through their interacting protein, RBP-JK/CBF1. The EBNA3s bind to the same site on RBP-JK/CBF1 as EBNA2 and can inhibit EBNA2-mediated activation of the latent promoter, Cp (Zimber-Strobl & Strobl, 2001). Since Cp is the promoter for initiation of all EBNA transcripts in LCLs, the EBNA3s may function in a negative-regulatory fashion. Consistent with this notion, EBNA3A and -3C interact with histone deacetylases and the transcription co-repressor, CtBP, which converts transcriptionally active chromatin to a silent state (Radkov *et al.*, 1999; Hickabottom *et al.*, 2002). Future work will be required to elucidate the target genes of EBNA3 and the CtBP transcription complex.

3.3. EBNA-LP

EBNA-LP has multiple copies of a 66-aa repeat encoded by the first two exons in the IRs of the EBV *Bam*H1 W fragment, W1 (22 aa) and W2 (44 aa) followed by a unique 45-aa domain encoded by two exons from *Bam*H1 Y fragment (Kieff & Rickinson, 2007). EBNA-LP is transcribed along with EBNA2 at the initiation of EBV infection in the primary B lymphocyte. EBNA-LP and EBNA2 coactivate EBNA2-regulated viral gene promoters such as Cp and LMP1 promoters (Peng *et al.*, 2000, 2005).

EBNA-LP interacts with several cellular factors including DNA-PK catalytic subunit, nuclear protein HA95, HSP70, and HSP27 (Han *et al.*, 2001). Association of these proteins may contribute to negative regulation of coactivation activity of EBNA2/EBNA-LP. EBNA-LP colocalizes with HA95 and causes HA95 to partially relocalize with EBNA-LP in promyelocytic leukemia nuclear bodies (PML NBs). EBNA-LP interacts with the PML NB-associated protein Sp100 and displaces Sp100 and heterochromatin protein 1 alpha (HP1alpha) from PML NBs (Ling *et al.*, 2005). EBNA-LP also indirectly associates with protein kinase A catalytic subunit alpha (PKAcsalpha) through HA95, which results in specific downregulation of the coactivating effects of EBNA-LP in B lymphoblasts (Han *et al.*, 2002). Thus, function of EBNA-LP as a coactivator is likely to be involved in EBV transformation of primary B lymphocytes into LCLs.

4. LMP1 and Its Variants

4.1. LMP1

Over the past two decades, various studies have collectively shown that latent membrane protein 1 (LMP1) is an important EBV oncoprotein. LMP1 is a classical oncogene that has been shown to induce anchorage-independent growth in rodent cells (Wang *et al.*, 1985), and is essential for B-lymphocyte transformation (Kaye *et al.*, 1993). Its expression has been correlated with proliferation, anti-apoptosis, and transformation both *in vitro* and in animal models (Wilson *et al.*, 1990; Shair *et al.*, 2007). LMP1 can be detected in EBV latency II and III, and it has been strongly associated with human malignancies, including NPC, HD, NHL, and PTLD (Rickinson & Kieff, 2007). Furthermore, LMP1 expression levels in NPC biopsies have been correlated to tumor processes, such as increased metastasis (Yoshizaki, 2002), invasion (Kondo *et al.*, 2005), and DNA methyltransferase (DNMT) activity (Tsai *et al.*, 2006), as well as downregulation of adhesion molecules (Yoshizaki, 2002). Overall, the presence of LMP1 increases transformation ability and enhances tumor survival.

Prototype LMP1 comprises 386 aa, although other subtypes isolated from NPC patients vary from 381–404 aa (Li & Chang, 2003). LMP1 localizes in the lipid raft or cell membrane (Higuchi *et al.*, 2001; Kaykas *et al.*, 2001). It mimics the function of tumor necrosis factor receptor (TNFR) family members, including TNFR1 and

CD40, even though there is little aa sequence homology among them. However, unlike TNFR1 and CD40, which activate upon ligand binding, LMP1 acts as a constitutively activated receptor-like molecule independent of ligand binding or regulation.

LMP1 is an integral protein that can be divided into three segments, as depicted in Fig. 3. A short N-terminus (1–23 aa) is responsible for membrane orientation (Izumi *et al.*, 1994) and ubiquitin attachment (Aviel *et al.*, 2000). A transmembrane domain (24–186 aa) consisting of six membrane-spanning regions induces LMP1 oligomerization (Gires *et al.*, 1997), initiates Cdc42-mediated cytoskeletal reorganization (Puls *et al.*, 1999), and enhances NF-κB signaling (Liu *et al.*, 2006). Lastly, the protein has a relatively long cytoplasmic tail (187–386 aa) that can be subdivided into three regions that have been designated C-terminal activating regions (CTARs) 1–3. CTAR1 and CTAR2 but not CTAR3 are necessary for B-lymphocyte transformation (Huen *et al.*, 1995; Kaye *et al.*, 1995; Izumi *et al.*, 1997, 1999a). The CTAR regions serve as docking sites for a number of cellular factors, most of which also associate with TNFR; these include the TNFR-associated factors (TRAFs) (Devergne *et al.*, 1996), the TNFR-associated death domain protein (TRADD) (Izumi & Kieff, 1997), and receptor interacting-protein (RIP) (Izumi *et al.*, 1999b). Once engaged to LMP1, the associated factors trigger several important downstream signaling cascades, including the nuclear factor (NF)-κB, p38/mitogen-activated protein kinase (MAPK), c-Jun N-terminal kinase (JNK), Janus kinase (JAK), and phosphatidylinositol 3 kinase (PI3-K) pathways, as indicated in Fig. 3 (Eliopoulos & Young, 2001; Tsao *et al.*, 2002; Lam & Sugden, 2003; Li & Chang, 2003; Young & Rickinson, 2004; Zheng *et al.*, 2007).

4.2. LMP1 Variants

LMP1 is one of the few latent genes expressed in NPC, and a variant form of LMP1 has been linked with this disease. In NPC tissues, a predominant 30-bp deletion (corresponding to aa 347–356 of the prototype B95-8 strain LMP1) within the C-terminal sequence was first reported in 50 out of 50 Taiwanese NPC samples (Chen *et al.*,

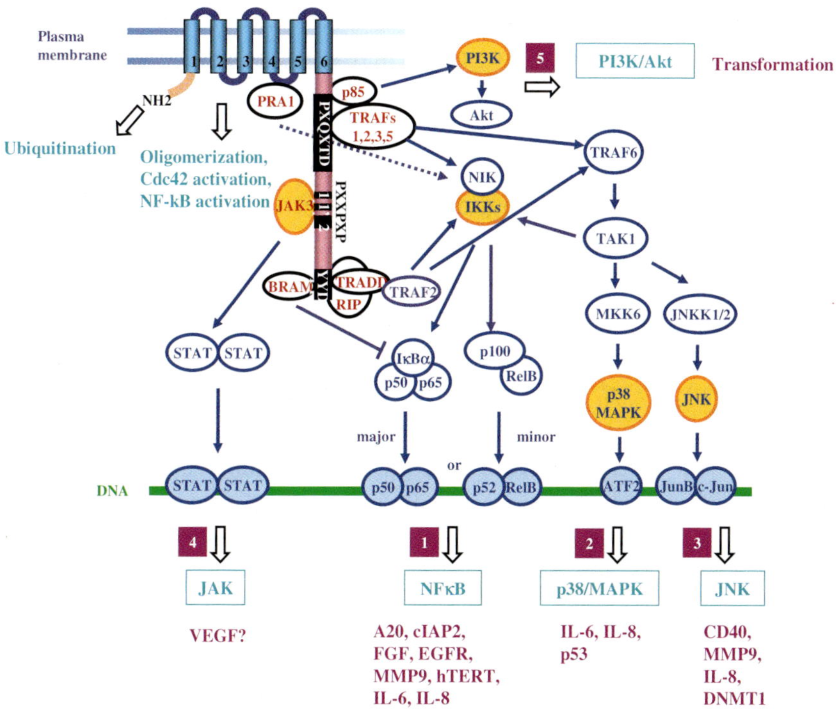

Fig. 3. Schematic diagram of LMP1 functional domains, associated factors and its major signaling pathways. LMP1 consists of a short cytoplasmic N-terminus tail (1–23 aa), six transmembrane domains (24–186 aa), and a long cytoplasmic C-terminus (187–386 aa) which contains three essential activating domains, namely, CTAR1 (194–232 aa), CTAR2 (351–386 aa), and CTAR3 (275–330 aa). Each CTAR domain has a consensus protein motif of aa sequences, which serves mainly as binding site for cellular adaptors. These cellular factors include TRAF1, -2, -3, -5, p85, TRADD, RIP, JAK3, BRAM, and PRA1, which activate a series of signaling pathways (indicated as open arrows) e.g. NF-κB, p38/MAPK, JNK, JAK, and PI3K/Akt (as shown in the box). These signaling pathways mostly activate protein kinases (in yellow) and downstream transcription factors; and eventually these activated transcription factors (in light blue) target their responsive elements resulting in gene expression modulation. Solid arrow represents direct target and dotted arrow as indicated in PRA1 represents NF-κB signaling enhancement.

1992) and in NPC samples from Southern China (Hu *et al.*, 1991). Further studies indicated that this variant is more pathogenic or tumorigenic than the prototype, as assayed in cultured cells and nude mouse model (Hu *et al.*, 1993; Li *et al.*, 1996; Yu *et al.*, 2002). Other reports have also supported that this deleted LMP1 was more prevalent in tumor biopsies than in normal counterpart (Chiang *et al.*, 1999; Hadhri-Guiga *et al.*, 2006). Moreover, this deleted form was found to be associated with other lymphoproliferative diseases in European and American EBV strains and this deletion may increase the risk of developing malignancies (Dolcetti *et al.*, 1997; Kershaw *et al.*, 1997; Knecht *et al.*, 1995). However, there are also reports arguing against the notion that the deleted LMP1 is a factor predisposing NPC development suggesting a geographic factor associated with Asian EBV strain (Sandvej *et al.*, 1997; Hahn *et al.*, 2001; Zhang *et al.*, 2002b). Therefore, the evidence that is more direct is required to settle this issue. The other consistent sequence variation is a point mutation in codon 17, which results in the loss of an XhoI restriction enzyme site in the first exon of the LMP1 gene (Hu *et al.*, 1991; Chen *et al.*, 1992). Although no direct functional change regarding to this point mutation have been reported to date, this polymorphism may be used to distinguish different LMP1 variants.

4.3. LMP1-Mediated Signaling Pathways

4.3.1. *NF-κB*

LMP1-mediated NF-κB activation (Huen *et al.*, 1995) has been linked to: (1) the association of TRAF1, -2, -3, and -5 at CTAR1 via the binding consensus sequence, $PXQXT_{208}$ (Devergne *et al.*, 1996; Kaye *et al.*, 1996; Brodeur *et al.*, 1997), and indirect association of TRAF2 and TRAF6 via TRADD at CTAR2 (Izumi & Kieff, 1997; Schultheiss *et al.*, 2001; Luftig *et al.*, 2003; Wu *et al.*, 2006); (2) the association of TRADD at CTAR2 via the last three aa, the YYD_{386} domain (Izumi *et al.*, 1999; Kieser *et al.*, 1999); and (3) the association of a newly recognized LMP1-interacting molecule, prenylated Rab acceptor 1 (PRA1), which interacts with LMP1 through transmembrane domains 3–6 (Liu *et al.*, 2006) (Fig. 3). The TRAFs are a family of cytoplasmic adaptor proteins that are responsible for coupling cell surface receptors, such as TNFR and CD40, with protein kinases in order to activate signaling pathways. TRAF2 on LMP1 CTAR1 further recruits NF-κB inducing kinase (NIK) (Sylla *et al.*, 1998). Activated NIK phosphorylates IKKα, which in turn induces processing of p100 and subsequent translocation of the transcription factor, p52/RelB, leading to mediation of a minor noncanonical NF-κB pathway (CTAR1: TRAF2 > NIK > IKKα > p100 > p52-RelB) (underlined factor represents activated transcription factor) (Eliopoulos *et al.*, 2003; Luftig *et al.*, 2003; Saito *et al.*, 2003). On the other hand, TRADD recruits TRAF6 (Schultheiss *et al.*, 2001), which then recruits TGF-β activated kinase 1 (TAK1), leading to phosphorylation of IKKβ and subsequent activation of the IκBα-bound transcription factor, p50/p65, triggering a major canonical NF-κB pathway in CTAR2 (CTAR2: TRADD > TRAF6 > TAK1 > IKKβ > IκBα > p50–p65) (Luftig *et al.*, 2003; Wu *et al.*, 2006; Soni *et al.*, 2007). Therefore, the two CTAR domains differentially interact with various TRAF molecules to confer distinct NF-κB activation. Another molecule that is associated with LMP1 and involved in NF-κB signaling is PRA1, an integral membrane protein localized in the Golgi and late endosome. Interactions between PRA1 and LMP1 may trigger or modulate the oligomerization or stabilization of LMP1, triggering trafficking of LMP1 to sites where it can elicit the full range of NF-κB signaling (Liu *et al.*, 2006). Disruption of their interaction was shown to result in LMP1 redistribution and NF-κB signaling impairment (Liu *et al.*, 2006).

LMP1-mediated NF-κB activation, which has been studied extensively, has been shown to stimulate cell survival through the activation of anti-apoptotic genes such as *A20*, *Bcl-2*, *Blf-1*, and *c-IAP2* (Laherty *et al.*, 1992; Rowe *et al.*, 1994; D'Souza *et al.*, 2000; Zhang *et al.*, 2002a). It also promotes cell proliferation through the induction of epidermal growth receptor (EGFR) (Thornburg *et al.*, 2003) and fibroblast growth factor (FGF) (Wakisaka *et al.*, 2002), increases metastasis through the upregulation of matrix metalloproteinases (MMPs) (Takeshita *et al.*, 1999), and supports cell immortality through induction of telomerase activity (Yang *et al.*, 2004). Therefore, it is conceivable that NF-κB signaling contributes significantly to LMP1-mediated tumor formation. Consistent with this, NF-κB activation has been shown to be a prevalent phenomenon in many cancers (Perkins & Gilmore, 2006; Inoue *et al.*, 2007).

4.3.2. *p38/MAPK*

LMP1 activates p38/MAPK, which upregulates the expression of the cytokines, IL-6 and IL-8, which are responsible for initiating and maintaining acute inflammatory responses (Eliopoulos *et al.*, 1999b). A TRAF2 dominant negative mutant blocked both the NF-κB and p38/MAPK pathways, indicating that TRAF2 is a common mediator of these two pathways. A p38-specific inhibitor (SB203580) and a constitutively active IκBα mutant (inhibitor of NF-κB) separately impaired the induction of IL-8 (Eliopoulos *et al.*, 1999b), indicating that the inductions of these two cytokines are coregulated by p38/MAPK and NF-κB signaling. Therefore, besides activating the NF-κB pathway, the interaction of TRAF2 and TRADD with the CTARs can also induce the p38/MAPK/ATF-2 signaling pathway (Eliopoulos *et al.*, 1999a; Schultheiss *et al.*, 2001). This in turn activates TAK1, MKK6, p38/MAPK, and its downstream transcription factor, ATF2 (CTAR1: TRAF2 > TRAF6 > TAK1 > MKK6 > p38/MAPK > ATF2; or CTAR2: TRADD > TRAF2 > TRAF6 > TAK1 > MKK6 > p38/MAPK > ATF2). These data further confirm that the two direct LMP1 interacting proteins, TRAF2 and TRADD, are key adaptors for LMP1-mediated signaling.

A recent study demonstrated that p53 phosphorylation is induced by LMP1 through the activation of p38/MAPK (Li *et al.*, 2007). LMP1-induced p53 phosphorylation was shown to trigger an increase in p53 transcription and protein levels. Further work will be required to examine the significance and consequence of this p53 accumulation, and/or whether p53 is correlated to NPC pathogenesis. It could also be useful to test whether other p38/MAPK-regulated cellular proteins are regulated by LMP1.

4.3.3. *JNK*

Activation of JNK has been well defined, particularly in TNFR signaling, where the TRAFs play an important role in linking the receptor to the MAPK kinase kinase (MAPKKK). In the context of LMP1, JNK signaling is mediated by the interaction of TRADD at the YYD domain (Kieser *et al.*, 1997, 1999; Eliopoulos *et al.*, 1999a). This interaction transmits the signal to the downstream interacting adaptors, TRAF2 and TRAF6, which further tether TAK1, a MAPKKK, which phosphorylates JNK kinases (JNKK 1/2) (Schultheiss *et al.*, 2001; Wan *et al.*, 2004). Subsequently, activated JNKK 1/2 phosphorylates JNK, which activates c-Jun (Wan *et al.*, 2004). In this way, LMP1 triggers JNK signaling via the following pathway: CTAR2/YYD: TRADD > TRAF2 > TRAF6 > TAK1 > JNKK1/2 > JNK > AP1. Accordingly, genes containing AP1 sites in their promoters may be potential targets for LMP1-JNK signaling. Genes that are known to be activated by the LMP1-mediated JNK pathway include CD40 (Kilger *et al.*, 1998), MMP9 (Takeshita *et al.*, 1999), IL-8 (Eliopoulos *et al.*, 1999b), DNA methyltransferase (DNMT) (Tsai *et al.*, 2006), and telomerase (Ding *et al.*, 2007).

4.3.4. *JAK3*

LMP1 activates JAK/STAT signaling by association of JAK3 with the CTAR3 domain, which includes a proline-rich (PXPXXP) cytoplasmic domain, the box1 domain (PHDPLP) and the box2 domain (PPQLTEEVENK) (Gires *et al.*, 1999). Although the LMP1 CTAR1 and -2 domains do not associate with JAK3, intact CTAR1 and CTAR2 are required for the ability of CTAR3 to mediate JAK3/STAT signaling (Brennan *et al.*, 2001; Liu *et al.*, 2008).

An important JAK/STAT signaling-regulated gene responsible for new blood vessel formation is vascular endothelial growth factor (VEGF) (Niu *et al.*, 2002; Xu *et al.*, 2005). A STAT3-binding site is present in the VEGF promoter, and a STAT3 inhibitor was shown to impair VEGF expression, thereby blocking tumor growth and angiogenesis *in vivo* (Xu *et al.*, 2005). These findings suggest that VEGF is transcriptionally regulated by Stat3. VEGF is a potent cytokine that regulates angiogenesis; and its expression is often detected in diverse cancer cells (Neufeld *et al.*, 1999). Studies have suggested that LMP1 expression may be correlated with VEGF expression; elevated VEGF levels have been detected in LMP1 transgenic mice (Stevenson *et al.*, 2005), in the serum of NPC patients (Li *et al.*, 2004), and in EBV-positive NPC tumors (Krishna *et al.*, 2006). LMP1 may upregulate VEGF production through its ability to activate the JAK/STAT pathway, although additional studies will be required to confirm this hypothesis. Another report indicated that the induction of VEGF by LMP1 was partly due to the overexpression of cyclooxygenase-2 (COX-2), which was induced by the LMP1-NF-κB pathway (Murono *et al.*, 2001). COX-2 is an enzyme capable of catalyzing essential fatty acids into prostanoids, which act as mediators of inflammation, vasoconstriction, and angiogenesis. Thus, COX-2 metabolites may also influence gene expression. Additional work is warranted to examine whether LMP1-mediated VEGF induction is a direct effect, or rather occurs indirectly via the downstream metabolites of COX-2.

4.3.5. *PI3K*

The CTAR1 domain of LMP1 associates with the phosphoinositide 3-kinase (PI3K) p85α subunit, which is the regulatory subunit of heterodimeric PI3K molecules (Dawson *et al.*, 2003). The association between LMP1 and the PI3K p85α subunit was shown to activate the downstream target, Akt/PKB, subsequently promoting cell survival and inducing actin-fiber formation (Dawson *et al.*, 2003). LMP1-mediated cell survival, stress-fiber formation, and colony formation in rodent cells were all blocked by dominant-negative mutants of p85, or by addition of the PI3K inhibitor, LY294002 (Dawson *et al.*, 2003; Mainou *et al.*, 2005). These results suggest that LMP1-induced PI3K/Akt signaling is an oncogenic pathway promoting cellular transformation and morphological change.

4.4. LMP1 and DNA Methylation

LMP1 has been shown to induce hypermethylation of the E-cadherin gene promoter through activation of cellular DNA methyltransferases at both transcriptional and translational levels (Tsai *et al.*, 2002). Experiments using various LMP1 deletion mutants, signaling transduction inhibitors, dominant negative mutants and siRNA knockdown revealed that this activation is modulated through LMP1 YYD domain-mediated JNK/AP1 signaling, but not by NF-κB or p38/MAPK signaling (Tsai *et al.*, 2006). LMP1-induced DNMT activation was blocked by either mutation of the AP1 site on the DNMT1 promoter, or a c-Jun dominant-negative mutation. Furthermore, immunohistochemical staining of NPC biopsy samples demonstrated a statistically significant correlation among the expression levels of LMP1, DNMT1, and phosphor-c-Jun (Tsai *et al.*, 2006), supporting the notion that LMP1 is capable of activating DNMTs via the JNK/AP1 signaling pathway.

DNA methylation is an epigenetic modification that does not alter the DNA sequence itself, but rather chemically and structurally changes the chromatin (Baylin *et al.*, 2001; Jones & Baylin, 2002; Herman & Baylin, 2003). Methylated DNA attracts the binding of protein factors such as methyl-CpG binding protein 2 (MeCP2), histone deacetylase (HDAC) and other chromatin remodeling complexes, and favors the binding of additional transcription repression complexes, yielding a more compact, inactive chromatin (Herman & Baylin, 2003). Aberrant methylation may mediate many abnormalities in various cancers, including loss of cell cycle control, dysfunction of transcription factors, disruption of normal cell–cell contact, loss of apoptotic signals, and genetic instability (Esteller & Herman, 2002; Jones, 2002; Baylin & Chen, 2005). Such aberrant DNA methylation can occur early in tumor progression and can be detrimental to cells, especially when the methylation status of tumor suppressor genes is deregulated. Intriguingly, the most frequent hypermethylated gene loci documented in NPC coincide with the locations of genes for which loss of heterozygosity (LOH) is commonly observed in NPC (Mutirangura *et al.*, 1996; Chan *et al.*, 2000; Shao *et al.*, 2001; Qiu *et al.*, 2004; Yi *et al.*, 2007). These frequently detected hypermethylation "hot spots" and/or LOH regions include chromosomes 3p, 9p, 9q, 11q, 12p, and 13q (Lo *et al.*, 2001; Lo & Huang, 2002; Chang *et al.*, 2003; Liu *et al.*, 2003; Wong *et al.*, 2004; Kwong *et al.*, 2005; Pan *et al.*, 2005; Zhou *et al.*, 2005; Lung *et al.*, 2006; Tan *et al.*, 2006). Interestingly, these "hot spots" are often situated within the tumor suppressor genes such as runt-related transcription factor 3 (RUNX3), mutL homolog 1, colon cancer (MLH1), retinoic acid receptor responder (tazarotene induced) 1 or tazarotene induced gene 1 (RARRES1/TIG1), Ras association domain family 1A (RASSF1A), deleted in liver cancer 1 (DLC1), p14, p16, death-associated protein kinase (DAPK), tumor suppressor in lung cancer 1 (TSLC1), checkpoint with forkhead and ring finger domains (CHFR), and endothelin receptor type B (EDNRB). It is possible that in addition to triggering hypermethylation of E-cadherin (CDH1), LMP1 may also be responsible for the hypermethylation of these reported tumor suppressor genes in NPC. This would be consistent with previous evidence showing that frequent hypermethylation on cellular promoters may be a common phenomenon in NPC. The fact that LMP1 activates DNMTs highlights the importance of a viral factor as an initiator/cofactor to induce epigenetic alterations. In fact, LMP1 was the first viral gene identified as being able to activate DNMTs via a defined signaling pathway. Thus, aberrant DNA hypermethylation induced by viral genes may be one of the methods through which the virus contributes to tumor development (Li *et al.*, 2005; Flanagan, 2007).

5. LMP2A and LMP2B

The LMP2 gene encodes two mRNAs using two different promoters. These highly spliced transcripts are transcribed across the terminal repeats of the circularized viral genome, resulting in two proteins, LMP2A (54 kDa) and LMP2B (40 kDa), sharing exons 2–9; exon 1 of LMP2A encodes a 119-aa hydrophilic cytoplasmic domain, whereas in LMP2B, exon 1 is a non-coding region, with translation starting in exon 2 prior to the first transmembrane sequence (Laux *et al.*, 1988; Sample *et al.*, 1989). The remaining exons encode 12 transmembrane domains and a 27-aa hydrophilic C-terminus. LMP2A, which has been detected in most EBV-associated tumors except for BL (Table 1), has potent transforming activities in epithelial cells.

LMP2A is one of the few proteins required for establishment and maintenance of EBV latency (Miyashita *et al.*, 1997) and the development of EBV-related diseases. It is also the most widely expressed EBV protein in the viral-related tumors (Brooks *et al.*, 1992; Busson *et al.*, 1992; Heussinger *et al.*, 2004). Overexpression of LMP2A can promote epithelial cell transformation, migration, and invasion (Pegtel *et al.*, 2005) and tumor formation in nude mice (Longnecker, 2000), suggesting that LMP2A plays a critical role in EBV-associated tumor development.

Although experimental data have suggested that LMP2A is dispensable for EBV-induced B-cell transformation, LMP2A mimics B-cell receptor (BCR)-mediated signal transduction and activates anti-apoptotic and cell-survival signals (Miller *et al.*, 1994; Dykstra *et al.*, 2001; Merchant *et al.*, 2001; Brinkmann & Schulz, 2006). To regulate its own function, LMP2A utilizes ubiquitin-dependent processes, which may allow it to modulate B cell differentiation and establish latent infection in memory B cells (Winberg *et al.*, 2000; Matskova *et al.*, 2001; Portis *et al.*, 2004). LMP2A consists of a 119-aa cytoplasmic N-terminal signaling domain, 12 putative membrane-spanning domains, and a cytoplasmic C-terminal domain composed of 27 aa (Longnecker & Kieff, 1990). LMP2A is the only EBV protein containing an immuno-receptor tyrosine-based activation motif (ITAM) domain, which associates with the protein tyrosine kinase (PTK), Syk, and activates the PI3K/Akt pathway. Phosphorylation of LMP2A at tyrosine 112 is important for its association with the Lyn PTK (Fruehling *et al.*, 1998), whereas phosphorylation at tyrosines 74 and 85 in the ITAM domain of LMP2A is required for activation of the Syk PTK (Fruehling & Longnecker, 1997). LMP2A also activates mTOR, a mediator of growth and proliferation signals, via the PI3K/Akt pathway (Moody *et al.*, 2005). ITAM-dependent PI3K and Akt activation and subsequent cell migration could be disrupted by mutation of tyrosine 74 and/or 85 of LMP2A (Scholle *et al.*, 2000). It has also been shown that LMP2A induces cell migration through ERK in the MAPK signaling pathway (Lu *et al.*, 2006).

LMP2B, on the other hand, has been shown to be colocalized with LMP2A in the membrane where the C-terminus of LMP2A and LMP2B can interact and regulate the activity of each other (Lynch *et al.*, 2002). LMP2B can also prevent LMP2A aggregation (Rovedo &

Longnecker, 2007), suggesting its antagonistic role in regulating LMP2A-mediated function. Recent report further demonstrates that LMP2B also regulates EBV entering lytic cycle upon BCR cross-linking through anti-immunoglobulin G, in which LMP2B reduces the degree of BCR cross-linking required to provoke this switching (Rechsteiner *et al.*, 2008). Moreover, LMP2B can restore calcium mobilization upon BCR cross-linking, a signaling process inhibited by LMP2A (Rechsteiner *et al.*, 2008). Taken together, LMP2B is likely to regulate susceptibility to induction of EBV lytic infection.

6. EBERs

The EBV-encoded small non-polyadenylated, non-coding RNAs (EBERs) are the most abundant viral transcripts (~10^7 copies per cell) in latently EBV-infected cells (Arrand & Rymo, 1982) and in NPC biopsies (Brousset *et al.*, 1992). EBERs contribute to the oncogenic process as demonstrated by EBERs-transfected cells which exhibited enhanced growth potential in soft agar, increased tumorigenicity in rodent models, resistance to apoptotic inducers, and induction of *bcl-2* gene (Komano *et al.*, 1999; Yamamoto *et al.*, 2000). EBERs confer resistance to interferon-induced apoptosis by directly binding to double-stranded RNA-activated protein kinase (PKR), and thereby inhibiting its phosphorylation (Wong *et al.*, 2005). EBER expression in immortalized nasopharyngeal epithelial cells may also confer an apoptosis-resistant phenotype, although these cells do not form colonies in soft agar or induce tumors in nude mice (Wong *et al.*, 2005). Alternatively, EBERs can also induce the expression of cellular growth factors such as insulin-like growth factor-1 in EBV-infected gastric carcinoma cells (Iwakiri *et al.*, 2003).

7. EBV-Encoded miRNA

miRNAs are a family of regulatory molecules that are involved in a wide variety of cellular processes and play critical roles in tissue development, metabolism, oncogenic transformation, and tumor suppression (Ambros, 2001; Dalmay & Edwards, 2006; Wilfred *et al.*, 2007).

The miRNA pathway is a prominent RNA regulatory mechanism that operates in differentiated mammalian cells. Given the extraordinary adaptation and imitating capability of viruses, it is not surprising that viruses encode their own miRNAs. Viral miRNAs were first discovered in EBV (Pfeffer *et al.*, 2004), and have since been found in KSHV, human cytomegalovirus (HCMV), mouse γ-herpesvirus 68 (MHV68), herpes simplex virus (HSV1) (Pfeffer *et al.*, 2005), and simian virus 40 (SV40) (Sullivan *et al.*, 2005). Recently, miRNAs have been implicated in the intricate cross talk between the host and pathogen in viral infections, suggesting that these regulatory molecules play a major role in viral pathogenesis (Qi *et al.*, 2006; Scaria *et al.*, 2006). Although miRNA production probably represents one of the many strategies used by viruses to divert or disrupt cellular mechanisms, it is striking that many of the miRNA-encoding viruses possess cellular transformation properties and have long-standing associations with cancer. It is possible that the viral miRNAs interact with or perturb existing miRNA-regulated pathways in mammalian cells, thereby promoting cancer.

7.1. Identification of EBV-encoded miRNAs

Using cloning methods, Pfeffer and colleagues (Pfeffer *et al.*, 2004) first identified five hairpin structures encoding six mature miRNAs in BL cells latently infected with the B95-8 EBV strain. Subsequent studies combining computational approaches and cloning methods (Grundhoff *et al.*, 2006; Cai *et al.*, 2006) identified additional EBV miRNAs in EBV-positive Jijoye and BC-1 cells. Recently, a large-scale cloning study (Landgraf *et al.*, 2007) determined the sequences of the most commonly cloned mature EBV miRNAs. To date, a total of 25 hairpin precursors and 44 potential mature miRNAs have been deposited in the miRBase miRNA registry database (*http://microrna.sanger.ac.uk/*).

Based on their genomic location, these EBV miRNAs can be generally categorized into two types, the *Bam*HI fragment H rightward open reading frame (BHRF) and the *Bam*HI-A region rightward transcript (BART) miRNAs, which can be further subdivided into four miRNA clusters (Table 2). The BHRF cluster, containing three

Table 2. EBV miRNAs Listed in miRBase (release 13.1)

EBVmiRNA	Sequence	Location	Expression
BHRF1 cluster			
BHRF1-1	UAACCUGAUCAGCCCCGGAGUU	41474	BL
BHRF1-2*	AAAUUCUGUUGCAGCAGAUAGC	42853	BL
BHRF1-2	UAUCUUUUGCGGCAGAAAUUGAA	42888	BL
BHRF1-3	UAACGGGAAGUGUGUAAGCACAC	42968	BL
BART cluster I			
BART3*	AACCTAGTGTTAGTGTTGTGC	139086	BL, NPC
BART3	CGCACCACTAGTCACCAGGTGT	139124	BL, NPC
BART4	GACCTGATGCTGCTGGTGTGCT	139228	BL, NPC
BART4*	CACATCACGTAGGCACCAGGTGT	139266	BL, NPC
BART1-5p	TCTTAGTGGAAGTGACGTGCTGTG	139351	BL, NPC
BART1-3p	TAGCACCGCTATCCACTATGTC	139387	BL, NPC
BART15	GTCAGTGGTTTTGTTTCCTTGA	139553	BL, NPC
BART5	CAAGGTGAATATAGCTGCCCATCG	139675	BL, NPC
BART5*	GTGGGCCGCTGTTCACCTAA	139717	BL, NPC
BART16	TTAGATAGAGTGGGTGTGTGCTC	139795	BL, NPC
BART17-5p	TAAGAGGACGCAGGCATACAA	139915	BL, NPC
BART17-3p	TGTATGCCTGGTGTCCCCTTAGT	139953	BL, NPC
BART6-5p	TAAGGTTGGTCCAATCCATAGG	140033	BL, NPC
BART6-3p	CGGGGATCGGACTAGCCTTAGA	140072	BL, NPC
BART cluster II			
BART21-5p	TCACTAGTGAAGGCAACTAAC	145514	NPC
BART21-3p	CTAGTTGTGCCCACTGGTGTTT	145548	NPC
BART18-5p	TCAAGTTCGCACTTCCTATACA	145962	BL, NPC
BART18-3p	TATCGGAAGTTTGGGCTTCGTC	145998	
BART7*	CCTGGACCTTGACTATGAAACA	146439	
BART7	CATCATAGTCCAGTGTCCAGGG	146475	BL, NPC
BART8	TACGGTTTCCTAGATTGTACAG	146772	BL, NPC
BART8*	GTCACAATCTATGGGGTCGTAGA	146807	BL, NPC
BART9*	TACTGGACCCTGAATTGGAAAC	146959	
BART9	TAACACTTCATGGGTCCCGTAGT	146997	BL, NPC
BART22	TTACAAAGTCATGGTCTAGTAGT	147203	NPC
BART10*	GCCACCTCTTTGGTTCTGTAC	147321	BL, NPC
BART10	TACATAACCATGGAGTTGGCTGT	147356	BL, NPC
BART11-5p	TCAGACAGTTTGGTGCGCTAGTTG	147537	BL, NPC
BART11-3p	ACGCACACCAGGCTGACTGCC	147575	BL, NPC
BART12	TCCTGTGGTGTTTGGTGTGGTT	147936	BL, NPC
BART19-5p	ACATTCCCCGCAAACATGACATG	148215	BL, NPC
BART19-3p	TTTTGTTTGCTTGGGAATGCT	148254	BL, NPC

(*Continued*)

Table 2. (*Continued*)

EBVmiRNA	Sequence	Location	Expression
BART20-5p	TAGCAGGCATGTCTTCATTCC	148339	
BART20-3p	CATGAAGGCACAGCCTGTTACC	148374	
BART13*	AACCGGCTCGTGGCTCGTACAG	148526	BL, NPC
BART13	TGTAACTTGCCAGGGACGGCTGA	148563	BL, NPC
BART14*	TACCCTACGCTGCCGATTTACA	148744	BL, NPC
BART14	TAAATGCTGCAGTAGTAGGGAT	148778	BL, NPC
BART2			
BART2-5p	TATTTTCTGCATTCGCCCTTGC	152747	BL, NPC
BART2-3p	AAGGAGCGATTTGGAGAAAATAA	152783	

precursors encoding four mature miRNAs, is located within the 5′- and 3′-untranslated regions (UTRs) of the BHRF1. The remaining 40 EBV miRNAs were mapped to the intronic regions of the BART gene and can be further divided into three clusters, which are BART cluster I (8 precursors for 14 mature miRNAs), BART cluster II (13 precursors for 24 mature miRNAs), and the BART2 cluster (one precursor for two mature miRNAs).

The genomic sequences of EBV strains from primary NPC tissues, cultured NPC cells and B cells exhibit a low degree of sequence variations in the mature miRNA of *BART8*, *BART17-5p*, and *BART19-5p* (unpublished data). One of the identified sequence variants, *BART19-5p* (17T/C), was found in the C6661 and Daudi cell lines, in three primary NPC tumor tissues, and may represent a polymorphism in EBV miRNAs. Several sequence variations were detected in the loop region or the flanking stem region of EBV miRNAs. The effects of these sequence variations on the biogenesis of EBV miRNAs remain to be determined.

Rhesus lymphocryptovirus, which is separated from EBV by more than 13 million years of evolution, expresses several miRNAs closely related to those of EBV, including homologs of *BHRF1-1*, *BART1*, *BART3*, *BART5*, *BART7*, and *BART11* (Cai *et al.*, 2006). The extensive sequence conservation suggests that these viral miRNAs may share similar cellular targets critical for viral infection.

7.2. Expression of EBV-encoded miRNAs

Various strategies have been utilized to document and quantify the expression of EBV miRNAs in EBV-infected cell lines and tissues. Studies using cloning and Northern blot analysis have revealed distinct expression patterns of EBV miRNAs in EBV-infected cell lines at different latency stages. The BHRF miRNAs, including *BHRF1-1* and *-2*, were found to be highly expressed in latency III-infected lymphoblasts (IM9, Raji, MUTU III, and Namalwa cells), but not in latency I-infected BL (MUTU I cells) or latency II-associated NPC cells (C666-1, BC-1, and C15 cells). On the other hand, BART miRNAs may be found at high levels in all stages of latency, as well as during lytic infection (Pfeffer *et al.*, 2004; Cai *et al.*, 2006).

Using a highly sensitive real-time PCR method, the expression levels of all 39 mature EBV miRNAs were determined in EBV-positive BL (B95-8, Jijoye, Namalwa, Daudi, and Raji) and NPC (HK1/EBV and C666-1) cells (Chen SJ, unpublished data). Both HK-1/EBV and C666-1 cells expressed at least 25 different EBV BART miRNAs but no BHRF miRNA. While the overall expression patterns were similar, the absolute expression levels of BART miRNAs were 8- to 10-fold higher in C666-1 cells. On the other hand, all of the tested BL cell lines expressed high levels of BHRF miRNAs. Compared to NPC cells, the expressions levels of BART miRNAs were relatively low in most BL cells, except for Jijoye cells, which expressed BART miRNAs at level comparable to those found in HK1/EBV cells.

A global expression profile of EBV miRNAs from 14 NPC tissues and 13 normal samples using the above sensitive real time Q-PCR assay revealed that 25 EBV miRNAs can be specifically detected in NPC samples, with a false positive rate <0.1% (unpublished data). No EBV miRNAs were detected in normal tissues or in non-NPC nasopharyngeal samples. While the levels of different EBV miRNAs varied significantly within individual samples, the overall expression profiles were similar across different NPC samples. The expression patterns of EBV miRNAs in NPC samples closely resembled those in the NPC cell lines. Several BART miRNAs, including *BART4*,

BART6-3p, *BART18-5p*, *BART7*, *BART9*, and *BART2-5p*, were detected at significant levels in NPC tissues, with expression levels 4- to 8-fold higher than that of the highly abundant human miRNA, hsa-miR-16. Correlation analysis revealed that EBV miRNAs within the same cluster were coordinately expressed. EBV miRNAs in BART clusters I and II were also highly correlated, and the level of BART miRNAs in NPC tissues showed significant correlation to the transcript levels of BART and EBER1.

In addition to BL and NPC, EBV is associated with about 6–16% of gastric carcinoma (EBVaGC) cases worldwide. The role of EBV in EBVaGC pathogenesis is unclear, especially given that the well-known EBV oncogenes, including LMP1, EBNA2, and the EBNA3s, are not expressed in EBVaGC. Recently, Kim do and colleagues (Kim do *et al.*, 2007) reported that several BART miRNAs were detected at high levels in tissues from EBV-positive gastric carcinoma. The authors found that BART miRNAs, but not *BHRF1* miRNAs, were expressed in EBV-infected gastric carcinoma cell lines, EBVaGC animal model, and EBV-positive gastric cancer tumor tissues. On the contrary, expression of EBV miRNA was not detected in EBV-negative gastric carcinoma cell lines and tissues.

7.3. Regulation of EBV miRNA Expression

Expression of the *BHRF1* miRNA cluster has been correlated with high activity levels at the Cp and Wp promoters, which are characteristic of stage III latency (Cai *et al.*, 2006). Latency III EBV gene expression causes continuous cell proliferation, which results in immortalization of primary B cells *in vitro* and lymphoproliferative diseases *in vivo*. Latency III-associated proteins are also detected with EBV replication in epithelial cells *in vivo* or late in EBV replication in latency I-infected BL cells. A recent study by Xing and Kieff suggested that *BHRF1-1*, *-2*, and *-3* are generated from the introns of EBNA transcripts (Xing & Kieff, 2007). The study also provided evidence indicating that *BHRF1-2* may negatively regulate the expression of *BHRF1*, an antiapoptotic *Bcl-2* homolog expressed early in

EBV replication. The physiological significance of this auto-regulation is unclear. Interestingly, induction of EBV replication in latency I-infected Akata cells was associated with a significant accumulation of *BHRF1-1*, *-2*, and *-3*, whereas EBV replication in preexisting latency III-infected cells (e.g. B95-8 cells) was not associated with changes in EBNA, *BHRF1-1*, *-2*, or *-3* (Xing & Kieff, 2007).

All BART miRNAs are located within the predicted introns of the alternatively spliced BART gene. Northern blot analysis and Q-PCR data indicated that the expression levels of various alternatively spliced BART mRNAs could be correlated with the expression levels of the BART miRNAs. Cai and colleagues reported that induction of EBV lytic replication in Daudi and MUTU I cells resulted in a significant increase in the expression of *BART1-3p*, *BART3-3p*, *BART7*, *BART10-3p*, and *BHRF1-2* (Cai *et al.*, 2006). However, a similar increase in BART miRNAs was not detected following the induction of EBV replication in latency I-infected Akata cells (Xing & Kieff, 2007). This apparent discrepancy in BART miRNA levels during lytic EBV replication remains to be clarified.

7.4. Functions of EBV miRNAs

A recent study showed that *BART2* regulates the expression of the viral *BALF5* gene. Sequence analysis revealed that *BART2*-miRNA overlaps with, and is expressed in the antisense orientation to, the 3′UTR of the EBV *BALF5* gene. A truncated *BALF5* mRNA has been identified (Furnari *et al.*, 1993), corresponding to the product of a *BART2*-miRNA-mediated degradation (Pfeffer *et al.*, 2004). Forced expression of *BART2* during lytic replication resulted in a reduction of *BALF5* and a decrease in viral particle release from EBV-infected cells (Barth *et al.*, 2007). Induction of the lytic viral replication cycle resulted in a reduction of both *BART2* and the cleavage product of *BALF5*. These results are consistent with the notion that *BART2* plays an inhibitory role in the transition from latent to lytic EBV replication, which is in agreement with the hypothesis that the *BART2* inhibits viral DNA replication through degradation of transcripts encoding the viral DNA polymerase, *BALF5*.

A close examination of the genomic organization of EBV reveals that EBV miRNAs encoded in BART clusters I and II may also regulate other EBV viral proteins in a similar auto-regulatory manner. EBV miRNAs in BART cluster I are transcribed in an antisense fashion to the LF3 transcript and are therefore perfectly complementary to the LF3 3′UTR (de Jesus *et al.*, 2003). The BART cluster II miRNAs are located in the complementary strand at the 3′UTR of three EBV genes, *LF1*, *LF2*, and *BILF-1*. *LF2* has been shown to interact with the EBV immediate early R transactivator (Rta) and was found to inhibit Rta transactivation (Calderwood *et al.*, 2007). *BILF-1*, a constitutively active G protein-coupled receptor exclusively encoded by γ1-herpesviruses, is expressed during the lytic EBV infection (Paulsen *et al.*, 2005). All of these potentially BART-miRNAs regulated viral genes are expressed during early infection stage (Calderwood *et al.*, 2007; Paulsen *et al.*, 2005; Xue & Griffin, 2007). Future work will be required to firmly establish whether EBV miRNAs encoded within BART clusters I and II play a role in regulating the viral lytic cycle in infected cells.

In addition to targeting lytic cycle genes, Lo and colleagues (Lo *et al.*, 2007) reported that three BART cluster I miRNAs (*BART1-5p*, *BART16*, and *BART17-5p*) suppressed the expression of LMP1 protein in EBV-infected cells. This observation provides an explanation for the discrepancy between LMP1 transcript and protein levels in NPC tissues. Expression of these BART miRNAs reduced the sensitivity of LMP1-expressing cells to cisplatin (Lo *et al.*, 2007). Although LMP1 is known to promote cellular transformation, overexpression of LMP1 has been shown to cause growth inhibition and potentiate cisplatin-induced apoptosis. By negatively regulating LMP1, these BART miRNAs may help to balance the growth advantage/disadvantage of LMP1 in EBV-infected cells.

The number of different BART miRNAs expressed in NPC tissues, as well as their levels, suggest that EBV miRNAs might play a critical role in the pathogenesis of viral infection. However, it is currently unknown whether these viral miRNAs are directed against viral target genes, host target genes, or both. Interestingly, several highly abundant BART miRNAs, including *BART1*, *BART3*, and

BART7, are highly conserved between EBV and rhesus lymphocryptovirus (Cai *et al.*, 2006), which is a simian equivalent to human EBV. The extensive miRNA conservation between related viruses may suggest that their targets are of predominantly cellular and not viral origin. As most of the EBV miRNAs are expressed in latently infected cells, it is conceivable that these EBV miRNAs may facilitate the viral life cycle by blocking innate or adaptive host immune responses or by interfering with the appropriate regulation of apoptosis, cell growth, DNA replication, or DNA repair in infected cells. Scanning the human genome for potential target sites for the EBV-encoded miRNAs yielded a list of genes, including those encoding a variety of cytokines and chemokines, as well as other factors involved in the regulation of cell proliferation and apoptosis, transcriptional regulators and components of signal transduction pathways (Pfeffer *et al.*, 2004). Future work will be required to examine whether these host genes are targeted by individual EBV miRNAs, and to elucidate the potential role(s) of this process in oncogenesis.

8. Perspectives

Since the initial discovery of EBV by Epstein and Barr more than 40 years ago, researchers have accumulated a great deal of knowledge regarding EBV-encoded genes and EBV-associated malignancies. However, several issues related to EBV-induced oncogenesis such as virus strain variations and virus–host interaction have not been fully understood, and animal models to validate the biochemical findings and clinical correlations have not been established.

The sequence of the entire EBV genome, which was reported in 1984 (Baer *et al.*, 1984), has become the basis for detailing the heterogeneity of EBV isolates. The differences across individual isolates or strains range from single nucleotide polymorphisms to large deletions. Some of the changes have been shown to result in altered biological functions; while others are silent mutation that can be used for strain identification. Among the studied sequence changes in EBV, those in the *LMP1* gene are the best studied. Although the link between the *LMP1* 30-bp C-terminal deletion and tumorigenesis has been supported by laboratory data, the molecular mechanism leading to a more oncogenic variant requires further study. On the other hand, even being the only viral protein detected in all EBV-associated tumors, there are far fewer studies on EBNA-1 sequence polymorphisms compared to LMP1 polymorphisms. Therefore, it will be useful to examine EBNA-1 sequences worldwide and examine whether particular EBNA-1 subtypes carry increased or decreased oncogenic potential.

Epigenetic alterations in various cancers are now becoming one of the most intensive studied areas. EBV utilizes the cellular DNA methylation machinery to regulate its own (Ambinder *et al.*, 1999; Klein, 1996; Li & Minarovits, 2003; Tao & Robertson, 2003) and cellular gene promoters (Tsai *et al.*, 2006). The occurrence of the aberrant DNA methylation due to the presence of EBV is likely genome wide; therefore, it is a challenge to identify the altered cellular "methylome" by high throughput screening due to the perturbation by EBV, in particular, LMP1. Hopefully, these signature methylome can be used as biomarkers to distinguish specific EBV-related cancers or stages. As the epigenetic alterations are reversible, drugs that can reverse such processes become the potential therapeutic agents for EBV-related cancers.

Studies have been carried out to identify cellular proteins that interact with EBV proteins, as well as cellular target genes or proteins of individual viral proteins and EBV miRNA. These cellular genes or proteins have provided a basis to examine the virus–host interaction or build up a hypothesis how this interaction might take place. An *in vivo* animal model that faithfully reproduces EBV biology should be considered in order to validate the significance of these interactions and downstream activities.

Our understanding of how EBV initiates infection of B- or epithelial cells is still limited. EBV is a highly (but not exclusively) lymphotropic virus that has variously been shown to infect macrophages, neutrophils, T cells, and natural killer cells (Faulkner *et al.*, 2000). However, the second major target of the virus is considered as the epithelial cell. EBV infects B lymphocytes through the surface CD21 molecules, and several key viral and cellular proteins involved in B-cell infection have been identified. Unlike infection of B lymphocytes, EBV infection of primary epithelial cells initiates lytic infection although the cell surface receptors remain to be identified and less is known about the important players in epithelial cell infection. Certainly, a very different picture as the one for B lymphocytes is gradually emerging. Epithelial cell malignancies comprise a large portion of EBV-associated disease worldwide, and epithelial cells may play an important role in spreading the virus both within and between hosts. In the future, it will be necessary to explore how EBV replication in each cell type may influence viral trafficking, transmission and persistence.

Developing drugs and prophylactic vaccines against EBV-associated diseases will be among the most important challenges for the future. Target molecules present on latency I, II, and III diseases have been well defined and the relative importance of both the cellular and the humoral responses are now understood at least in the broad sense. The continued expression of EBV proteins provides multiple opportunities to target the viral proteins and their properties using immunotherapy, inhibitors of critical activated pathways, or specific molecular therapy directed toward the viral functions. Besides EBV, some herpesviruses and SV40 are the few known DNA viruses that encode miRNA. The miRNA-mediated regulation appears to occur mainly at the post-transcription level. Although the relative abundance of EBV miRNAs in different tumors has not been carefully compared, the abundance of EBV miRNAs in NPC samples suggests that these molecules may be ideal targets for therapeutic intervention. Future work aimed at understanding their roles in tumorigenesis and immune modulation may help researchers design new potential therapeutic strategies for NPC and other EBV-associated diseases. Moreover, the RNA interference (RNAi) approaches targeting individual viral proteins or EBV miRNA is only now beginning to support the rational development of potential drugs against EBV.

In sum, this chapter has sought to survey the various EBV-encoded gene/proteins, examine their biological functions related to oncogenesis, highlight our current understanding of EBV biology and disease pathogenesis, and consider the most important challenges for the future.

References

Aiyar A, Tyree C, Sugden B (1998) The plasmid replicon of EBV consists of multiple *cis*-acting elements that facilitate DNA synthesis by the cell and a viral maintenance element. *EMBO J* **17**: 6394–6403.

Allday MJ, Crawford DH, Griffin BE (1989) Epstein-Barr virus latent gene expression during the initiation of B cell immortalization. *J Gen Virol* **70**(Pt 7): 1755–1764.

Ambinder RF, Browning PJ, Lorenzana I, Leventhal BG, Cosenza H, Mann RB, MacMahon EM, Medina R, Cardona V, Grufferman S *et al.* (1993) Epstein-Barr virus and childhood Hodgkin's disease in Honduras and the United States. *Blood* **81**: 462–467.

Ambinder RF, Mullen MA, Chang YN, Hayward GS, Hayward SD (1991) Functional domains of Epstein-Barr virus nuclear antigen EBNA-1. *J Virol* **65**: 1466–1478.

Ambinder RF, Robertson KD, Tao Q (1999) DNA methylation and the Epstein-Barr virus. *Semin Cancer Biol* **9**: 369–375.

Ambros V (2001) MicroRNAs: tiny regulators with great potential. *Cell* **107**: 823–826.

Anderton E, Yee J, Smith P, Crook T, White RE, Allday MJ (2008) Two Epstein-Barr virus (EBV) oncoproteins cooperate to repress expression of the proapoptotic tumour-suppressor Bim: clues to the pathogenesis of Burkitt's lymphoma. *Oncogene* **27**: 421–433.

Arrand JR, Rymo L (1982) Characterization of the major Epstein-Barr virus-specific RNA in Burkitt lymphoma-derived cells. *J Virol* **41**: 376–389.

Aviel S, Winberg G, Massucci M, Ciechanover A (2000) Degradation of the Epstein-Barr virus latent membrane protein 1 (LMP1) by the ubiquitin-proteasome pathway. Targeting via ubiquitination of the N-terminal residue. *J Biol Chem* **275**: 23491–23499.

Baer R, Bankier AT, Biggin MD, Deininger PL, Farrell PJ, Gibson TJ, Hatfull G, Hudson GS, Satchwell SC, Seguin C *et al.* (1984) DNA sequence and expression of the B95-8 Epstein-Barr virus genome. *Nature* **310**: 207–211.

Barth S, Pfuhl T, Mamiani A, Ehses C, Roemer K, Kremmer E, Jaker C, Hock J, Meister G, Grasser FA (2008) Epstein-Barr virus-encoded microRNA miR-BART2 down-regulates the viral DNA polymerase *BALF5*. *Nucleic Acids Res* **36**: 666–675.

Baylin SB, Chen WY (2005) Aberrant gene silencing in tumor progression: implications for control of cancer. *Cold Spring Harb Symp Quant Biol* **70**: 427–433.

Baylin SB, Esteller M, Rountree MR, Bachman KE, Schuebel K, Herman JG (2001) Aberrant patterns of DNA methylation, chromatin formation and gene expression in cancer. *Hum Mol Genet* **10**: 687–692.

Bhatia K, Raj A, Guitierrez MI, Judde JG, Spangler G, Venkatesh H, Magrath IT (1996) Variation in the sequence of Epstein Barr virus nuclear antigen 1 in normal peripheral blood lymphocytes and in Burkitt's lymphomas. *Oncogene* **13**: 177–181.

Bochkarev A, Barwell JA, Pfuetzner RA, Furey W Jr, Edwards AM, Frappier L (1995) Crystal structure of the DNA-binding domain of the Epstein-Barr virus origin-binding protein EBNA 1. *Cell* **83**: 39–46.

Bochkarev A, Bochkareva E, Frappier L, Edwards AM (1998) The 2.2 A structure of a permanganate-sensitive DNA site bound by the Epstein-Barr virus origin binding protein, EBNA1. *J Mol Biol* **284**: 1273–1278.

Brennan P, Floettmann JE, Mehl A, Jones M, Rowe M (2001) Mechanism of action of a novel latent membrane protein-1 dominant negative. *J Biol Chem* **276**: 1195–1203.

Brinkmann MM, Schulz TF (2006) Regulation of intracellular signalling by the terminal membrane proteins of members of the Gammaherpesvirinae. *J Gen Virol* **87**: 1047–1074.

Brodeur SR, Cheng G, Baltimore D, Thorley-Lawson DA (1997) Localization of the major NF-kappaB-activating site and the sole TRAF3 binding site of LMP-1 defines two distinct signaling motifs. *J Biol Chem* **272**: 19777–19784.

Brooks L, Yao QY, Rickinson AB, Young LS (1992) Epstein-Barr virus latent gene transcription in nasopharyngeal carcinoma cells: coexpression of EBNA1, LMP1, and LMP2 transcripts. *J Virol* **66**: 2689–2697.

Brousset P, Butet V, Chittal S, Selves J, Delsol G (1992) Comparison of *in situ* hybridization using different nonisotopic probes for detection of Epstein-Barr virus in nasopharyngeal carcinoma and immunohistochemical correlation with anti-latent membrane protein antibody. *Lab Invest* **67**: 457–464.

Busson P, McCoy R, Sadler R, Gilligan K, Tursz T, Raab-Traub N (1992) Consistent transcription of the Epstein-Barr virus LMP2 gene in nasopharyngeal carcinoma. *J Virol* **66**: 3257–3262.

Cai X, Schafer A, Lu S, Bilello JP, Desrosiers RC, Edwards R, Raab-Traub N, Cullen BR (2006) Epstein-Barr virus microRNAs are evolutionarily conserved and differentially expressed. *PLoS Pathog* **2**: e23.

Calderwood MA, Venkatesan K, Xing L, Chase MR, Vazquez A, Holthaus AM, Ewence AE, Li N, Hirozane-Kishikawa T, Hill DE, Vidal M, Kieff E, Johannsen E (2007) Epstein-Barr virus and virus human protein interaction maps. *Proc Natl Acad Sci USA* **104**: 7606–7611.

Chan AS, To KF, Lo KW, Mak KF, Pak W, Chiu B, Tse GM, Ding M, Li X, Lee JC, Huang DP (2000) High frequency of chromosome 3p deletion in histologically normal nasopharyngeal epithelia from southern Chinese. *Cancer Res* **60**: 5365–5370.

Chang HW, Chan A, Kwong DL, Wei WI, Sham JS, Yuen AP (2003) Evaluation of hypermethylated tumor suppressor genes as tumor markers in mouth and throat rinsing fluid, nasopharyngeal swab and peripheral blood of nasopharygeal carcinoma patient. *Int J Cancer* **105**: 851–855.

Chang Y, Sheen TS, Lu J, Huang YT, Chen JY, Yang CS, Tsai CH (1998) Detection of transcripts initiated from two viral promoters (Cp and Wp) in Epstein-Barr virus-infected nasopharyngeal carcinoma cells and biopsies. *Lab Invest* **78**: 715–726.

Chen ML, Tsai CN, Liang CL, Shu CH, Huang CR, Sulitzeanu D, Liu ST, Chang YS (1992) Cloning and characterization of the latent membrane protein (LMP) of a specific Epstein-Barr virus variant derived from the nasopharyngeal carcinoma in the Taiwanese population. *Oncogene* 7: 2131–2140.

Chen MR, Tsai CH, Wu FF, Kan SH, Yang CS, Chen JY (1999) The major immunogenic epitopes of Epstein-Barr virus (EBV) nuclear antigen 1 are encoded by sequence domains which vary among nasopharyngeal carcinoma biopsies and EBV-associated cell lines. *J Gen Virol* **80**(Pt 2): 447–455.

Chiang AK, Wong KY, Liang AC, Srivastava G (1999) Comparative analysis of Epstein-Barr virus gene polymorphisms in nasal T/NK-cell lymphomas and normal nasal tissues: implications on virus strain selection in malignancy. *Int J Cancer* **80**: 356–364.

Cohen JI, Wang F, Mannick J, Kieff E (1989) Epstein-Barr virus nuclear protein 2 is a key determinant of lymphocyte transformation. *Proc Natl Acad Sci USA* **86**: 9558–9562.

Cordier M, Calender A, Billaud M, Zimber U, Rousselet G, Pavlish O, Banchereau J, Tursz T, Bornkamm G, Lenoir GM (1990) Stable transfection of Epstein-Barr virus (EBV) nuclear antigen 2 in lymphoma cells containing the EBV P3HR1 genome induces expression of B-cell activation molecules CD21 and CD23. *J Virol* **64**: 1002–1013.

D'Souza B, Rowe M, Walls D (2000) The bfl-1 gene is transcriptionally upregulated by the Epstein-Barr virus LMP1, and its expression promotes the survival of a Burkitt's lymphoma cell line. *J Virol* **74**: 6652–6658.

Dalmay T, Edwards DR (2006) MicroRNAs and the hallmarks of cancer. *Oncogene* **25**: 6170–6175.

Dawson CW, Tramountanis G, Eliopoulos AG, Young LS (2003) Epstein-Barr virus latent membrane protein 1 (LMP1) activates the phosphatidylinositol 3-kinase/Akt pathway to promote cell survival and induce actin filament remodeling. *J Biol Chem* **278**: 3694–3704.

de Jesus O, Smith PR, Spender LC, Elgueta Karstegl C, Niller HH, Huang D, Farrell PJ (2003) Updated Epstein-Barr virus (EBV) DNA sequence and analysis of a promoter for the BART (CST, BARF0) RNAs of EBV. *J Gen Virol* **84**: 1443–1450.

Deng Z, Atanasiu C, Zhao K, Marmorstein R, Sbodio JI, Chi NW, Lieberman PM (2005) Inhibition of Epstein-Barr virus *OriP* function by tankyrase, a telomere-associated poly-ADP ribose polymerase that binds and modifies EBNA1. *J Virol* 79: 4640–4650.

Deng Z, Lezina L, Chen CJ, Shtivelband S, So W, Lieberman PM (2002) Telomeric proteins regulate episomal maintenance of Epstein-Barr virus origin of plasmid replication. *Mol Cell* 9: 493–503.

Devergne O, Hatzivassiliou E, Izumi KM, Kaye KM, Kleijnen MF, Kieff E, Mosialos G (1996) Association of TRAF1, TRAF2, and TRAF3 with an Epstein-Barr virus LMP1 domain important for B-lymphocyte transformation: role in NF-kappaB activation. *Mol Cell Biol* **16**: 7098–7108.

Dhar SK, Yoshida K, Machida Y, Khaira P, Chaudhuri B, Wohlschlegel JA, Leffak M, Yates J, Dutta A (2001) Replication from *oriP* of Epstein-Barr virus requires human ORC and is inhibited by geminin. *Cell* **106**: 287–296.

Dillner J, Sternas L, Kallin B, Alexander H, Ehlin-Henriksson B, Jornvall H, Klein G, Lerner R (1984) Antibodies against a synthetic peptide identify the Epstein-Barr virus-determined nuclear antigen. *Proc Natl Acad Sci USA* **81**: 4652–4656.

Ding L, Li L, Yang J, Zhou S, Li W, Tang M, Shi Y, Yi W, Cao Y (2007) Latent membrane protein 1 encoded by Epstein-Barr virus induces telomerase activity via p16INK4A/Rb/E2F1 and JNK signaling pathways. *J Med Virol* **79**: 1153–1163.

Do NV, Ingemar E, Phi PT, Jenny A, Chinh TT, Zeng Y, Hu L (2008) A major EBNA1 variant from Asian EBV isolates shows enhanced transcriptional activity compared to prototype B95.8. *Virus Res* **132**: 15–24.

Dolcetti R, Zancai P, De Re V, Gloghini A, Bigoni B, Pivetta B, De Vita S, Carbone A, Boiocchi M (1997) Epstein-Barr virus strains with latent membrane protein-1 deletions: prevalence in the Italian population and high association with human immunodeficiency virus-related Hodgkin's disease. *Blood* **89**: 1723–1731.

Dolyniuk M, Pritchett R, Kieff E (1976a) Proteins of Epstein-Barr virus. I. Analysis of the polypeptides of purified enveloped Epstein-Barr virus. *J Virol* **17**: 935–949.

Dolyniuk M, Wolff E, Kieff E (1976b) Proteins of Epstein-Barr virus. II. Electrophoretic analysis of the polypeptides of the nucleocapsid and the glucosamine- and polysaccharide-containing components of enveloped virus. *J Virol* **18**: 289–297.

Dykstra ML, Longnecker R, Pierce SK (2001) Epstein-Barr virus coopts lipid rafts to block the signaling and antigen transport functions of the BCR. *Immunity* **14**: 57–67.

Eliopoulos AG, Blake SM, Floettmann JE, Rowe M, Young LS (1999a) Epstein-Barr virus-encoded latent membrane protein 1 activates the JNK pathway through its extreme C terminus via a mechanism involving TRADD and TRAF2. *J Virol* **73**: 1023–1035.

Eliopoulos AG, Caamano JH, Flavell J, Reynolds GM, Murray PG, Poyet JL, Young LS (2003) Epstein-Barr virus-encoded latent infection membrane protein 1 regulates the processing of p100 NF-kappaB2 to p52 via an IKKgamma/NEMO-independent signalling pathway. *Oncogene* **22**: 7557–7569.

Eliopoulos AG, Gallagher NJ, Blake SM, Dawson CW, Young LS (1999b) Activation of the p38 mitogen-activated protein kinase pathway by Epstein-Barr virus-encoded latent membrane protein 1 coregulates interleukin-6 and interleukin-8 production. *J Biol Chem* **274**: 16085–16096.

Eliopoulos AG, Young LS (2001) LMP1 structure and signal transduction. *Semin Cancer Biol* **11**: 435–444.

Epstein MA, Achong BG, Barr YM (1964) Virus particles in cultured lymphoblasts from Burkitt's lymphoma. *Lancet* **1**: 702–703.

Epstein MA, Barr YM (1964) Cultivation *in vitro* of human lymphoblasts from Burkitt's Malignant lymphoma. *Lancet* **1**: 252–253.

Epstein MA, Henle G, Achong BG, Barr YM (1965) Morphological and biological studies on a virus in cultured lymphoblasts from Burkitt's lymphoma. *J Exp Med* **121**: 761–770.

Esteller M, Herman JG (2002) Cancer as an epigenetic disease: DNA methylation and chromatin alterations in human tumours. *J Pathol* **196**: 1–7.

Faulkner GC, Krajewski AS, Crawford DH (2000) The ins and outs of EBV infection. *Trends Microbiol* **8**: 185–189.

Fischer N, Kremmer E, Lautscham G, Mueller-Lantzsch N, Grasser FA (1997) Epstein-Barr virus nuclear antigen 1 forms a complex with the nuclear transporter karyopherin alpha2. *J Biol Chem* **272**: 3999–4005.

Flanagan JM (2007) Host epigenetic modifications by oncogenic viruses. *Br J Cancer* **96**: 183–188.

Fruehling S, Longnecker R (1997) The immunoreceptor tyrosine-based activation motif of Epstein-Barr virus LMP2A is essential for blocking BCR-mediated signal transduction. *Virology* **235**: 241–251.

Fruehling S, Swart R, Dolwick KM, Kremmer E, Longnecker R (1998) Tyrosine 112 of latent membrane protein 2A is essential for protein tyrosine kinase loading and regulation of Epstein-Barr virus latency. *J Virol* **72**: 7796–7806.

Furnari FB, Adams MD, Pagano JS (1993) Unconventional processing of the 3′ termini of the Epstein-Barr virus DNA polymerase mRNA. *Proc Natl Acad Sci USA* **90**: 378–382.

Gal AA, Unger ER, Koss MN, Yen TS (1991) Detection of Epstein-Barr virus in lymphoepithelioma-like carcinoma of the lung. *Mod Pathol* **4**: 264–268.

Gires O, Kohlhuber F, Kilger E, Baumann M, Kieser A, Kaiser C, Zeidler R, Scheffer B, Ueffing M, Hammerschmidt W (1999) Latent membrane protein 1 of Epstein-Barr virus interacts with JAK3 and activates STAT proteins. *EMBO J* **18**: 3064–3073.

Gires O, Zimber-Strobl U, Gonnella R, Ueffing M, Marschall G, Zeidler R, Pich D, Hammerschmidt W (1997) Latent membrane protein 1 of Epstein-Barr virus mimics a constitutively active receptor molecule. *EMBO J* **16**: 6131–6140.

Given D, Kieff E (1979) DNA of Epstein-Barr virus. VI. Mapping of the internal tandem reiteration. *J Virol* **31**: 315–324.

Goldsmith K, Bendell L, Frappier L (1993) Identification of EBNA1 amino acid sequences required for the interaction of the functional elements of the Epstein-Barr virus latent origin of DNA replication. *J Virol* **67**: 3418–3426.

Grundhoff A, Sullivan CS, Ganem D (2006) A combined computational and microarray-based approach identifies novel microRNAs encoded by human gamma-herpesviruses. *RNA* **12**: 733–750.

Gutierrez MI, Raj A, Spangler G, Sharma A, Hussain A, Judde JG, Tsao SW, Yuen PW, Joab I, Magrath IT, Bhatia K (1997) Sequence variations in EBNA-1 may dictate restriction of tissue distribution of Epstein-Barr virus in normal and tumour cells. *J Gen Virol* **78**(Pt 7): 1663–1670.

Gutierrez MI, Spangler G, Kingma D, Raffeld M, Guerrero I, Misad O, Jaffe ES, Magrath IT, Bhatia K (1998) Epstein-Barr virus in nasal lymphomas contains multiple ongoing mutations in the EBNA-1 gene. *Blood* **92**: 600–606.

Habeshaw G, Yao QY, Bell AI, Morton D, Rickinson AB (1999) Epstein-Barr virus nuclear antigen 1 sequences in endemic and sporadic Burkitt's lymphoma reflect virus strains prevalent in different geographic areas. *J Virol* **73**: 965–975.

Hadhri-Guiga B, Khabir AM, Mokdad-Gargouri R, Ghorbel AM, Drira M, Daoud J, Frikha M, Jlidi R, Gargouri A (2006) Various 30 and 69 bp deletion variants of the Epstein-Barr virus LMP1 may arise by homologous recombination in nasopharyngeal carcinoma of Tunisian patients. *Virus Res* **115**: 24–30.

Hahn P, Novikova E, Scherback L, Janik C, Pavlish O, Arkhipov V, Nicholls J, Muller-Lantzsch N, Gurtsevitch V, Grasser FA (2001) The LMP1 gene isolated from Russian nasopharyngeal carcinoma has no 30-bp deletion. *Int J Cancer* **91**: 815–821.

Hammerschmidt W, Sugden B (1989) Genetic analysis of immortalizing functions of Epstein-Barr virus in human B lymphocytes. *Nature* **340**: 393–397.

Han I, Harada S, Weaver D, Xue Y, Lane W, Orstavik S, Skalhegg B, Kieff E (2001) EBNA-LP associates with cellular proteins including DNA-PK and HA95. *J Virol* **75**: 2475–2481.

Han I, Xue Y, Harada S, Orstavik S, Skalhegg B, Kieff E (2002) Protein kinase A associates with HA95 and affects transcriptional coactivation by Epstein-Barr virus nuclear proteins. *Mol Cell Biol* **22**: 2136–2146.

Harrison S, Fisenne K, Hearing J (1994) Sequence requirements of the Epstein-Barr virus latent origin of DNA replication. *J Virol* **68**: 1913–1925.

Hayward SD, Kieff E (1977) DNA of Epstein-Barr virus. II. Comparison of the molecular weights of restriction endonuclease fragments of the DNA of Epstein-Barr virus strains and identification of end fragments of the B95-8 strain. *J Virol* **23**: 421–429.

Hearing JC, Levine AJ (1985) The Epstein-Barr virus nuclear antigen (BamHI K antigen) is a single-stranded DNA binding phosphoprotein. *Virology* **145**: 105–116.

Henkel T, Ling PD, Hayward SD, Peterson MG (1994) Mediation of Epstein-Barr virus EBNA2 transactivation by recombination signal-binding protein J kappa. *Science* **265**: 92–95.

Henle G, Henle W (1966) Studies on cell lines derived from Burkitt's lymphoma. *Trans NY Acad Sci* **29**: 71–79.

Hennessy K, Heller M, van Santen V, Kieff E (1983) Simple repeat array in Epstein-Barr virus DNA encodes part of the Epstein-Barr nuclear antigen. *Science* **220**: 1396–1398.

Herman JG, Baylin SB (2003) Gene silencing in cancer in association with promoter hypermethylation. *N Engl J Med* **349**: 2042–2054.

Heussinger N, Buttner M, Ott G, Brachtel E, Pilch BZ, Kremmer E, Niedobitek G (2004) Expression of the Epstein-Barr virus (EBV)-encoded latent membrane protein 2A (LMP2A) in EBV-associated nasopharyngeal carcinoma. *J Pathol* **203**: 696–699.

Hickabottom M, Parker GA, Freemont P, Crook T, Allday MJ (2002) Two nonconsensus sites in the Epstein-Barr virus oncoprotein EBNA3A cooperate to bind the co-repressor carboxyl-terminal-binding protein (CtBP). *J Biol Chem* **277**: 47197–47204.

Higuchi M, Izumi KM, Kieff E (2001) Epstein-Barr virus latent-infection membrane proteins are palmitoylated and raft-associated: protein 1 binds to the cytoskeleton through TNF receptor cytoplasmic factors. *Proc Natl Acad Sci USA* **98**: 4675–4680.

Holowaty MN, Sheng Y, Nguyen T, Arrowsmith C, Frappier L (2003a) Protein interaction domains of the ubiquitin-specific protease, USP7/HAUSP. *J Biol Chem* **278**: 47753–47761.

Holowaty MN, Zeghouf M, Wu H, Tellam J, Athanasopoulos V, Greenblatt J, Frappier L (2003b) Protein profiling with Epstein-Barr nuclear antigen-1 reveals an interaction with the herpesvirus-associated ubiquitin-specific protease HAUSP/USP7. *J Biol Chem* **278**: 29987–29994.

Hu LF, Chen F, Zheng X, Ernberg I, Cao SL, Christensson B, Klein G, Winberg G (1993) Clonability and tumorigenicity of human epithelial cells expressing the EBV encoded membrane protein LMP1. *Oncogene* **8**: 1575–1583.

Hu LF, Zabarovsky ER, Chen F, Cao SL, Ernberg I, Klein G, Winberg G (1991) Isolation and sequencing of the Epstein-Barr virus BNLF-1 gene (LMP1) from a Chinese nasopharyngeal carcinoma. *J Gen Virol* **72**(Pt 10): 2399–2409.

Huen DS, Henderson SA, Croom-Carter D, Rowe M (1995) The Epstein-Barr virus latent membrane protein-1 (LMP1) mediates activation of NF-kappaB and cell surface phenotype via two effector regions in its carboxy-terminal cytoplasmic domain. *Oncogene* **10**: 549–560.

Inoue J, Gohda J, Akiyama T, Semba K (2007) NF-kappaB activation in development and progression of cancer. *Cancer Sci* **98**: 268–274.

Ito S, Ikeda M, Kato N, Matsumoto A, Ishikawa Y, Kumakubo S, Yanagi K (2000) Epstein-Barr virus nuclear antigen-1 binds to nuclear transporter karyopherin alpha1/NPI-1 in addition to karyopherin alpha2/Rch1. *Virology* **266**: 110–119.

Iwakiri D, Eizuru Y, Tokunaga M, Takada K (2003) Autocrine growth of Epstein-Barr virus-positive gastric carcinoma cells mediated by an Epstein-Barr virus-encoded small RNA. *Cancer Res* **63**: 7062–7067.

Izumi KM, Cahir McFarland ED, Riley EA, Rizzo D, Chen Y, Kieff E (1999a) The residues between the two transformation effector sites of Epstein-Barr virus latent membrane protein 1 are not critical for B lymphocyte growth transformation. *J Virol* **73**: 9908–9916.

Izumi KM, Cahir McFarland ED, Ting AT, Riley EA, Seed B, Kieff ED (1999b) The Epstein-Barr virus oncoprotein latent membrane protein 1 engages the tumor necrosis factor receptor-associated proteins TRADD and receptor-interacting protein (RIP) but does not induce apoptosis or require RIP for NF-kappaB activation. *Mol Cell Biol* **19**: 5759–5767.

Izumi KM, Kaye KM, Kieff ED (1994) Epstein-Barr virus recombinant molecular genetic analysis of the LMP1 amino-terminal cytoplasmic domain reveals a probable structural role, with no component essential for primary B lymphocyte growth transformation. *J Virol* **68**: 4369–4376.

Izumi KM, Kaye KM, Kieff ED (1997) The Epstein-Barr virus LMP1 amino acid sequence that engages tumor necrosis factor receptor associated factors is critical for primary B lymphocyte growth transformation. *Proc Natl Acad Sci USA* **94**: 1447–1452.

Izumi KM, Kieff ED (1997) The Epstein-Barr virus oncogene product latent membrane protein 1 engages the tumor necrosis factor receptor-associated death domain protein to mediate B lymphocyte growth transformation and activate NF-kappaB. *Proc Natl Acad Sci USA* **94**: 12592–12597.

Jin XW, Speck SH (1992) Identification of critical *cis* elements involved in mediating Epstein-Barr virus nuclear antigen 2-dependent activity of an enhancer located upstream of the viral BamHI C promoter. *J Virol* **66**: 2846–2852.

Johannsen E, Koh E, Mosialos G, Tong X, Kieff E, Grossman SR (1995) Epstein-Barr virus nuclear protein 2 transactivation of the latent membrane protein 1 promoter is mediated by J kappa and PU.1. *J Virol* **69**: 253–262.

Jones JF, Shurin S, Abramowsky C, Tubbs RR, Sciotto CG, Wahl R, Sands J, Gottman D, Katz BZ, Sklar J (1988) T-cell lymphomas containing Epstein-Barr viral DNA in patients with chronic Epstein-Barr virus infections. *N Engl J Med* **318**: 733–741.

Jones PA (2002) DNA methylation and cancer. *Oncogene* **21**: 5358–5360.

Jones PA, Baylin SB (2002) The fundamental role of epigenetic events in cancer. *Nat Rev Genet* **3**: 415–428.

Kang MS, Lu H, Yasui T, Sharpe A, Warren H, Cahir-McFarland E, Bronson R, Hung SC, Kieff E (2005) Epstein-Barr virus nuclear antigen 1 does not induce lymphoma in transgenic FVB mice. *Proc Natl Acad Sci USA* **102**: 820–825.

Kapoor P, Lavoie BD, Frappier L (2005) EBP2 plays a key role in Epstein-Barr virus mitotic segregation and is regulated by aurora family kinases. *Mol Cell Biol* **25**: 4934–4945.

Kaul R, Murakami M, Choudhuri T, Robertson ES (2007) Epstein-Barr virus latent nuclear antigens can induce metastasis in a nude mouse model. *J Virol* **81**: 10352–10361.

Kaye KM, Devergne O, Harada JN, Izumi KM, Yalamanchili R, Kieff E, Mosialos G (1996) Tumor necrosis factor receptor associated factor 2 is a mediator of NF-kappaB activation by latent infection membrane protein 1, the Epstein-Barr virus transforming protein. *Proc Natl Acad Sci USA* **93**: 11085–11090.

Kaye KM, Izumi KM, Kieff E (1993) Epstein-Barr virus latent membrane protein 1 is essential for B lymphocyte growth transformation. *Proc Natl Acad Sci USA* **90**: 9150–9154.

Kaye KM, Izumi KM, Mosialos G, Kieff E (1995) The Epstein-Barr virus LMP1 cytoplasmic carboxy terminus is essential for B-lymphocyte transformation; fibroblast cocultivation complements a critical function within the terminal 155 residues. *J Virol* **69**: 675–683.

Kaykas A, Worringer K, Sugden B (2001) CD40 and LMP-1 both signal from lipid rafts but LMP-1 assembles a distinct, more efficient signaling complex. *EMBO J* **20**: 2641–2654.

Kennedy G, Komano J, Sugden B (2003) Epstein-Barr virus provides a survival factor to Burkitt's lymphomas. *Proc Natl Acad Sci USA* **100**: 14269–14274.

Kerr BM, Lear AL, Rowe M, Croom-Carter D, Young LS, Rookes SM, Gallimore PH, Rickinson AB (1992) Three transcriptionally distinct forms of Epstein-Barr virus latency in somatic cell hybrids: cell phenotype dependence of virus promoter usage. *Virology* **187**: 189–201.

Kershaw GR, Berger C, McQuain C, al-Homsi AS, Pihan G, Quesenberry PJ, Woda BA, Knecht H (1997) Selective outgrowth of a posttransplant B-immunoblastic lymphoma expressing a latent membrane protein-1 deletion variant. *Transplantation* **64**: 1079–1081.

Kieff E, Rickinson AB (2007) Epstein-Barr virus and its replication. In: Knipe DM, Howley PM, Griffin DE, Lamb RA, Martin MA, Roizman B, Straus SE (eds.), *Fields Virology*. Philadelphia: Lippincott, Williams & Wilkins.

Kieser A, Kaiser C, Hammerschmidt W (1999) LMP1 signal transduction differs substantially from TNF receptor 1 signaling in the molecular functions of TRADD and TRAF2. *EMBO J* **18**: 2511–2521.

Kieser A, Kilger E, Gires O, Ueffing M, Kolch W, Hammerschmidt W (1997) Epstein-Barr virus latent membrane protein-1 triggers AP-1 activity via the c-Jun N-terminal kinase cascade. *EMBO J* **16**: 6478–6485.

Kilger E, Kieser A, Baumann M, Hammerschmidt W (1998) Epstein-Barr virus-mediated B-cell proliferation is dependent upon latent membrane protein 1, which simulates an activated CD40 receptor. *EMBO J* **17**: 1700–1709.

Kim AL, Maher M, Hayman JB, Ozer J, Zerby D, Yates JL, Lieberman PM (1997) An imperfect correlation between DNA replication activity of Epstein-Barr virus nuclear antigen 1 (EBNA1) and binding to the nuclear import receptor, Rch1/importin alpha. *Virology* **239**: 340–351.

Kim do N, Chae HS, Oh ST, Kang JH, Park CH, Park WS, Takada K, Lee JM, Lee WK, Lee SK (2007) Expression of viral microRNAs in Epstein-Barr virus-associated gastric carcinoma. *J Virol* **81**: 1033–1036.

Kitamura R, Sekimoto T, Ito S, Harada S, Yamagata H, Masai H, Yoneda Y, Yanagi K (2006) Nuclear import of Epstein-Barr virus nuclear antigen 1 mediated by NPI-1 (Importin alpha5) is up- and down-regulated by phosphorylation of the nuclear localization signal for which Lys379 and Arg380 are essential. *J Virol* **80**: 1979–1991.

Klein E, Kis LL, Klein G (2007) Epstein-Barr virus infection in humans: from harmless to life endangering virus-lymphocyte interactions. *Oncogene* **26**: 1297–1305.

Klein G (1976) The biology and serology of Epstein-Barr virus (EBV) infections. *Bull Cancer* **63**: 399–410.

Klein G (1996) EBV-B cell interactions: immortalization, rescue from apoptosis, tumorigenicity (a short review). *Acta Microbiol Immunol Hung* **43**: 97–105.

Knecht H, Bachmann E, Brousset P, Rothenberger S, Einsele H, Lestou VS, Delsol G, Bachmann F, Ambros PF, Odermatt BF (1995) Mutational hot spots within the carboxy terminal region of the LMP1 oncogene of Epstein-Barr virus are frequent in lymphoproliferative disorders. *Oncogene* **10**: 523–528.

Komano J, Maruo S, Kurozumi K, Oda T, Takada K (1999) Oncogenic role of Epstein-Barr virus-encoded RNAs in Burkitt's lymphoma cell line Akata. *J Virol* **73**: 9827–9831.

Kondo S, Wakisaka N, Schell MJ, Horikawa T, Sheen TS, Sato H, Furukawa M, Pagano JS, Yoshizaki T (2005) Epstein-Barr virus latent membrane protein 1 induces the matrix metalloproteinase-1 promoter via an Ets binding site formed by a single nucleotide polymorphism: enhanced susceptibility to nasopharyngeal carcinoma. *Int J Cancer* **115**: 368–376.

Krishna SM, James S, Balaram P (2006) Expression of VEGF as prognosticator in primary nasopharyngeal cancer and its relation to EBV status. *Virus Res* **115**: 85–90.

Kwong J, Lo KW, Chow LS, To KF, Choy KW, Chan FL, Mok SC, Huang DP (2005) Epigenetic silencing of cellular retinol-binding proteins in nasopharyngeal carcinoma. *Neoplasia* **7**: 67–74.

Laherty CD, Hu HM, Opipari AW, Wang F, Dixit VM (1992) The Epstein-Barr virus LMP1 gene product induces A20 zinc finger protein expression by activating nuclear factor kappa B. *J Biol Chem* **267**: 24157–24160.

Lam N, Sugden B (2003) CD40 and its viral mimic, LMP1: similar means to different ends *Cell Signal* **15**: 9–16.

Landgraf P, Rusu M, Sheridan R, Sewer A, Iovino N, Aravin A, Pfeffer S, Rice A, Kamphorst AO, Landthaler M, Lin C, Socci ND, Hermida L, Fulci V, Chiaretti S, Foa R, Schliwka J, Fuchs U, Novosel A, Muller RU, Schermer B, Bissels U, Inman J, Phan Q, Chien M, Weir DB, Choksi R, De Vita G, Frezzetti D, Trompeter HI, Hornung V, Teng G, Hartmann G, Palkovits M, Di Lauro R, Wernet P, Macino G, Rogler CE, Nagle JW, Ju J, Papavasiliou FN, Benzing T, Lichter P, Tam W, Brownstein MJ, Bosio A, Borkhardt A, Russo JJ, Sander C, Zavolan M, Tuschl T (2007) A mammalian microRNA expression atlas based on small RNA library sequencing. *Cell* **129**: 1401–1414.

Laux G, Adam B, Strobl LJ, Moreau-Gachelin F (1994) The Spi-1/PU.1 and Spi-B ets family transcription factors and the recombination signal binding protein RBP-J kappa interact with an Epstein-Barr virus nuclear antigen 2 responsive *cis*-element. *EMBO J* **13**: 5624–5632.

Laux G, Perricaudet M, Farrell PJ (1988) A spliced Epstein-Barr virus gene expressed in immortalized lymphocytes is created by circularization of the linear viral genome. *EMBO J* 7: 769–774.

Levitskaya J, Coram M, Levitsky V, Imreh S, Steigerwald-Mullen PM, Klein G, Kurilla MG, Masucci MG (1995) Inhibition of antigen processing by the internal repeat region of the Epstein-Barr virus nuclear antigen-1. *Nature* **375**: 685–688.

Levitskaya J, Sharipo A, Leonchiks A, Ciechanover A, Masucci MG (1997) Inhibition of ubiquitin/proteasome-dependent protein degradation by the Gly-Ala repeat domain of the Epstein-Barr virus nuclear antigen 1. *Proc Natl Acad Sci USA* **94**: 12616–12621.

Li H, Minarovits J (2003) Host cell-dependent expression of latent Epstein-Barr virus genomes: regulation by DNA methylation. *Adv Cancer Res* **89**: 133–156.

Li HP, Chang YS (2003) Epstein-Barr virus latent membrane protein 1: structure and functions. *J Biomed Sci* **10**: 490–504.

Li HP, Leu YW, Chang YS (2005) Epigenetic changes in virus-associated human cancers. *Cell Res* **15**: 262–271.

Li L, Guo L, Tao Y, Zhou S, Wang Z, Luo W, Hu D, Li Z, Xiao L, Tang M, Yi W, Tsao SW, Cao Y (2007) Latent membrane protein 1 of Epstein-Barr virus regulates p53 phosphorylation through MAP kinases. *Cancer Lett* **255**: 219–231.

Li M, Chen D, Shiloh A, Luo J, Nikolaev AY, Qin J, Gu W (2002) Deubiquitination of p53 by HAUSP is an important pathway for p53 stabilization. *Nature* **416**: 648–653.

Li SN, Chang YS, Liu ST (1996) Effect of a 10-amino acid deletion on the oncogenic activity of latent membrane protein 1 of Epstein-Barr virus *Oncogene* **12**: 2129–2135.

Li YH, Shao JY, Li S, Zou BY, Huang HQ, Guan ZZ (2004) [Clinical significance of quantitative analysis of serum VEGF, CD44s, and MMP-3 protein in nasopharyngeal carcinoma]. *Ai Zheng* **23**: 1060–1064.

Ling PD, Peng RS, Nakajima A, Yu JH, Tan J, Moses SM, Yang WH, Zhao B, Kieff E, Bloch KD, Bloch DB (2005) Mediation of Epstein-Barr virus EBNA-LP transcriptional coactivation by Sp100. *EMBO J* **24**: 3565–3575.

Liu HP, Wu CC, Chang YS (2006) PRA1 promotes the intracellular trafficking and NF-kappaB signaling of EBV latent membrane protein 1. *EMBO J* **25**: 4120–4130.

Liu XQ, Chen HK, Zhang XS, Pan ZG, Li A, Feng QS, Long QX, Wang XZ, Zeng YX (2003) Alterations of BLU, a candidate tumor suppressor gene on chromosome 3p21.3, in human nasopharyngeal carcinoma. *Int J Cancer* **106**: 60–65.

Liu YP, Tan YN, Wang ZL, Zeng L, Lu ZX, Li LL, Luo W, Tang M, Cao Y (2008) Phosphorylation and nuclear translocation of STAT3 regulated by the Epstein-Barr virus latent membrane protein 1 in nasopharyngeal carcinoma. *Int J Mol Med* **21**: 153–162.

Lo AK, To KF, Lo KW, Lung RW, Hui JW, Liao G, Hayward SD (2007) Modulation of LMP1 protein expression by EBV-encoded microRNAs. *Proc Natl Acad Sci USA* **104**: 16164–16169.

Lo KW, Huang DP (2002) Genetic and epigenetic changes in nasopharyngeal carcinoma. *Semin Cancer Biol* **12**: 451–462.

Lo KW, Kwong J, Hui AB, Chan SY, To KF, Chan AS, Chow LS, Teo PM, Johnson PJ, Huang DP (2001) High frequency of promoter hypermethylation of RASSF1A in nasopharyngeal carcinoma. *Cancer Res* **61**: 3877–3881.

Longnecker R (2000) Epstein-Barr virus latency: LMP2, a regulator or means for Epstein-Barr virus persistence? *Adv Cancer Res* **79**: 175–200.

Longnecker R, Kieff E (1990) A second Epstein-Barr virus membrane protein (LMP2) is expressed in latent infection and colocalizes with LMP1. *J Virol* **64**: 2319–2326.

Lu J, Lin WH, Chen SY, Longnecker R, Tsai SC, Chen CL, Tsai CH (2006) Syk tyrosine kinase mediates Epstein-Barr virus latent membrane protein 2A-induced cell migration in epithelial cells. *J Biol Chem* **281**: 8806–8814.

Luftig M, Prinarakis E, Yasui T, Tsichritzis T, Cahir-McFarland E, Inoue J, Nakano H, Mak TW, Yeh WC, Li X, Akira S, Suzuki N, Suzuki S, Mosialos G, Kieff E (2003) Epstein-Barr virus latent membrane protein 1 activation of NF-kappaB through IRAK1 and TRAF6. *Proc Natl Acad Sci USA* **100**: 15595–15600.

Lung HL, Cheung AK, Xie D, Cheng Y, Kwong FM, Murakami Y, Guan XY, Sham JS, Chua D, Protopopov AI, Zabarovsky ER, Tsao SW, Stanbridge EJ, Lung ML (2006) TSLC1 is a tumor suppressor gene associated with metastasis in nasopharyngeal carcinoma. *Cancer Res* **66**: 9385–9392.

Lynch DT, Zimmerman JS, Rowe DT (2002) Epstein-Barr virus latent membrane protein 2B (LMP2B) co-localizes with LMP2A in perinuclear regions in transiently transfected cells. *J Gen Virol* **83**: 1025–1035.

Mackey D, Middleton T, Sugden B (1995) Multiple regions within EBNA1 can link DNAs. *J Virol* **69**: 6199–6208.

Mai SJ, Ooka T, Li DJ, Zeng MS, Jiang RC, Yu XJ, Zhang RH, Chen SP, Zeng YX (2007) Functional advantage of NPC-related V-val subtype of Epstein-Barr virus nuclear antigen 1 compared with prototype in epithelial cell line. *Oncol Rep* **17**: 141–146.

Mainou BA, Everly DN Jr, Raab-Traub N (2005) Epstein-Barr virus latent membrane protein 1 CTAR1 mediates rodent and human fibroblast transformation through activation of PI3K. *Oncogene* **24**: 6917–6924.

Marechal V, Dehee A, Chikhi-Brachet R, Piolot T, Coppey-Moisan M, Nicolas JC (1999) Mapping EBNA-1 domains involved in binding to metaphase chromosomes. *J Virol* **73**: 4385–4392.

Matskova L, Ernberg I, Pawson T, Winberg G (2001) C-terminal domain of the Epstein-Barr virus LMP2A membrane protein contains a clustering signal. *J Virol* **75**: 10941–10949.

Merchant M, Swart R, Katzman RB, Ikeda M, Ikeda A, Longnecker R, Dykstra ML, Pierce SK (2001) The effects of the Epstein-Barr virus latent membrane protein 2A on B cell function. *Int Rev Immunol* **20**: 805–835.

Miller CL, Lee JH, Kieff E, Burkhardt AL, Bolen JB, Longnecker R (1994) Epstein-Barr virus protein LMP2A regulates reactivation from latency by negatively regulating tyrosine kinases involved in sIg-mediated signal transduction. *Infect Agents Dis* **3**: 128–136.

Milman G, Hwang ES (1987) Epstein-Barr virus nuclear antigen forms a complex that binds with high concentration dependence to a single DNA-binding site. *J Virol* **61**: 465–471.

Miyashita EM, Yang B, Babcock GJ, Thorley-Lawson DA (1997) Identification of the site of Epstein-Barr virus persistence *in vivo* as a resting B cell. *J Virol* **71**: 4882–4891.

Moody CA, Scott RS, Amirghahari N, Nathan CA, Young LS, Dawson CW, Sixbey JW (2005) Modulation of the cell growth regulator mTOR by Epstein-Barr virus-encoded LMP2A. *J Virol* **79**: 5499–5506.

Murakami M, Lan K, Subramanian C, Robertson ES (2005) Epstein-Barr virus nuclear antigen 1 interacts with Nm23-H1 in lymphoblastoid cell lines and inhibits its ability to suppress cell migration. *J Virol* **79**: 1559–1568.

Murono S, Inoue H, Tanabe T, Joab I, Yoshizaki T, Furukawa M, Pagano JS (2001) Induction of cyclooxygenase-2 by Epstein-Barr virus latent membrane protein 1 is involved in vascular endothelial growth factor production in nasopharyngeal carcinoma cells. *Proc Natl Acad Sci USA* **98**: 6905–6910.

Mutirangura A, Tanunyutthawongese C, Kerekhanjanarong V, Sriuranpong V, Pornthanakasem W, Yenrudi S, Supiyaphun P, Voravud N (1996) Loss of heterozygosity for chromosome 11 in Epstein-Barr-virus associated nasopharyngeal carcinoma. *J Med Assoc Thai* **79**(1): S65–S70.

Neri A, Barriga F, Inghirami G, Knowles DM, Neequaye J, Magrath IT, Dalla-Favera R (1991) Epstein-Barr virus infection precedes clonal expansion in Burkitt's and acquired immunodeficiency syndrome-associated lymphoma. *Blood* 77: 1092–1095.

Neufeld G, Cohen T, Gengrinovitch S, Poltorak Z (1999) Vascular endothelial growth factor (VEGF) and its receptors. *Faseb J* **13**: 9–22.

Niedobitek G, Young LS, Lau R, Brooks L, Greenspan D, Greenspan JS, Rickinson AB (1991) Epstein-Barr virus infection in oral hairy leukoplakia: virus replication in the absence of a detectable latent phase. *J Gen Virol* **72** (Pt 12): 3035–3046.

Niu G, Wright KL, Huang M, Song L, Haura E, Turkson J, Zhang S, Wang T, Sinibaldi D, Coppola D, Heller R, Ellis LM, Karras J, Bromberg J, Pardoll D, Jove R, Yu H (2002) Constitutive Stat3 activity up-regulates VEGF expression and tumor angiogenesis. *Oncogene* **21**: 2000–2008.

Pan ZG, Kashuba VI, Liu XQ, Shao JY, Zhang RH, Jiang JH, Guo C, Zabarovsky E, Ernberg I, Zeng YX (2005) High frequency somatic mutations in RASSF1A in nasopharyngeal carcinoma. *Cancer Biol Ther* **4**: 1116–1122.

Parker GA, Touitou R, Allday MJ (2000) Epstein-Barr virus EBNA3C can disrupt multiple cell cycle checkpoints and induce nuclear division divorced from cytokinesis. *Oncogene* **19**: 700–709.

Paulsen SJ, Rosenkilde MM, Eugen-Olsen J, Kledal TN, Beisser PS, Verzijl D, Gruijthuijsen YK, Beuken E, Smit MJ, Leurs R, Bruggeman CA, Vink C (2005) Epstein-Barr virus-encoded BILF1 is a constitutively active G protein-coupled receptor. *J Virol* **79**: 536–546.

Pear WS, Aster JC, Scott ML, Hasserjian RP, Soffer B, Sklar J, Baltimore D (1996) Exclusive development of T cell neoplasms in mice transplanted with bone marrow expressing activated Notch alleles. *J Exp Med* **183**: 2283–2291.

Pegtel DM, Subramanian A, Sheen TS, Tsai CH, Golub TR, Thorley-Lawson DA (2005) Epstein-Barr-virus-encoded LMP2A induces primary epithelial cell migration and invasion: possible role in nasopharyngeal carcinoma metastasis. *J Virol* **79**: 15430–15442.

Peh SC, Looi LM, Pallesen G (1997) Epstein-Barr virus (EBV) and Hodgkin's disease in a multi-ethnic population in Malaysia. *Histopathology* **30**: 227–233.

Peng R, Gordadze AV, Fuentes Panana EM, Wang F, Zong J, Hayward GS, Tan J, Ling PD (2000) Sequence and functional analysis of EBNA-LP and EBNA2 proteins from nonhuman primate lymphocryptoviruses. *J Virol* **74**: 379–389.

Peng R, Moses SC, Tan J, Kremmer E, Ling PD (2005) The Epstein-Barr virus EBNA-LP protein preferentially coactivates EBNA2-mediated stimulation of latent membrane proteins expressed from the viral divergent promoter. *J Virol* **79**: 4492–4505.

Perkins N, Gilmore T (2006) Good cop, bad cop: the different faces of NF-kappaB. *Cell Death Differ* **13**: 759–772.

Pfeffer S, Sewer A, Lagos-Quintana M, Sheridan R, Sander C, Grasser FA, van Dyk LF, Ho CK, Shuman S, Chien M, Russo JJ, Ju J, Randall G, Lindenbach BD, Rice CM, Simon V, Ho DD, Zavolan M, Tuschl T (2005) Identification of microRNAs of the herpesvirus family. *Nat Methods* **2**: 269–276.

Pfeffer S, Zavolan M, Grasser FA, Chien M, Russo JJ, Ju J, John B, Enright AJ, Marks D, Sander C, Tuschl T (2004) Identification of virus-encoded microRNAs. *Science* **304**: 734–736.

Portis T, Ikeda M, Longnecker R (2004) Epstein-Barr virus LMP2A: regulating cellular ubiquitination processes for maintenance of viral latency? *Trends Immunol* **25**: 422–426.

Puls A, Eliopoulos AG, Nobes CD, Bridges T, Young LS, Hall A (1999) Activation of the small GTPase Cdc42 by the inflammatory cytokines TNF(alpha) and IL-1, and by the Epstein-Barr virus transforming protein LMP1. *J Cell Sci* **112**(Pt 17): 2983–2992.

Qi P, Han JX, Lu YQ, Wang C, Bu FF (2006) Virus-encoded microRNAs: future therapeutic targets? *Cell Mol Immunol* **3**: 411–419.

Qiu GH, Tan LK, Loh KS, Lim CY, Srivastava G, Tsai ST, Tsao SW, Tao Q (2004) The candidate tumor suppressor gene BLU, located at the commonly deleted region 3p21.3, is an E2F-regulated, stress-responsive gene and inactivated by both epigenetic and genetic mechanisms in nasopharyngeal carcinoma. *Oncogene* **23**: 4793–4806.

Radkov SA, Touitou R, Brehm A, Rowe M, West M, Kouzarides T, Allday MJ (1999) Epstein-Barr virus nuclear antigen 3C interacts with histone deacetylase to repress transcription. *J Virol* **73**: 5688–5697.

Rawlins DR, Milman G, Hayward SD, Hayward GS (1985) Sequence-specific DNA binding of the Epstein-Barr virus nuclear antigen (EBNA-1) to clustered sites in the plasmid maintenance region. *Cell* **42**: 859–868.

Rechsteiner MP, Berger C, Zauner L, Sigrist JA, Weber M, Longnecker R, Bernasconi M, Nadal D (2008) Latent membrane protein 2B regulates susceptibility to induction of lytic Epstein-Barr virus infection. *J Virol* **82**: 1739–1747.

Reisman D, Sugden B (1986) *trans* activation of an Epstein-Barr viral transcriptional enhancer by the Epstein-Barr viral nuclear antigen 1. *Mol Cell Biol* **6**: 3838–3846.

Reisman D, Yates J, Sugden B (1985) A putative origin of replication of plasmids derived from Epstein-Barr virus is composed of two *cis*-acting components. *Mol Cell Biol* **5**: 1822–1832.

Rezk SA, Weiss LM (2007) Epstein-Barr virus-associated lymphoproliferative disorders. *Hum Pathol* **38**: 1293–1304.

Rickinson A, Kieff E (2007) Epstein-Barr virus; in Knipe DM, Howley PM, Griffin DE, Lamb RA, Martin MA, Roizman B, Straus SE (eds.), *Fields Virology*. Philadelphia: Lippincott, Williams & Wilkins.

Rickinson AB, Young LS, Rowe M (1987) Influence of the Epstein-Barr virus nuclear antigen EBNA 2 on the growth phenotype of virus-transformed B cells. *J Virol* **61**: 1310–1317.

Rovedo M, Longnecker R (2007) Epstein-Barr virus latent membrane protein 2B (LMP2B) modulates LMP2A activity. *J Virol* **81**: 84–94.

Rowe M, Lear AL, Croom-Carter D, Davies AH, Rickinson AB (1992) Three pathways of Epstein-Barr virus gene activation from EBNA1-positive latency in B lymphocytes. *J Virol* **66**: 122–131.

Rowe M, Peng-Pilon M, Huen DS, Hardy R, Croom-Carter D, Lundgren E, Rickinson AB (1994) Upregulation of bcl-2 by the Epstein-Barr virus latent membrane protein LMP1: a B-cell-specific response that is delayed relative to NF-kappaB activation and to induction of cell surface markers. *J Virol* **68**: 5602–5612.

Rowe M, Rowe DT, Gregory CD, Young LS, Farrell PJ, Rupani H, Rickinson AB (1987) Differences in B cell growth phenotype reflect novel patterns of Epstein-Barr virus latent gene expression in Burkitt's lymphoma cells. *EMBO J* **6**: 2743–2751.

Saito N, Courtois G, Chiba A, Yamamoto N, Nitta T, Hironaka N, Rowe M, Yamamoto N, Yamaoka S (2003) Two carboxyl-terminal activation regions of Epstein-Barr virus latent membrane protein 1 activate NF-kappaB through distinct signaling pathways in fibroblast cell lines. *J Biol Chem* **278**: 46565–46575.

Sample J, Brooks L, Sample C, Young L, Rowe M, Gregory C, Rickinson A, Kieff E (1991) Restricted Epstein-Barr virus protein expression in Burkitt lymphoma is due to a different Epstein-Barr nuclear antigen 1 transcriptional initiation site. *Proc Natl Acad Sci USA* **88**: 6343–6347.

Sample J, Henson EB, Sample C (1992) The Epstein-Barr virus nuclear protein 1 promoter active in type I latency is autoregulated. *J Virol* **66**: 4654–4661.

Sample J, Liebowitz D, Kieff E (1989) Two related Epstein-Barr virus membrane proteins are encoded by separate genes. *J Virol* **63**: 933–937.

Sandvej K, Gratama JW, Munch M, Zhou XG, Bolhuis RL, Andresen BS, Gregersen N, Hamilton-Dutoit S (1997) Sequence analysis of the Epstein-Barr virus (EBV) latent membrane protein-1 gene and promoter region: identification of four variants among wild-type EBV isolates. *Blood* **90**: 323–330.

Saridakis V, Sheng Y, Sarkari F, Holowaty MN, Shire K, Nguyen T, Zhang RG, Liao J, Lee W, Edwards AM, Arrowsmith CH, Frappier L (2005) Structure of the p53 binding domain of HAUSP/USP7 bound to Epstein-Barr nuclear antigen 1 implications for EBV-mediated immortalization. *Mol Cell* **18**: 25–36.

Scaria V, Hariharan M, Maiti S, Pillai B, Brahmachari SK (2006) Host-virus interaction: a new role for microRNAs. *Retrovirology* **3**: 68.

Schepers A, Ritzi M, Bousset K, Kremmer E, Yates JL, Harwood J, Diffley JF, Hammerschmidt W (2001) Human origin recognition complex binds to the region of the latent origin of DNA replication of Epstein-Barr virus. *EMBO J* **20**: 4588–4602.

Scholle F, Bendt KM, Raab-Traub N (2000) Epstein-Barr virus LMP2A transforms epithelial cells, inhibits cell differentiation, and activates Akt. *J Virol* **74**: 10681–10689.

Schultheiss U, Püschner S, Kremmer E, Mak TW, Engelmann H, Hammerschmidt W, Kieser A (2001) TRAF6 is a critical mediator of signal transduction by the viral oncogene latent membrane protein 1. *EMBO J* **20**: 5678–5691.

Shair KH, Bendt KM, Edwards RH, Bedford EC, Nielsen JN, Raab-Traub N (2007) EBV latent membrane protein 1 activates Akt, NFkappaB, and Stat3 in B cell lymphomas. *PLoS Pathog* **3**: e166.

Shao JY, Huang XM, Yu XJ, Huang LX, Wu QL, Xia JC, Wang HY, Feng QS, Ren ZF, Ernberg I, Hu LF, Zeng YX (2001) Loss of heterozygosity and its correlation with clinical outcome and Epstein-Barr virus infection in nasopharyngeal carcinoma. *Anticancer Res* **21**: 3021–3029.

Sharipo A, Imreh M, Leonchiks A, Branden C, Masucci MG (2001) *cis*-Inhibition of proteasomal degradation by viral repeats: impact of length and amino acid composition. *FEBS Lett* **499**: 137–142.

Sharipo A, Imreh M, Leonchiks A, Imreh S, Masucci MG (1998) A minimal glycine-alanine repeat prevents the interaction of ubiquitinated I kappaB alpha with the proteasome: a new mechanism for selective inhibition of proteolysis. *Nat Med* **4**: 939–944.

Shibata D, Weiss LM (1992) Epstein-Barr virus-associated gastric adenocarcinoma. *Am J Pathol* **140**: 769–774.

Shire K, Ceccarelli DF, Avolio-Hunter TM, Frappier L (1999) EBP2, a human protein that interacts with sequences of the Epstein-Barr virus nuclear antigen 1 important for plasmid maintenance. *J Virol* **73**: 2587–2595.

Shire K, Kapoor P, Jiang K, Hing MN, Sivachandran N, Nguyen T, Frappier L (2006) Regulation of the EBNA1 Epstein-Barr virus protein by serine phosphorylation and arginine methylation. *J Virol* **80**: 5261–5272.

Sjoblom A, Jansson A, Yang W, Lain S, Nilsson T, Rymo L (1995) PU box-binding transcription factors and a POU domain protein cooperate in the Epstein-Barr virus (EBV) nuclear antigen 2-induced transactivation of the EBV latent membrane protein 1 promoter. *J Gen Virol* 76 (Pt 11): 2679–2692.

Snudden DK, Smith PR, Lai D, Ng MH, Griffin BE (1995) Alterations in the structure of the EBV nuclear antigen, EBNA1, in epithelial cell tumours. *Oncogene* **10**: 1545–1552.

Soni V, Cahir-McFarland E, Kieff E (2007) LMP1 Trafficking activates growth and survival pathways. *Adv Exp Med Biol* **597**: 173–187.

Stevenson D, Charalambous C, Wilson JB (2005) Epstein-Barr virus latent membrane protein 1 (CAO) up-regulates VEGF and TGF alpha concomitant with hyper[p]lasia, with subsequent up-regulation of p16 and MMP9. *Cancer Res* **65**: 8826–8835.

Su W, Middleton T, Sugden B, Echols H (1991) DNA looping between the origin of replication of Epstein-Barr virus and its enhancer site: stabilization of an origin complex with Epstein-Barr nuclear antigen 1. *Proc Natl Acad Sci USA* **88**: 10870–10874.

Sullivan CS, Grundhoff AT, Tevethia S, Pipas JM, Ganem D (2005) SV40-encoded microRNAs regulate viral gene expression and reduce susceptibility to cytotoxic T cells. *Nature* **435**: 682–686.

Sylla BS, Hung SC, Davidson DM, Hatzivassiliou E, Malinin NL, Wallach D, Gilmore TD, Kieff E, Mosialos G (1998) Epstein-Barr virus-transforming protein latent infection membrane protein 1 activates transcription factor NF-kappaB through a pathway that includes the NF-kappaB-inducing kinase and the IkappaB kinases IKKalpha and IKKbeta. *Proc Natl Acad Sci USA* **95**: 10106–10111.

Takeshita H, Yoshizaki T, Miller W, Sato H, Furukawa M, Pagano J, Raab-Traub N (1999) Matrix metalloproteinase 9 expression is induced by Epstein-Barr virus latent membrane protein 1 C-terminal activation regions 1 and 2. *J Virol* **73**: 5548–5555.

Tamura K, Taniguchi Y, Minoguchi S, Sakai T, Tun T, Furukawa T, Honjo T (1995) Physical interaction between a novel domain of the receptor Notch and the transcription factor RBP-J kappa/Su(H). *Curr Biol* **5**: 1416–1423.

Tan SH, Ida H, Goh BC, Hsieh W, Loh M, Ito Y (2006) Analyses of promoter hypermethylation for RUNX3 and other tumor suppressor genes in nasopharyngeal carcinoma. *Anticancer Res* **26**: 4287–4292.

Tao Q, Robertson KD (2003) Stealth technology: how Epstein-Barr virus utilizes DNA methylation to cloak itself from immune detection. *Clin Immunol* **109**: 53–63.

Thornburg NJ, Pathmanathan R, Raab-Traub N (2003) Activation of nuclear factor-kappaB p50 homodimer/Bcl-3 complexes in nasopharyngeal carcinoma. *Cancer Res* **63**: 8293–8301.

Tierney RJ, Steven N, Young LS, Rickinson AB (1994) Epstein-Barr virus latency in blood mononuclear cells: analysis of viral gene transcription during primary infection and in the carrier state. *J Virol* **68**: 7374–7385.

Tomkinson B, Robertson E, Kieff E (1993) Epstein-Barr virus nuclear proteins EBNA-3A and EBNA-3C are essential for B-lymphocyte growth transformation *J Virol* **67**: 2014–2025.

Tsai CL, Li HP, Lu YJ, Hsueh C, Liang Y, Chen CL, Tsao SW, Tse KP, Yu JS, Chang YS (2006) Activation of DNA methyltransferase 1 by EBV LMP1 Involves c-Jun NH(2)-terminal kinase signaling. *Cancer Res* **66**: 11668–11676.

Tsai CN, Liu ST, Chang YS (1995) Identification of a novel promoter located within the Bam HI Q region of the Epstein-Barr virus genome for the EBNA 1 gene. *DNA Cell Biol* **14**: 767–776.

Tsai CN, Tsai CL, Tse KP, Chang HY, Chang YS (2002) The Epstein-Barr virus oncogene product, latent membrane protein 1, induces the down-regulation of E-cadherin gene expression via activation of DNA methyltransferases. *Proc Natl Acad Sci USA* **99**: 10084–10089.

Tsao SW, Tramoutanis G, Dawson CW, Lo AK, Huang DP (2002) The significance of LMP1 expression in nasopharyngeal carcinoma. *Semin Cancer Biol* **12**: 473–487.

Wakisaka N, Murono S, Yoshizaki T, Furukawa M, Pagano JS (2002) Epstein-Barr virus latent membrane protein 1 induces and causes release of fibroblast growth factor-2. *Cancer Res* **62**: 6337–6344.

Waltzer L, Logeat F, Brou C, Israel A, Sergeant A, Manet E (1994) The human J kappa recombination signal sequence binding protein (RBP-J kappa) targets the Epstein-Barr virus EBNA2 protein to its DNA responsive elements. *EMBO J* **13**: 5633–5638.

Wan J, Sun L, Mendoza JW, Chui YL, Huang DP, Chen ZJ, Suzuki N, Suzuki S, Yeh WC, Akira S, Matsumoto K, Liu ZG, Wu Z (2004) Elucidation of the c-Jun N-terminal kinase pathway mediated by Epstein-Barr virus-encoded latent membrane protein 1 *Mol Cell Biol* **24**: 192–199.

Wang D, Liebowitz D, Kieff E (1985) An EBV membrane protein expressed in immortalized lymphocytes transforms established rodent cells. *Cell* **43**: 831–840.

Wang JT, Sheeng TS, Su IJ, Chen JY, Chen MR (2003) EBNA-1 sequence variations reflect active EBV replication and disease status or quiescent latency in lymphocytes. *J Med Virol* **69**: 417–425.

Wang WY, Chien YC, Jan JS, Chueh CM, Lin JC (2002) Consistent sequence variation of Epstein-Barr virus nuclear antigen 1 in primary tumor and peripheral blood cells of patients with nasopharyngeal carcinoma. *Clin Cancer Res* **8**: 2586–2590.

Wang Y, Finan JE, Middeldorp JM, Hayward SD (1997) P32/TAP, a cellular protein that interacts with EBNA-1 of Epstein-Barr virus. *Virology* **236**: 18–29.

Wilfred BR, Wang WX, Nelson PT (2007) Energizing miRNA research: a review of the role of miRNAs in lipid metabolism, with a prediction that miR-103/107 regulates human metabolic pathways. *Mol Genet Metab* **91**: 209–217.

Wilson JB, Bell JL, Levine AJ (1996) Expression of Epstein-Barr virus nuclear antigen-1 induces B cell neoplasia in transgenic mice. *EMBO J* **15**: 3117–3126.

Wilson JB, Weinberg W, Johnson R, Yuspa S, Levine AJ (1990) Expression of the BNLF-1 oncogene of Epstein-Barr virus in the skin of transgenic mice induces hyperplasia and aberrant expression of keratin 6. *Cell* **61**: 1315–1327.

Winberg G, Matskova L, Chen F, Plant P, Rotin D, Gish G, Ingham R, Ernberg I, Pawson T (2000) Latent membrane protein 2A of Epstein-Barr virus binds WW domain E3 protein-ubiquitin ligases that ubiquitinate B-cell tyrosine kinases *Mol Cell Biol* **20**: 8526–8535.

Wong HL, Wang X, Chang RC, Jin DY, Feng H, Wang Q, Lo KW, Huang DP, Yuen PW, Takada K, Wong YC, Tsao SW (2005) Stable expression of EBERs in immortalized nasopharyngeal epithelial cells confers resistance to apoptotic stress. *Mol Carcinog* **44**: 92–101.

Wong TS, Kwong DL, Sham JS, Wei WI, Kwong YL, Yuen AP (2004) Quantitative plasma hypermethylated DNA markers of undifferentiated nasopharyngeal carcinoma. *Clin Cancer Res* **10**: 2401–2406.

Wrightham MN, Stewart JP, Janjua NJ, Pepper SD, Sample C, Rooney CM, Arrand JR (1995) Antigenic and sequence variation in the C-terminal unique domain of the Epstein-Barr virus nuclear antigen EBNA-1. *Virology* **208**: 521–530.

Wu H, Ceccarelli DF, Frappier L (2000) The DNA segregation mechanism of Epstein-Barr virus nuclear antigen 1. *EMBO Rep* **1**: 140–144.

Wu H, Kapoor P, Frappier L (2002) Separation of the DNA replication, segregation, and transcriptional activation functions of Epstein-Barr nuclear antigen 1. *J Virol* **76**: 2480–2490.

Wu L, Nakano H, Wu Z (2006) The C-terminal activating region 2 of the Epstein-Barr virus-encoded latent membrane protein 1 activates NF-kappaB through TRAF6 and TAK1. *J Biol Chem* **281**: 2162–2169.

Xing L, Kieff E (2007) Epstein-Barr virus BHRF1 micro and stable RNAs in latency III and after induction of replication. *J Virol* **81**: 9967–9975.

Xu Q, Briggs J, Park S, Niu G, Kortylewski M, Zhang S, Gritsko T, Turkson J, Kay H, Semenza GL, Cheng JQ, Jove R, Yu H (2005) Targeting Stat3 blocks both HIF-1 and VEGF expression induced by multiple oncogenic growth signaling pathways. *Oncogene* **24**: 5552–5560.

Xue SA, Griffin BE (2007) Complexities associated with expression of Epstein-Barr virus (EBV) lytic origins of DNA replication. *Nucleic Acids Res* **35**: 3391–3406.

Yalamanchili R, Tong X, Grossman S, Johannsen E, Mosialos G, Kieff E (1994) Genetic and biochemical evidence that EBNA 2 interaction with a 63-kDa cellular GTG-binding protein is essential for B lymphocyte growth transformation by EBV. *Virology* **204**: 634–641.

Yamamoto N, Takizawa T, Iwanaga Y, Shimizu N, Yamamoto N (2000) Malignant transformation of B lymphoma cell line BJAB by Epstein-Barr virus-encoded small RNAs. *FEBS Lett* **484**: 153–158.

Yang J, Deng X, Deng L, Gu H, Fan W, Cao Y (2004) Telomerase activation by Epstein-Barr virus latent membrane protein 1 is associated with c-Myc expression in human nasopharyngeal epithelial cells. *J Exp Clin Cancer Res* **23**: 495–506.

Yates JL, Warren N, Sugden B (1985) Stable replication of plasmids derived from Epstein-Barr virus in various mammalian cells. *Nature* **313**: 812–815.

Yi HM, Ren CP, Peng D, Zhou L, Li H, Yao KT (2007) [Expression, loss of heterozygosity, and methylation of GNAT1 gene in nasopharyngeal carcinoma]. *Ai Zheng* **26**: 9–14.

Yoshizaki T (2002) Promotion of metastasis in nasopharyngeal carcinoma by Epstein-Barr virus latent membrane protein-1. *Histol Histopathol* **17**: 845–850.

Young LS, Rickinson AB (2004) Epstein-Barr virus: 40 years on. *Nat Rev Cancer* **4**: 757–768.

Yu JS, Tsai HC, Wu CC, Weng LP, Li HP, Chung PJ, Chang YS (2002) Induction of inducible nitric oxide synthase by Epstein-Barr virus B95-8-derived LMP1 in Balb/3T3 cells promotes stress-induced cell death and impairs LMP1-mediated transformation. *Oncogene* **21**: 8047–8061.

Zhang D, Frappier L, Gibbs E, Hurwitz J, O'Donnell M (1998) Human RPA (hSSB) interacts with EBNA1, the latent origin binding protein of Epstein-Barr virus. *Nucleic Acids Res* **26**: 631–637.

Zhang X, Hu L, Fadeel B, Ernberg IT (2002a) Apoptosis modulation of Epstein-Barr virus-encoded latent membrane protein 1 in the epithelial cell line HeLa is stimulus-dependent. *Virology* **304**: 330–341.

Zhang XS, Song KH, Mai HQ, Jia WH, Feng BJ, Xia JC, Zhang RH, Huang LX, Yu XJ, Feng QS, Huang P, Chen JJ, Zeng YX (2002b) The 30-bp deletion variant: a polymorphism of latent membrane protein 1 prevalent in endemic and non-endemic areas of nasopharyngeal carcinomas in China. *Cancer Lett* **176**: 65–73.

Zheng H, Li LL, Hu DS, Deng XY, Cao Y (2007) Role of Epstein-Barr virus encoded latent membrane protein 1 in the carcinogenesis of nasopharyngeal carcinoma. *Cell Mol Immunol* **4**: 185–196.

Zhou L, Jiang W, Ren C, Yin Z, Feng X, Liu W, Tao Q, Yao K (2005) Frequent hypermethylation of RASSF1A and TSLC1, and high viral load of Epstein-Barr Virus DNA in nasopharyngeal carcinoma and matched tumor-adjacent tissues. *Neoplasia* 7: 809–815.

Zimber-Strobl U, Kremmer E, Grasser F, Marschall G, Laux G, Bornkamm GW (1993) The Epstein-Barr virus nuclear antigen 2 interacts with an EBNA2 responsive *cis*-element of the terminal protein 1 gene promoter. *EMBO J* **12**: 167–175.

Zimber-Strobl U, Strobl LJ (2001) EBNA2 and Notch signalling in Epstein-Barr virus mediated immortalization of B lymphocytes. *Semin Cancer Biol* **11**: 423–434.

Chapter 6

Human Kaposi's Sarcoma-associated Herpesvirus: Molecular Biology and Oncogenesis

Patrick J. Dillon* and Blossom Damania*

Abstract: Both RNA and DNA viruses have been linked to human cancers and an estimated 15–20% of cancers in humans are caused by viruses. Viral infection alone is generally not sufficient to induce cancer. Other events such as immunosuppression or genetic predisposition, also play a role. Kaposi's sarcoma-associated herpesvirus (KSHV) has been well defined as a virus associated with three neoplastic diseases. Here we describe KSHV viral proteins that play important roles in the viral lifecycle and potentially in the transformation process. From binding its target receptors to the establishment of latency, KSHV alters cellular processes and the intracellular environment in favor of the virus instituting a life-long infection. Much work is being done to determine which viral proteins are critical for inducing cellular transformation and oncogenesis as well as to get a better understanding of the paracrine mechanisms involved in KSHV-associated diseases. This research will be important for the design of KSHV vaccines as well as treatments for KSHV-related disease.

*Department of Microbiology & Immunology and Lineberger Comprehensive Cancer Center, University of North Carolina at Chapel Hill, Chapel Hill, North Carolina.

1. Introduction

The herpesviruses are a large family of viruses that are ubiquitous in nature with many animal species harboring at least one herpesvirus (Pellett & Roizman, 2007). Members of the *Herpesviridae* family exhibit many differences with respect to their biological processes, but one commonality is that they have adapted very well to their hosts. It seems an ideal strategy for a virus to keep its host viable to allow for continual dissemination to other cells and hosts. While infections of immunocompetent individuals with herpesviruses may be symptomatic, it very rarely results in fatality. Typically, it is when the immune system of the host is compromised by another infectious agent or immunosuppressive drugs, that herpesviruses cause severe disease or death.

During a viral infection, there is a battle being waged between the host cell and the virus and the winner determines the overall outcome of the infection. If the host cell defenses prove too strong for the virus, the virus is cleared and the infection is aborted. If the virus is able to circumvent the host response or inhibit the host cell from eliciting a potent antiviral response, the virus can establish a productive, persistent infection. Herpesviruses have coevolved with their hosts for millions of years and they have garnered the ability to modify normal cellular processes and establish lifelong latent infections of their host.

KSHV has developed a very complex viral gene expression program that alters the cellular environment to facilitate lifelong infection. Many of the viral proteins, some of which are hijacked cellular homologs, serve to suppress the host antiviral response through modulating signal transduction pathways, inhibiting apoptosis, and altering cell cycle progression. This allows KSHV to establish latency and shut down viral gene expression to successfully evade detection by the host immunosurveillance machinery. When cells harboring latent KSHV undergo reactivation, the lytic cycle is initiated and new viral progenies are produced and released from the cell. These new virions can then infect neighboring cells, starting the infection process anew. Both the latent and lytic phases of KSHV replication are believed to be important in the development of KSHV-associated neoplasia.

This chapter will discuss the diseases linked to KSHV, many of the interactions between viral and host proteins during KSHV infection, and the potential roles these proteins have in the progression of KSHV-associated malignancies.

2. Clinical Disease

Kaposi's sarcoma (KS) is a highly vascularized spindle-cell tumor characterized by the dysregulated growth of endothelial cells (Dupin *et al.*, 1995; Wang *et al.*, 2004). KS often presents as a red, purple, or brown cutaneous lesion, but can also present on internal organs such as the liver, lungs, and intestines. KS was originally described by Dr. Moritz Kaposi, a Hungarian dermatologist practicing at the University of Vienna in 1872. Five of his patients presented with what he termed "idiopathic multiple pigmented sarcomas of the skin" (Kaposi, 1872). While there was suspicion of a viral cause to KS, it was not until 1994 that KS was linked to infection with KSHV, also known as human herpesvirus-8 (HHV-8). Through use of representational difference analysis, Chang and his colleagues were able to detect DNA fragments of a previously unidentified herpesvirus, KSHV, from KS lesions of AIDS patients (Chang *et al.*, 1994). Since then, greater than 95% of all KS lesions have been found to contain KSHV viral DNA, further linking KS to KSHV infection.

There are four subtypes of KS that differ in their clinical manifestations. They are classic, endemic or African, iatrogenic or transplant-related, and epidemic or AIDS-associated. Classic KS is a rare disease that primarily affects elderly men between the ages of 50 and 70 of Mediterranean or Eastern European descent. It is a slowly growing cancer that typically forms lesions on the hands or soles of the feet. Additional lesions may appear on the arms and legs over the course of years to decades but very rarely spread to other parts of the body. While the lesions can be painful at times, classic KS is generally not considered life threatening. Endemic KS is found in parts of equatorial Africa and accounted for 3–9% of reported cancers in Uganda in 1971 (Taylor *et al.*, 1971). Unlike classic KS, endemic KS often develops at a much younger age and tends to be more aggressive. In the aggressive cases, the tumors may penetrate the underlying bone or spread to the lymph nodes or other organs with the median survival time being just months to years.

Another population at risk for KS are those receiving immunosuppressive therapy following organ transplantation or for another medical condition. Dampening of the host immune response by immunosuppressive drugs increases KSHV replication and pathogenesis. Additionally, KSHV can be transmitted from the donor organ to the transplant recipient (Barozzi *et al.*, 2003). Iatrogenic KS tends to be more aggressive than classic KS with about half of the patients having involvement of the lymph nodes, mucosa, and other organs.

In the early stages of the AIDS epidemic, physicians began to see a marked rise in the number of patients presenting with KS. For a while, upwards of 30–40% of patients with AIDS also had KS (Beral *et al.*, 1990), and in 1981 KS was recognized as an AIDS-defining illness. A patient is deemed to have epidemic KS if they also have AIDS. Epidemic KS results in the appearance of lesions on many parts of the body soon after AIDS develops. It is a highly aggressive cancer that generally spreads to the skin, lymph nodes, and internal organs. Without treatment, persons with epidemic KS have a survival time of just weeks to months. The advent of Highly Active Anti-Retroviral Therapy (HAART) has significantly decreased the incidence of epidemic KS and increased life expectancy, but KS still has the highest incidence rates among the AIDS-defining or AIDS-associated cancers (Mbulaiteye *et al.*, 2003).

Besides its strong causal association with KS, KSHV is also associated with the B-cell lymphoproliferative diseases, primary effusion lymphoma (PEL) and multicentric Castleman's disease (MCD). PEL is a rare, aggressive type of B-cell non-Hodgkin lymphoma characterized by an abnormal build-up of fluids in a body cavity such as the pleural space or pericardium without an identifiable contiguous tumor mass (Nador *et al.*, 1996). PELs are also sometimes referred to as body cavity-based lymphomas (BCBLs). It most commonly arises in patients with suppressed immune systems, such as patients with AIDS (Chen *et al.*, 2007; Mbulaiteye *et al.*, 2002). It is generally resistant to cancer chemotherapy drugs that are active against other lymphomas, and carries a very poor prognosis. The majority of PELs are KSHV-positive and some are also infected with Epstein-Barr virus (EBV) (Cesarman *et al.*, 1995).

MCD, also referred to as multicentric angiofollicular hyperplasia, is characterized by vascular proliferation of the germinal centers of lymph nodes. Patients with MCD often present with widespread lymphadenopathy and sometimes hepatosplenomegaly. There are two forms of MCD: a plasmablastic variant that is associated with lymphadenopathy and immunological abnormalities (Frizzera *et al.*, 1983) and a hyaline vascular form that presents as a solid mass. KSHV infection is present in nearly 100% of MCD cases associated with HIV-1 infection, and in about 50% of cases that are HIV-1 negative (Dupin *et al.*, 1999; Soulier *et al.*, 1995). The plasmablastic form is most closely associated with KSHV. Patients with AIDS-associated MCD often go on to develop KS. MCD is a polyclonal tumor with the disease likely due to hypersecretion of cytokines such as interleukin-6 (IL-6). In KSHV positive tumors, this is most likely due to expression of the viral homolog of IL-6, viral IL-6 (vIL-6) (Parravicini *et al.*, 1997).

There have been several other reports of diseases linked to KSHV such as multiple myeloma (Chauhan *et al.*, 1999; Rettig *et al.*, 1997), sarcoidosis (DiAlberti *et al.*, 1997), and pulmonary hypertension (Cool *et al.*, 2003) but other investigators have been unable to confirm these results (Brander *et al.*, 2002; Henke-Gendo *et al.*, 2004; Maeda *et al.*, 2000; Olsen *et al.*, 1998; Perna *et al.*, 1998).

3. KSHV Genome

The *Herpesviridae* family of viruses are grouped into three subfamilies: *Alphaherpesvirinae* (e.g. HSV-1/2 and VZV), *Betaherpesvirinae* (e.g. HCMV), and *Gammaherpesvirinae* (e.g. KSHV and EBV). The γ-herpesviruses are grouped into two genera: *Lymphocryptovirus* (or γ_1 group) and *Rhadinovirus* (or γ_2 group). The lymphocryptoviruses include EBV and its primate relatives while KSHV is the only known human rhadinovirus. Rhadinoviruses are even further subdivided into the classification of Old World and New World viruses with KSHV belonging to the Old World virus group (reviewed in McGeoch *et al.*, 2005).

The KSHV virion, like all of the herpesviruses, has a lipid bilayer envelope containing about a dozen viral glycoproteins and a tegument that surrounds the icosahedral capsid. The capsid comprises 12 pentons, 150 hexons, and 320 triplexes as determined by cryo-electron microscopy (Wu *et al.*, 2000). KSHV capsids exhibit very similar structural features compared to HSV-1 and HCMV (Trus *et al.*, 2001). The capsid contains the linear, double-stranded DNA, which is wrapped around a toroid-like protein core. Following infection of a host cell, the DNA forms a double-stranded episome in the nucleus. Between the envelope and the nucleocapsid lies the viral tegument, which is a cluster of RNA and proteins. Little is known about the KSHV tegument structure and function but at least some of the tegument proteins and binding partners have recently been identified (Bechtel *et al.*, 2005; Rozen *et al.*, 2008; Zhu *et al.*, 2005). The tegument proteins are released into the cell at the very initial stage of infection and are believed to exert important regulatory functions and play roles in virion assembly, envelopment, or budding.

The KSHV genome is estimated to be approximately 165 kb in length with a 145-kb long unique coding region (LUR) that is flanked by multiple 801-bp terminal repeats (TR) with high G/C content (Russo *et al.*, 1996; Zhong *et al.*, 1996). There are over 85 open reading frames (ORFs) within the LUR, designated ORFs 4 to 75 based on their shared amino acid sequence identity to the prototype γ_2-herpesvirus, herpesvirus saimiri (HVS) (Neipel *et al.*, 1997). The genome is organized into seven highly conserved gene blocks separated by regions containing unique or subfamily-specific ORFs, as seen in other herpesviruses (McGeoch, 2005). The conserved genes are often found at similar locations in the viral genome between KSHV and HVS. There are currently 20 known KSHV-specific genes that are denoted by the prefix "K." Many of the unique KSHV genes are homologs to known cellular genes and have functions, which include modulating the immune response, regulating the cell cycle, and inhibiting apoptosis (Moore & Chang, 2003; Wong & Damania, 2005). Some of these will be discussed later in this chapter.

While expression patterns of KSHV genes have many similarities to other herpesviruses, there have been several interesting features of KSHV viral gene expression uncovered through studies on its transcription. KSHV appears to use mRNA splicing to express different coding domains from the same precursor mRNA more than any other herpesvirus. There are upwards of 25 KSHV genes (over one-quarter of the total number of KSHV genes) that are spliced with 15 of them expressing bicistronic or tricistronic RNA (Zheng, 2003). For the KSHV mRNAs that are polycistronic, usually only the 5′ ORF is translated (Dittmer *et al.*, 1998). The downstream ORFs are expressed by other mechanisms such as use of a different transcriptional start site (Lin *et al.*, 1999) and use of an internal ribosome entry site (IRES) (Low *et al.*, 2001).

4. Life Cycle

While not yet fully characterized, KSHV appears to have a very broad *in vivo* host range with viral DNA and mRNA being recovered from B-cells from the peripheral blood, B-cells in PEL and MCD, KS spindle cells, monocytes, macrophages, keratinocytes, endothelial, and epithelial cells (Ambroziak *et al.*, 1995; Antman & Chang, 2000; Ganem, 1998; Henry *et al.*, 1999; Schulz *et al.*, 2002). It is believed that the primary reservoir for KSHV is $CD19^+$ B-cells due to the harboring of viral DNA in seropositive individuals (Dourmishev *et al.*, 2003; Schulz *et al.*, 2002). There is also recent evidence that $CD34^+$ hematopoietic progenitor cells may also serve as a viral reservoir (Wu *et al.*, 2006).

Entry of herpesviruses into cells typically occurs through direct attachment and fusion of the virion and target cell membrane, but receptor-mediated endocytosis is also used (reviewed in Spear & Longnecker, 2003). Endocytosis may be the primary entry mechanism of KSHV, as it has been shown to use endocytosis to enter BJABs (Akula *et al.*, 2001), endothelial cells (Akula *et al.*, 2002), human foreskin fibroblast cells (Akula *et al.*, 2003), and epithelial cells (Inoue *et al.*, 2003; Liao *et al.*, 2003). On the other hand, it has been shown that a variety of cell types are susceptible to KSHV glycoprotein-mediated cell fusion and entry (Kaleeba & Berger, 2006b; Pertel, 2002).

Most herpesviruses use a two-step entry process where the virus first binds to glycosaminoglycan(s) on the cell surface followed by binding of the viral ligand to an entry receptor. Heparin sulfate is a commonly used cell receptor by herpesviruses and this appears to be true for KSHV as well. The K8.1A viral glycoprotein has been shown to bind heparin sulfate with an affinity very similar to HSV gC (Birkmann *et al.*, 2001; Wang *et al.*, 2001) and contains a putative heparin-binding domain (Wang *et al.*, 2001). The KSHV glycoprotein gB also contains a heparin-binding domain and can interact with heparin sulfate (Akula *et al.*, 2001). While binding of heparin sulfate greatly aids in viral entry into a cell, it appears not to be essential. Binding to heparin sulfate probably increases the efficiency of entry by concentrating the virus on the cell surface and increasing the binding to other host cell molecules required for entry.

Recent investigations have revealed several cellular receptors used by KSHV for entry into adherent cells; integrin $\alpha3\beta1$ (CD49c/29) and the cysteine transporter xCT (Akula *et al.*, 2002; Kaleeba & Berger, 2006a). The gB protein of KSHV contains an integrin-binding RGD motif, which binds to integrin $\alpha3\beta1$ (Akula *et al.*, 2002; Wang *et al.*, 2003). Soluble $\alpha3\beta1$ integrin, antibodies against $\alpha3$ and $\beta1$ integrins, and RGD peptides all inhibited infection by KSHV, but did not block binding to the target cell. This suggests that $\alpha3\beta1$ integrin is just one of the receptors used for entry by KSHV.

Using functional complementary DNA selection for a receptor mediating KSHV cell fusion, the xCT cystine transporter was identified as an entry receptor (Kaleeba & Berger, 2006a). Expression of recombinant xCT in otherwise non-permissive cells allowed for fusion and entry of KSHV virions into the cells. Antibodies against xCT blocked virion entry and fusion. Interestingly, since xCT is upregulated in response to glutathione depletion (Qiang *et al.*, 2004; Sasaki *et al.*, 2002) and HIV Tat reduces glutathione levels (Choi *et al.*, 2000a), the authors suggest that HIV coinfection may promote clinically aggressive HIV/AIDS-associated KS by upregulating the xCT KSHV receptor (Kaleeba & Berger, 2006a).

For entry into myeloid dendritic cells and macrophages, it has been shown that KSHV utilizes DC-SIGN as a receptor (Rappocciolo *et al.*, 2006). In similar experiments, as described for $\alpha3\beta1$ integrin and xCT, antibodies against DC-SIGN significantly decreased virus binding and infection and expression of DC-SIGN on non-permissive cells enabled viral penetration. The viral ligand that bound xCT and DC-SIGN was not examined but in another report, a cell-based assay was used, which showed that the glycoproteins gB, gH, and gL were needed to fuse to human embryonic kidney (HEK) cells and B-cells (Pertel, 2002).

Upon binding to cell surface $\alpha3\beta1$ integrin, KSHV induces activation and phosphorylation of focal adhesion kinase (FAK), which is a critical component to the outside-in signaling pathway of integrins that leads to the activation of several downstream signaling molecules (Krishnan *et al.*, 2006). Use of $FAK^{-/-}$ cells or a FAK dominant negative mutant resulted in about a 70% reduction of viral entry, demonstrating an important role of FAK signaling for internalization of KSHV DNA into cells (Krishnan *et al.*, 2006). One of the important downstream effectors activated by FAK signaling is PI3K. PI3K can activate multiple signaling molecules such as Akt, Rho-GTPases, and mitogen-activated protein kinase (MAPK) that have a variety of cellular functions including antiapoptosis, remodeling of actin cytoskeleton, and altering cellular transcription, respectively (Giancotti & Ruoslahti, 1999).

After the virion has fused with the cellular membrane and is released into the cytoplasm, it traffics through the cytoplasm and the viral DNA is delivered into the nucleus. This process may be facilitated by the activation of the signaling pathways following virion binding mentioned above. There is a lot that happens between the time the virus enters the cell and the viral genome is injected into the nucleus and this area has not been studied in great detail. It is known that KSHV, like HSV, uses the dynein motors to achieve delivery of the viral DNA to the nucleus and this is severely inhibited by depolymerization of microtubules (Naranatt *et al.*, 2005). The Rho GTPases seem to play a critical role in capsid trafficking since their inactivation significantly reduces the amount of viral DNA transported to the nucleus (Naranatt *et al.*, 2005).

4.1. Latency

Like the classic herpesviruses, KSHV exhibits both latent and lytic replications, each of which is defined by specific and distinct expression of viral genes. The majority of KSHV infections lead to the establishment of latency. The virus infects the cell, undergoes an initial propagation of the virus, then establishes latency in a subset of $CD19^+$ B-cells. The exact mechanism for the establishment of latency is poorly understood. Latency is considered to be established when only a very few viral genes are expressed and no progeny virus is produced. Maintenance of latency is achieved by the circularization of the viral DNA, which is tethered to the host cell chromosome. The copy number of viral DNA varies per cell with different PEL cell lines containing between 20 and 100 copies (Cesarman *et al.*, 1995; Renne *et al.*, 1996; Staudt *et al.*, 2004). Interestingly, it may be that the establishment of latency may depend upon lytic gene expression. One study has shown that following *de novo* infection, early lytic genes as well as latency genes were being expressed, but during the course of the infection the majority of the lytic genes expressed dramatically reduced (Krishnan *et al.*, 2004). Several of these lytic genes are known to counteract the antiviral response suggesting that the function of the lytic genes expressed immediately after initial infection is to alter the immune response to provide a favorable environment for the virus to establish latency.

Latency plays a key role in viral pathogenesis (Chaudhary *et al.*, 1999; Katano *et al.*, 2001). Several studies have proposed that latent gene expression contributes to the tumorigenic process in KSHV-associated cancers (Garber *et al.*, 2001; Hyun *et al.*, 2001; Renne *et al.*, 2001). Virtually all PEL, KS, and MCD lesions harbor KSHV DNA and the vast majority of these are latently infected (Dupin *et al.*, 1999; Parravicini *et al.*, 1997; Soulier *et al.*, 1995; Staskus *et al.*, 1997). The products of the latently expressed genes affect cell proliferation, survival, and transformation, promoting the idea that they are critical to the generation of KSHV-associated malignancies.

The KSHV proteins that are expressed during latency are latency-associated nuclear antigen (LANA), viral FLICE inhibitory protein (vFLIP), viral cyclin (v-cyclin), the kaposins, K15, and viral interferon regulatory factor 3 (vIRF3) in PEL. LANA is the universal marker of KSHV latency and has a wide variety of functions that make it critical in the establishment and maintenance of latency (reviewed in Nicholas, 2007). LANA is encoded by ORF73, which is part of the major latency locus situated at the right-hand end of the linear genome. The major latency locus also encodes vFLIP and v-cyclin (ORFs K13 and 72, respectively) as a tricistronic transcription unit (Dittmer *et al.*, 1998; Sarid *et al.*, 1999; Talbot *et al.*, 1999). A significant obstacle for episomal viruses to overcome is maintaining its DNA in proliferating cells. It appears that LANA is able to answer that challenge as it has been shown to promote latent viral DNA replication (Grundhoff & Ganem, 2003) as well as tether the newly replicated episomal DNA to the host cell chromosome to allow for proper segregation of the viral genomes during cell division (Cotter & Robertson, 1999). Along the same lines, LANA also promotes proliferation via binding and inactivating the tumor suppressor Rb, thus preventing it from negatively regulating entry into S phase of the cell cycle (Radkov *et al.*, 2000). Another of the many functional properties of LANA is that it can also inhibit p53-mediated cell death by inhibiting the transcriptional activator function of p53 (Friborg *et al.*, 1999).

While LANA promotes latent replication of viral DNA, it suppresses lytic viral replication and has been shown to suppress transcription of lytic viral genes and cellular genes (Garber *et al.*, 2001; Lan *et al.*, 2004; Lim *et al.*, 2000; Schwam *et al.*, 2000). This suggests that LANA may control the switch between latency and lytic replication or inhibit expression of antiviral cellular genes. A key event in the establishment of latency may be the association of LANA with the protein critical for the switch to viral lytic replication, Rta (replication and transcription activator). Recent work has revealed that LANA and Rta work in a feedback loop, as illustrated in Fig. 1. Rta is associated with the virion particle and expressed early during infection where it can activate LANA, which then leads to the downregulation of Rta by LANA through transcriptional repression of the Rta promoter (Lan *et al.*, 2004, 2005).

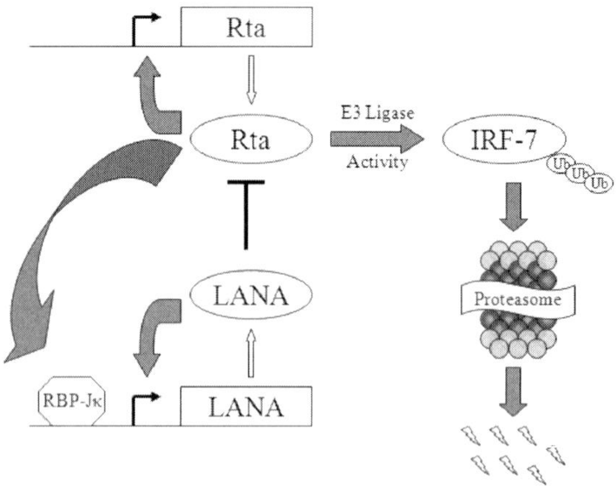

Fig. 1. Feedback loops of LANA and Rta to control the switch between latency and lytic replication. Depiction of the regulation of LANA and Rta via positive and negative feedback loops. Both Rta and LANA transactivate their own promoters while Rta also induces LANA expression through interactions with RBP-Jκ. LANA can repress Rta-mediated transactivation through binding of Rta. Rta encodes ubiquitin E3 ligase activity and regulates its own expression through self-ubiquitination and also targets IRF-7 for degradation by the proteasome.

As mentioned above, the other two genes encoded in the major latency locus along with LANA are *vFLIP* and *v-cyclin*. *vFLIP* is encoded by ORF K13 and is expressed from the *v-cyclin* mRNA through use of an IRES located at the 3′-end of the *v-cyclin* message (Bieleski & Talbot, 2001; Low *et al.*, 2001). *vFLIP* is a homolog of cellular FLIPs (cFLIPs), which are inhibitors of the extrinsic apoptotic-signaling pathway by blocking the interaction of Fas-associated protein with death domain (FADD) with caspase-8 (Inohara *et al.*, 1997; Irmler *et al.*, 1997). Similarly, *vFLIP* can inhibit death receptor signaling-induced apoptosis (Thome *et al.*, 1997). It also can upregulate NF-κB signaling and IL-6 expression, both of which may play a significant role in the disease caused by KSHV (An *et al.*, 2003; Liu *et al.*, 2002).

V-cyclin is expressed from a spliced mRNA from which the upstream LANA gene has been removed (Dittmer *et al.*, 1998). As its name implies, v-cyclin is a homolog to the cellular cyclins with

sequence similarity to the D-type cyclins. Cyclins are a family of proteins that regulate control of the cell cycle and replication through interaction with cyclin-dependent kinases (CDKs) and subsequent phosphorylation of specific cell cycle components (reviewed in Sanchez & Dynlacht, 2005). The D-type cyclins associate with CDK4 and CDK6 and phosphorylate pRb, thereby releasing Rb from its inhibition of E2F-induced transcription. V-cyclin associates almost exclusively with CDK6 and promotes G1–S cell cycle transition and DNA replication (Laman *et al.*, 2001; Li *et al.*, 1997). Unlike cellular cyclins, v-cyclin is resistant to the inhibitory effects of the CDK inhibitors p16, p21, and p27 (Chang *et al.*, 1996; Li *et al.*, 1997; Swanton *et al.*, 1997). V-cyclin transgenic mice have been generated and it was observed that about 10% of them developed lymphoma around seven months of age (Verschuren *et al.*, 2002). Crossing the v-cyclin transgenics with $p53^{-/-}$ mice resulted in dysregulated DNA synthesis and all of the v-cyclin/$p53^{-/-}$ mice developed lymphoma within four months (Vershuren *et al.*, 2002). This suggests a role for v-cyclin in viral tumorigenesis *in vivo* but this has proven to be difficult to determine as of yet.

The K12 locus encodes the kaposin family of proteins, termed kaposin A, B, and C, which are expressed via differential initiation of translation. Kaposin A translation uses the AUG codon that defines the start of ORF K12 while kaposins B and C use a non-AUG codon upstream of K12 (Sadler *et al.*, 1999). Expression of kaposin A in Rat-3 cells resulted in focal transformation and upon injection into athymic *nu/nu* mice, high-grade, highly vascular, undifferentiated sarcomas developed (Muralidhar *et al.*, 1998). With the detection of kaposin A protein in several PEL cell lines, it is suggestive that it may play a role in the development of KSHV-associated neoplasia. Kaposin B has been reported to activate MK2 (MAPK-associated kinase 2) whose activity is controlled by phosphorylation by p38 (McCormick & Ganem, 2005). Increases in MK2 activity leads to the stabilization of the normally quick turnover cytokine transcripts that contain AU-rich elements (AREs) such as IL-6 and GM-CSF (McCormick & Ganem, 2005; Winzen *et al.*, 1999). Cytokines such as IL-6 are believed to play a very important role in KSHV-associated disease and stabilization of IL-6 transcripts by kaposin B hint at its potential role in tumorigenesis. Currently, there is no known function of kaposin C, which contains the same C-terminal sequence as kaposin A.

ORF K15 is located at the far right of the linear genome neighboring the terminal repeat region (Choi *et al.*, 2000b; Glenn *et al.*, 1999). K15 is a multiply-spliced transcript resulting in four known variants with the most prominent transcript encoding eight exons and the protein containing 12 membrane-spanning regions (Choi *et al.*, 2000b; Glenn *et al.*, 1999). Two different isoforms of K15 have been identified, which are predominant (P) and minor (M) that have almost identical splicing patterns and protein structure but as little as 33% amino acid identity (Choi *et al.*, 2000b; Glenn *et al.*, 1999; Poole *et al.*, 1999). While there is low sequence identity, the putative signaling motifs of the two isoforms are highly conserved (Brinkmann & Schulz, 2006). Low levels of K15 are seen in uninduced PEL cells and this increases dramatically upon chemical stimulation of lytic reactivation, suggesting that K15 may play a role in both latent and lytic infections (Choi *et al.*, 2000b; Glenn *et al.*, 1999; Poole *et al.*, 1999). The K15 promoter transactivation is mediated by Rta, which is consistent with expression during lytic replication (Wong & Damania, 2006). K15 has been shown to activate several signaling transduction pathways, which may contribute to cellular transformation and disease progression of KSHV (Brinkmann & Schulz, 2006). This will be discussed in further detail later in this chapter.

The KSHV genome contains four genes that are homologous to the cellular IRFs, *vIRFs 1–4*, but just *vIRF3* is latently expressed in B-cells. *vIRF3* is localized to the nucleus so it has also been termed *LANA-2*. It is not expressed in all cell types *in vivo*, as it is found in the nucleus of latently infected B-cells but not KS spindle cells (Rivas *et al.*, 2001). Cellular IRFs play a central role in antiviral defense and immune regulation following viral infection (Honda & Taniguchi, 2006). IRF-3 and -7 are known to play critical roles in the activation of the type I interferon pathway (Hiscott *et al.*, 1999; Levy *et al.*, 2002) and there is data to support that *vIRF3* can act as a dominant-negative IRF to inhibit their functions (Lubyova & Pitha, 2000). *vIRF3* has been shown to have a variety of functions including inhibition of IFNα (Joo *et al.*, 2007), p53-mediated apoptosis (Rivas *et al.*, 2001), NF-κB activation (Seo *et al.*, 2004), and PKR activity (Esteban *et al.*, 2003). The increased survival of latently infected B-cells due to *vIRF3* definitely could contribute to the development of PEL or MCD.

Recently, it was discovered that KSHV latently expresses up to 17 micro RNAs (miRNAs) encoded by 12 miRNA genes that are located within the latency-associated region of the viral genome (Cai *et al.*, 2005; Pfeffer *et al.*, 2005; Samols *et al.*, 2005). Two of the miRNAs are found in the K12 ORF and the other 10 are in the intergenic region between vFLIP and kaposin. The main function of miRNAs is the downregulation of gene expression by either degradation of mRNA or inhibition of translation (reviewed in Bartel, 2004). miRNAs and miRNA processing have recently been shown to play an important role in tumorigenesis (Kumar *et al.*, 2007; Ma *et al.*, 2007; Voorhoeve *et al.*, 2006). For KSHV-encoded miRNAs, there have been three cellular targets currently described whose expression is repressed, which are osteopontin, thrombospondin-1, and plasticity-related gene 1 (Samols *et al.*, 2007). Other candidate targets have been proposed through use of computational methods (Cai *et al.*, 2005). Thrombospondin-1 has previously been reported to be downregulated in KS lesions (Taraboletti *et al.*, 1999) and has known activity as a tumor suppressor, anti-angiogenic factor, and immune stimulator (de Fraipont *et al.*, 2001; Lawler, 2002; Li *et al.*, 2005; Narizhneva *et al.*, 2005). Thus, KSHV-encoded miRNAs may play critical roles in establishment/maintenance of latency, immune evasion, pathogenesis, and oncogenesis.

4.2. Reactivation and Lytic Replication

While the majority of KSHV infections result in the virus establishing latency, there is always a small percentage of cells that harbor lytically replicating virus both *in vitro* and *in vivo*. The natural ligands and physiological conditions that spur reactivation of KSHV are poorly understood, but chemical induction of lytic replication is commonly used to study the molecular events associated with reactivation.

Currently, one of the best systems used to study viral gene expression and the switch between latent and lytic replication are PEL cell lines, which are latently infected with KSHV. Chemical treatment with phorbol esters or butyrate is known to initiate the reactivation process in up to 20–30% of the cells.

Following reactivation of the virus from latency, the virus undergoes the characteristic herpesvirus temporal regulation of viral gene expression. Lytic replication is classically broken down into three phases: immediate early, delayed early, and late gene expression. Genes were categorized as immediate early or late by their expression or lack thereof following chemical induction in the presence of certain inhibitors of translation and replication. The immediate early genes do not require *de novo* protein synthesis as shown by their transcription in the presence of the translation inhibitors such as cycloheximide. Late genes are defined by their requirement of prior DNA replication. Their transcription is inhibited by cidofovir, a nucleoside analog that inhibits replication (Lu *et al.*, 2004). By default, the genes that require new protein synthesis but not DNA replication for maximal expression are termed delayed early genes.

The protein product of ORF50, Rta, has been shown to be critical in the switch from latency to lytic reactivation (Gradoville *et al.*, 2000; Lukac *et al.*, 1998; Sun *et al.*, 1998). Transfection of a plasmid that constitutively expressed Rta was able to activate viral DNA replication and promote release of encapsidated KSHV virions in cultured PEL cells indicating that Rta is sufficient to drive the lytic cycle to completion (Gradoville *et al.*, 2000). Rta is expressed very early (<4 hrs) in reactivation, prior to the other lytic genes (Lukac *et al.*, 1999; Sun *et al.*, 1998).

Rta is a 691-amino-acid-long protein that shares two regions of relatively high amino acid homology at the C- and N-termini with its gammaherpesvirus homologs (Damania *et al.*, 2004; Lukac *et al.*, 1998). The N-terminus is a DNA-binding domain (Lukac *et al.*, 2001; Song *et al.*, 2002) while the C-terminus contains a transactivation domain (Wang *et al.*, 2001). Deletion of the activation domain results in the formation of an Rta mutant that acts as a dominant negative inihibitor of Rta transactivation (Lukac *et al.*, 1999).

This dominant negative inhibitor can actually block reactivation following treatment with the chemical inducers TPA, sodium butyrate, and ionomycin (Lukac *et al.*, 1999). While Rta can directly bind to KSHV promoters (Chang *et al.*, 2002; Liang *et al.*, 2002; Song *et al.*, 2002), it requires interactions with other cellular proteins such as RBP-Jκ (recombination signal binding protein Jκ), AP-1, and Oct-1 for transactivation of promoters (Carroll *et al.*, 2006; Sakakibara *et al.*, 2001; Wang *et al.*, 2004).

RBP-Jκ is particularly interesting since it is a transcriptional repressor that is involved in the Notch-signaling pathway. The Notch-signaling pathway functions in a wide variety of developmental processes and regulates the fate of cells and its dysregulation is implicated in many cancers (Radtke & Raj, 2003; Weng *et al.*, 2004). Once activated, Notch is cleaved and its intracellular domain interacts with RBP-Jκ and converts it from a transcriptional repressor to an activator. This complex then activates expression of specific target genes, much like that seen for KSHV Rta-RBP-Jκ (Bray, 2006; He & Pear, 2003; Liang *et al.*, 2002). The interaction of Rta and RBP-Jκ has been shown to be essential for the switch from viral latent replication to lytic replication in rodent cells, as reactivation is severely limited in RBP-Jκ null cells (Liang & Ganem, 2003). In a recent paper, it was determined that the association of Rta with RBP-Jκ and the subsequent binding of the complex to DNA were not sufficient to activate RBP-Jκ and induce KSHV lytic replication, suggesting that another cofactor(s) is required (Papugani *et al.*, 2008).

Rta activity can be inhibited by a number of viral and cellular factors, which can limit the switch to lytic replication and promote latency and persistent infection. Some of these factors are IRF-7, KSHV Rta-binding protein (K-RBP), poly(ADP-ribose) polymerase 1 (PARP-1), NF-κB, histone deacetylase 1 (HDAC1), KbZIP (ORF K8), and LANA (Brown *et al.*, 2003; Gwack *et al.*, 2001, 2003; Izumiya *et al.*, 2003; Lan *et al.*, 2004; Wang *et al.*, 2005; Yang & Wood, 2007). The question arises as to how Rta can transactivate genes and induce lytic replication when there are so many repressors of Rta present in the cell. It turns out that Rta is able to promote the degradation of all of these factors except for HDAC1 via proteosome-dependent and -independent mechanisms (Yang *et al.*, 2008). Interestingly, Rta also regulates its own degradation through self-ubiquitination (Yu *et al.*, 2005). This suggests that there is a balance between repression of viral lytic genes and degradation of repressors to control the switch between latency and lytic replication (see Fig. 1).

While latency is thought to play a very important part in herpesvirus-induced oncogenesis through enhanced survival and proliferation of infected cells, there is evidence that lytic replication also has an active role in tumorigenesis. One puzzling question to this idea is since lytic replication ultimately leads to cell death, how could expression of lytic genes in cells that are going to die result in cancer? First, the main latent reservoir of KSHV is the B lymphocyte. In order to spread to the previously uninfected cells such as endothelial cells, the virus must enter the lytic phase and produce new viral progeny. Second, the lytic cycle encodes a variety of signaling proteins that are secreted or induce secretion of proangiogenic and mitogenic factors that act in a paracrine fashion and have been shown to play important roles in disease progression (Cesarman *et al.*, 2000). Just a couple of these are vIL-6 and viral G-protein-coupled receptor (vGPCR), both of which have tumorigenic properties and will be discussed in more detail later. vIL-6 expression is frequently detected in clinical samples of PEL, MCD, and KS in the absence of other lytic genes (Brousset *et al.*, 2001; Parravicini *et al.*, 2000; Staskus *et al.*, 1999). These lytically expressed proteins can also induce the expression of host proteins that can mediate angiogenesis and inflammation (Bais *et al.*, 1998; Polson *et al.*, 2002). It has also been theorized that dysregulated expression of lytic genes during latent phase or during abortive lytic cycles may trigger KSHV tumorigenesis (Grisotto *et al.*, 2006; Montaner *et al.*, 2003; Sodhi *et al.*, 2004). Finally, it has been shown that patients developing KS have significantly elevated levels of antibodies to lytically expressed proteins in their sera (Goudsmit *et al.*, 2000) and treatment with gancyclovir, a drug that targets actively replicating herpesvirus, dramatically reduces the incidence of KS development in HIV-1 infected individuals (Martin *et al.*, 1999).

5. Viral Proteins Involved in Signal Transduction

The interruption or alteration of cell-signaling cascades is a common property among oncogenic DNA viruses. Cellular transformation by tumor viruses is often achieved by targeting cell-signaling pathways. The goal of oncogenic viruses is to prolong the life of the cell through inhibition of apoptosis and to promote cellular proliferation. Viral oncoproteins often target key transcription factors to activate or repress their function in order to obtain the desired outcome. KSHV is no exception to this general rule. It encodes numerous proteins that modify cell-signaling pathways, many of which are homologous to cellular proteins (Fig. 2). One advantage to these viral homologs is

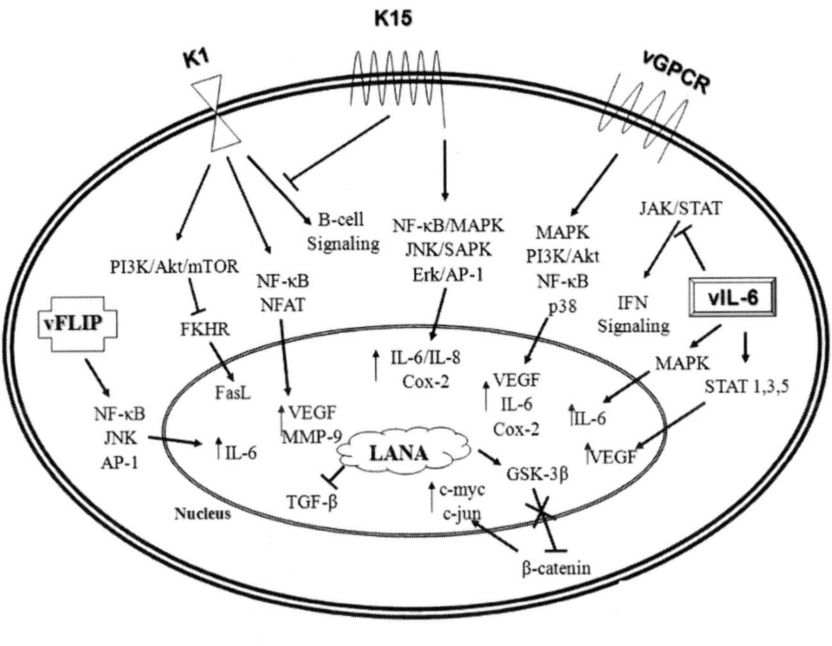

Fig. 2. Modulation of signaling cascades by KSHV proteins. Summary of the signal transduction pathways altered by the KSHV viral proteins described in this chapter. Many of the pathways activated lead to the induction of proangiogenic and mitogenic factors important in disease progression.

that they can escape the normal regulatory mechanisms put in place to prevent uncontrolled cell growth and proliferation. Just a few of these KSHV proteins and their potential roles in tumorigenesis will be described in detail below.

5.1. K1

The K1 protein is encoded by the very first ORF in the viral genome. It is a 46-kDa transmembrane glycoprotein that is mainly expressed during lytic replication (Jenner *et al.*, 2001; Lee *et al.*, 1998a; Nakamura *et al.*, 2003). K1 has an N-terminal extracellular domain and a short cytoplasmic C-terminus, which contains an immunoreceptor tyrosine-based activation motif (ITAM) with two SH2-binding motifs that are similar to the one found in the B- and T-cell receptor proteins as well as EBV LMP2A (Lagunoff & Ganem, 1997; Lee *et al.*, 1998b). ITAMs are found in a variety of immune receptor complexes and play central roles in signal transduction events, leading to cell proliferation, differentiation, and death. In B lymphocytes, the K1 ITAM recruits the SH2-containing signaling kinases NFAT (nuclear factor of activated T-cells), syk, and vav, which lead to the activation of the PI3K/Akt/mTOR pathway (Lagunoff *et al.*, 1999; Lee *et al.*, 1998b, 2005; Tomlinson & Damania, 2004; Wang *et al.*, 2004, 2006). Activation of Akt leads to the phosphorylation of its downstream targets with the net result being cell survival via inactivation of the forkhead transcription factor (FKHR) family and Fas signaling in B-cells and inactivation of Akt's pro-apoptotic targets in endothelial cells (Tomlinson & Damania, 2004; Wang *et al.*, 2004, 2006). K1 expression also leads to the activation of NF-κB-dependent promoters (Samaniego *et al.*, 2001). Due to its mitogenic signaling properties, the K1 protein has transforming capabilities, as it has been shown to produce morphological changes and foci formation in Rat-1 fibroblasts and primary human umbilical vein endothelial cells (Lee *et al.*, 1998a; Wang *et al.*, 2006).

K1 is expressed in KS lesions as well as MCD and PEL (Lee *et al.*, 2003; Samaniego *et al.*, 2001; Wang *et al.*, 2006). Expression of K1 in endothelial and epithelial cells results in the upregulation and secretion of the angiogenic factors vascular endothelial growth factor

(VEGF) and matrix metalloproteinase-9 (MMP-9) (Wang *et al.*, 2004), suggesting that K1 might contribute to KSHV pathogenesis through a paracrine mechanism that promotes tumor progression and growth. K1 protein can also downregulate B-cell receptor (BCR) expression on the cell surface via retention of the BCR in the endoplasmic reticulum (ER) and subsequent degradation (Lee *et al.*, 2000). Since K1 is structurally similar to the BCR, it is a possibility that the K1 protein acts as a decoy molecule.

5.2. vGPCR

G-protein-coupled receptors (GPCRs) are the largest family of signaling molecules and bind a wide variety of ligands. KSHV encodes a viral homolog termed vGPCR that is expressed from ORF74, has seven transmembrane domains, and is expressed early in lytic replication (Cesarman *et al.*, 1996). vGPCR is a constitutively active CXC receptor that has greatest sequence similarity to the cellular IL-8 receptor (Cesarman *et al.*, 1996; Chiou *et al.*, 2002; Guo *et al.*, 1997). While constitutive signaling is not dependent upon ligand binding, its signaling is up- or downregulated by the binding of various chemokines (Geras-Raaka *et al.*, 1998; Ho *et al.*, 1999; Rosenkilde *et al.*, 1999). vGPCR is known to activate the MAPK, PI3K/Akt, NF-κB, and p38 pathways, which results in the expression of the angiogenic factor VEGF and other cytokines (Bais *et al.*, 1998; Montaner, 2007; Schwarz & Murphy, 2001). This also leads to transformation of fibroblasts and endothelial cells (Arvanitakis *et al.*, 1997; Bais *et al.*, 2003). Furthermore, it has been shown that vGPCR induces cyclooxygenase-2 (Cox-2)-mediated prostaglandin production in endothelial cells, which is found at elevated levels in KS lesions (Ambrus *et al.*, 1992; Shelby *et al.*, 2007).

One of the most interesting findings concerning vGPCR was that transgenic mice that expressed vGPCR in hematopoietic cells developed angioproliferative lesions in multiple organs that pathologically resembled KS lesions (Montaner *et al.*, 2003; Yang *et al.*, 2000). Also in these mouse models, only a small percentage of cells in the lesion expressed detectable levels of vGPCR, very similar to what is seen in early KS lesions where only about 10% of endothelial and spindle cells are infected by KSHV (Dupin *et al.*, 1999). This and other data suggest that paracrine mechanisms triggered by vGPCR play an important role in the development of angioproliferative diseases such as KS. In KS, proliferation of latently infected cells may depend on paracrine factors released by neighboring cells that are undergoing lytic replication (Kirshner *et al.*, 1999). vGPCR has been shown to promote tumor formation in cells expressing KSHV latent genes, indicating that there is a cooperation between lytic and latent genes in the development of KS (Montaner *et al.*, 2003).

5.3. vIL-6

Another homolog of a cellular protein encoded by KSHV is vIL-6, which has about 25% identity to human IL-6 and also shares several biological properties with its cellular counterpart (Moore *et al.*, 1996; Neipel *et al.*, 1997; Nicholas *et al.*, 1997). Even before the discovery of KSHV and vIL-6, secreted cellular IL-6 had been linked to KS and MCD (Miles *et al.*, 1990; Yoshizaki *et al.*, 1989). Human IL-6 is an autocrine growth factor that has been implicated in several lymphoproliferative disorders including multiple myeloma (Catlett-Falcone *et al.*, 1999). vIL-6 activates IL-6-signaling pathways by binding to gp130, a signal transducer molecule, but does not require binding to gp80, the IL-6 specific receptor (Molden *et al.*, 1997; Mullberg *et al.*, 2000). Downregulation of the gp80 subunit is a normal cellular response to IL-6-signaling, thus the requirement of vIL-6 for only gp130 most likely allows for vIL-6 to circumvent this regulatory feedback loop and continue transmitting growth stimulatory signals.

vIL-6 has been shown to have a variety of functions. It is able to induce phosphorylation of signal transducers and activators of transcription (STATs) 1, 3, and 5 as well as activating the MAP kinase-signaling cascade (Hideshima *et al.*, 2000; Molden *et al.*, 1997; Osborne *et al.*, 1999). Phosphorylation and activation of STAT-3 is particularly interesting, as it has been shown to have numerous oncogenic properties such as induction of cell transformation and tumorigenesis (Bromberg *et al.*, 1999), inhibiting apoptosis (Bromberg *et al.*, 1999; Catlett-Falcone *et al.*, 1999; Grandis *et al.*, 2000), and inducing mitogenesis by upregulating c-myc (Bowman *et al.*, 2001). The activation of STAT-3 by vIL-6 has also been demonstrated to induce VEGF expression (Aoki *et al.*, 1999; Liu *et al.*, 2001). Furthermore, mice injected with vIL-6-transfected NIH-3T3 cells developed highly vascularized tumors, elevated VEGF levels, and increased hematopoiesis (Aoki *et al.*, 1999).

In contrast to cellular IL-6, vIL-6 is able to protect PEL cells from the antiproliferative effects of interferon (IFN) α (Chatterjee *et al.*, 2002). During viral infection, host cells activate the IFN pathway, which can lead to p21 upregulation, initiation of cell cycle arrest, and inhibition of virus replication. vIL-6 can block the IFNα-signaling pathway and is actually upregulated in response to IFNα (Chatterjee *et al.*, 2002). This creates a negative feedback loop that can prevent infected cells from undergoing cell cycle arrest. Based on the data above, vIL-6 seems to be a very good candidate in contributing to progression of KSHV-related malignancies. In the context of disease, vIL-6 expression can be detected in PEL cells and to very high levels in MCD, but it is found at very low levels in KS (Jones *et al.*, 1999; Parravicini *et al.*, 1997, 2000).

5.4. K15

The genome location, splicing pattern, and predicted protein structure of K15 are very similar to EBV LMP2A while C-terminal sequence and binding motifs resemble the EBV LMP1 protein (Damania, 2004). K15 has a short cytoplasmic N-terminus that has no known function associated with it, and a longer cytoplasmic C-terminal domain that contains the signal transduction activity. The K15 cytoplasmic tail is constitutively tyrosine phosphorylated (Choi *et al.*, 2000b). The phosphorylation of Y^{481} in the YEEVL SH2-binding motif is necessary for activation of the Ras/MAPK, NF-κB, and JNK/SAPK pathways and results in the induction of IL-6, IL-8, and Cox-2 (Brinkmann *et al.*, 2003, 2007). The phosphorylation of Y^{481} is performed through interactions with the tyrosine kinases Src, Lck, Yes, Hck, and Fyn (Brinkmann *et al.*, 2003). There is also a putative

TRAF binding site in the K15 cytoplasmic tail that, along with the YEEVL motif, binds TRAFs 1–3 and is involved in NF-κB, AP-1, and Erk2 signaling (Brinkmann *et al.*, 2003; Glenn *et al.*, 1999).

A CD8-K15 chimeric protein was able to downregulate BCR signaling following antibody cross-linking via its SH2 (YEEVL) and SH3 (PPLP) binding motifs (Choi *et al.*, 2000b). This is similar to that seen with LMP2A of EBV (Fruehling & Longnecker, 1997). Inhibition of BCR signaling by K15 may be due to increased BCR internalization. The PPLP motif has been shown to interact with intersectin-2, an adaptor protein involved in endocytic trafficking (Lim *et al.*, 2007). Activation of B-cells through BCR signaling is one possible mechanism for viral reactivation, thus antagonizing BCR signaling may play a role in maintaining viral latency and/or preventing apoptosis. The C-terminus may also play a role in preventing apoptosis as the SH2-binding YASIL motif of K15 has been found to bind to the antiapoptotic protein HAX-1 (Sharp *et al.*, 2002). HAX-1 can inhibit Bax-induced apoptosis of B-cells, but co-transfection of K15 with Bax and HAX-1 had no effect, positive or negative, on HAX-1 blocking of Bax-induced apoptosis (Sharp *et al.*, 2002).

5.5. vFLIP

As mentioned previously, the latent protein vFLIP can inhibit caspase-8-dependent death receptor signaling to promote cell survival (Thome *et al.*, 1997). In addition to regulating caspase-8 activity, vFLIP can also induce NF-κB signaling by both the classical and alternative pathways through interaction with IKKγ (Field *et al.*, 2003; Liu *et al.*, 2002; Matta & Chaudhary, 2004). There is a TRAF-interacting motif within vFLIP that has been shown to directly bind TRAF2 (Guasparri *et al.*, 2006). While TRAF3 was not shown to bind vFLIP, both TRAF2 and TRAF3 were essential for NF-κB signaling (Guasparri *et al.*, 2006). This activity is critical for the survival of KSHV-infected PEL cells as inhibitors of NF-κB quickly induces PEL cell apoptosis (Guasparri *et al.*, 2004; Keller *et al.*, 2000). The importance of vFLIP for PEL cell survival *in vivo* has been demonstrated as well (Godfrey *et al.*, 2005). vFLIP-mediated activation of NF-κB also protects cells against apoptosis induced by growth factor withdrawal (Sun *et al.*, 2003). There is some question as to the effect vFLIP has on the JNK/AP-1 pathway. One group reported that vFLIP activates JNK/AP-1 in a TRAF2-dependent manner while others found that vFLIP did not bind TRAF2 and had either no effect or suppressed AP-1 activity (An *et al.*, 2003; Matta *et al.*, 2007; Sun *et al.*, 2006; Ye *et al.*, 2008). Clearly, more studies need to be performed to explain the discrepancies in these works. The activation of NF-κB has been shown to inhibit lytic replication (Brown *et al.*, 2003; Ye *et al.*, 2008) and vFLIP has been found to inhibit Rta expression (Ye *et al.*, 2008). Thus, by promoting persistent latent infection, vFLIP may contribute to tumor development.

5.6. LANA

KSHV LANA is a multifunctional protein that is critical to the establishment and maintenance of latency following viral infection. To perform its many functions, LANA deregulates a variety of cellular-signaling pathways. LANA induces IL-6 expression through stimulating a c-Jun-Fos heterodimer to bind and activate the AP-1 response element within the IL-6 promoter (An *et al.*, 2004). The Wnt pathway is also activated by LANA through its interaction with glycogen synthase kinase-3 beta (GSK-3β) (Fujimuro *et al.*, 2005). GSK-3β normally phosphorylates β-catenin causing its cytoplasmic sequestration and subsequent degradation by the proteasome. By binding to GSK-3β, LANA allows for the accumulation of β-catenin in the cytoplasm, which then translocates to the nucleus to stimulate the transcription of many proliferation-associated genes. An increase in β-catenin production has been noted in people with basal cell carcinoma and leads to the increase in proliferation of related tumors (Saldanha *et al.*, 2004). β-Catenin is also found at elevated levels in PEL cells and KS tumor cells. LANA has been shown to target the Notch pathway as well. RBP-Jκ is the primary mediator of the Notch-signaling pathway and is a sequence-specific transcriptional repressor (Dou *et al.*, 1994) and the KSHV Rta promoter contains an RBP-Jκ binding site (Liang *et al.*, 2002). LANA binds RBP-Jκ and represses

Rta expression by targeting the RBP-Jκ binding sites in the Rta promoter (Lan *et al.*, 2004, 2005). Recently, it has been discovered that LANA blocks the transforming growth factor β (TGF-β) pathway, thus inhibiting growth arrest and apoptosis (Di Bartolo *et al.*, 2008). Through subversion of these different cell-signaling cascades, LANA promotes viral latency and likely the progression of KSHV-associated neoplasia.

6. Summary

KSHV is a relatively new virus in terms of its discovery, but in the 15 years since it was first identified there has been an ever-increasing wealth of information uncovered regarding its life cycle and its effects on the host response. While a lot is known about KSHV, there are still gaps in our knowledge with regard to every step of the viral life cycle from binding and fusion to capsid trafficking to the nucleus to reactivation. Studies on the biology and pathogenesis of KSHV have been hindered by the lack of an animal model that reproduces the human diseases caused by KSHV since KSHV does not infect mice or macaques. The most reliable animal model uses rhesus rhadinovirus (RRV), which is a close simian relative of KSHV.

From the moment the KSHV virion binds to its receptor(s) on the cell surface, it modulates cellular processes to increase its chance of a successful infection. Just the binding of the virion to integrins induces a signaling cascade that modifies the intracellular environment in favor of the virus. This potentially means that by the time the nucleocapsid is released into the cytoplasm, cellular gene expression has been altered to suppress antiviral responses and cytoskeletal rearrangement has occurred to promote translocation of the KSHV genome to the nucleus. The establishment of latency and lifelong infection soon follows. This is indicative of how well KSHV has evolved over the millions of years and the challenge that we face in finding ways to prevent infection and subsequent disease.

KSHV encodes a plethora of proteins that appear to induce cellular transformation and oncogenesis. In all probability, only a few of theses proteins play a primary role in tumorigenesis, but as of yet it is unknown which ones are the major contributors. Such information would be very important for the design of potential vaccines or treatments for KSHV-related diseases. Latency genes appear to be the leading factors for promoting oncogenesis, but even that idea has been challenged by the recent findings that some lytic genes are expressed very early in infection during abortive lytic replication and during the establishment of latency (Krishnan *et al.*, 2004). Morever, it is becoming apparent that paracrine mechanisms, such as the action of secreted IL-6 and VEGF, play a substantial role in the development of KSHV-associated neoplasia. In conclusion, more research is needed to generate a clearer understanding of the various mechanisms involved in KSHV-induced tumorigenesis.

Acknowledgments

Work carried out in the authors' laboratory is supported by grants from the NIH (CA096500, HL083469, and DE018281) to BD. PJD was supported by the basic mechanisms of viral and chemical carcinogenesis training grant (CA009156). BD is a Leukemia & Lymphoma Society Scholar and Burroughs Wellcome Fund Investigator in Infectious Disease.

References

Akula SM, Pramod NP, Wang FZ, Chandran B (2001) Human herpesvirus 8 envelope-associated glycoprotein B interacts with heparan sulfate-like moieties. *Virology* **284**: 235–249.

Akula SM, Pramod NP, Wang FZ, Chandran B (2002) Integrin alpha3beta1 (CD 49c/29) is a cellular receptor for Kaposi's sarcoma-associated herpesvirus (KSHV/HHV-8) entry into the target cells. *Cell* **108**: 407–419.

Akula SM, Naranatt PP, Walia NS, Wang FZ, Fegley B, Chandran B (2003) Kaposi's sarcoma-associated herpesvirus (human herpesvirus 8) infection of human fibroblast cells occurs through endocytosis. *J Virol* **77**: 7978–7990.

Ambroziak JA, Blackbourn DJ, Herndier BG, Glogau RG, Gullett JH, McDonald AR, Lennette ET, Levy JA (1995) Herpes-like sequences in

HIV-infected and uninfected Kaposi's sarcoma patients. *Science* **268**: 582–583.

Ambrus JL, Stoll HL, Klein EA, Karakousis CP, Stadler S (1992) Increased prostaglandin E2 and cAMP phosphodiesterase levels in Kaposi's sarcoma — a virus against host defense mechanism. *Res Commun Chem Pathol Pharmacol* **78**: 249–252.

An J, Sun Y, Sun R, Rettig MB (2003) Kaposi's sarcoma-associated herpesvirus encoded vFLIP induces cellular IL-6 expression: the role of the NF-kappaB and JNK/AP1 pathways. *Oncogene* **22**: 3371–3385.

An J, Sun Y, Rettig MB (2004) Transcriptional coactivation of c-Jun by the KSHV-encoded LANA. *Blood* **103**: 222–228.

Antman K, Chang Y (2000) Kaposi's sarcoma. *N Engl J Med* **342**: 1027–1038.

Aoki Y, Jaffe ES, Chang Y, Jones K, Teruya-Feldstein J, Moore PS, Tosato G (1999) Angiogenesis and hematopoiesis induced by Kaposi's sarcoma-associated herpesvirus-encoded interleukin-6. *Blood* **93**: 4034–4043.

Arvanitakis L, Geras-Raaka E, Varma A, Gershengorn MC, Cesarman E (1997) Human herpesvirus KSHV encodes a constitutively active G-protein-coupled receptor linked to cell proliferation. *Nature* **385**: 347–350.

Bais C, Santomasso B, Coso O, Arvanitakis L, Raaka EG, Gutkind JS, Asch AS, Cesarman E, Gershengorn MC, Mesri EA (1998) G-protein-coupled receptor of Kaposi's sarcoma-associated herpesvirus is a viral oncogene and angiogenesis activator. *Nature* **391**: 86–89.

Bais C, Van Geelen A, Eroles P, Mutlu A, Chiozzini C, Dias S, Silverstein RL, Rafii S, Mesri EA (2003) Kaposi's sarcoma associated herpesvirus G protein-coupled receptor immortalizes human endothelial cells by activation of the VEGF receptor-2/KDR. *Cancer Cell* **3**: 131–143.

Barozzi P, Luppi M, Facchetti F, Mecucci C, Alù M, Sarid R, Rasini V, Ravazzini L, Rossi E, Festa S, Crescenzi B, Wolf DG, Schulz TF, Torelli G (2003) Post-transplant Kaposi sarcoma originates from the seeding of donor-derived progenitors. *Nat Med* **9**: 554–561.

Bartel DP (2004) MicroRNAs: genomics, biogenesis, mechanism, and function. *Cell* **116**: 281–297.

Bechtel JT, Winant RC, Ganem D (2005) Host and viral proteins in the virion of Kaposi's sarcoma-associated herpesvirus. *J Virol 79*: 4952–4964.

Beral V, Peterman TA, Berkelman RL, Jaffe HW (1990) Kaposi's sarcoma among persons with AIDS: a sexually transmitted infection? *Lancet* **335**: 123–128.

Bieleski L, Talbot SJ (2001) Kaposi's sarcoma-associated herpesvirus vCyclin open reading frame contains an internal ribosome entry site. *J Virol* **75**: 1864–1869.

Birkmann A, Mahr K, Ensser A, Yağuboğlu S, Titgemeyer F, Fleckenstein B, Neipel F (2001) Cell surface heparan sulfate is a receptor for human herpesvirus 8 and interacts with envelope glycoprotein K8.1. *J Virol* **75**: 11583–11593.

Bowman T, Broome MA, Sinibaldi D, Wharton W, Pledger WJ, Sedivy JM, Irby R, Yeatman T, Courtneidge SA, Jove R (2001) Stat3-mediated Myc expression is required for Src transformation and PDGF-induced mitogenesis. *Proc Natl Acad Sci USA* **98**: 7319–7324.

Brander C, Raje N, O'Connor PG, Davies F, Davis J, Chauhan D, Hideshima T, Martin J, Osmond D, Kedes DH, Walker BD, Scadden DT, Anderson KC (2002) Absence of biologically important Kaposi sarcoma-associated herpesvirus gene products and virus-specific cellular immune responses in multiple myeloma. *Blood* **100**: 698–700.

Bray SJ (2006) Notch signalling: a simple pathway becomes complex. *Nat Rev Mol Cell Biol* **7**: 678–689.

Brinkmann MM, Glenn M, Rainbow L, Kieser A, Henke-Gendo C, Schulz TF (2003) Activation of mitogen-activated protein kinase and NF-kappaB pathways by a Kaposi's sarcoma-associated herpesvirus K15 membrane protein. *J Virol* **77**: 9346–9358.

Brinkmann MM, Schulz TF (2006) Regulation of intracellular signalling by the terminal membrane proteins of members of the *Gammaherpesvirinae*. *J Gen Virol* **87**: 1047–1074.

Brinkmann MM, Pietrek M, Dittrich-Breiholz O, Kracht M, Schulz TF (2007) Modulation of host gene expression by the K15 protein of Kaposi's sarcoma-associated herpesvirus. *J Virol* **81**: 42–58.

Bromberg JF, Wrzeszczynska MH, Devgan G, Zhao Y, Pestell RG, Albanese C, Darnell JE Jr (1999) Stat3 as an oncogene. *Cell* **98**: 295–303.

Brousset P, Cesarman E, Meggetto F, Lamant L, Delsol G (2001) Colocalization of the viral interleukin-6 with latent nuclear antigen-1 of human herpesvirus-8 in endothelial spindle cells of Kaposi's sarcoma and lymphoid cells of multicentric Castleman's disease. *Hum Pathol* **32**: 95–100.

Brown HJ, Song MJ, Deng H, Wu TT, Cheng G, Sun R (2003) NF-kappaB inhibits gammaherpesvirus lytic replication. *J Virol* **77**: 8532–8540.

Cai X, Lu S, Zhang Z, Gonzalez CM, Damania B, Cullen BR (2005) Kaposi's sarcoma-associated herpesvirus expresses an array of viral microRNAs in latently infected cells. *Proc Natl Acad Sci USA* **102**: 5570–5575.

Carroll KD, Bu W, Palmeri D, Spadavecchia S, Lynch SJ, Marras SA, Tyagi S, Lukac DM (2006) Kaposi's Sarcoma-associated herpesvirus lytic switch protein stimulates DNA binding of RBP-Jk/CSL to activate the Notch pathway. *J Virol* **80**: 9697–9709.

Catlett-Falcone R, Landowski TH, Oshiro MM, Turkson J, Levitzki A, Savino R, Ciliberto G, Moscinski L, Fernández-Luna JL, Nuñez G, Dalton WS, Jove R (1999) Constitutive activation of Stat3 signaling confers resistance to apoptosis in human U266 myeloma cells. *Immunity* **10**: 105–115.

Cesarman E, Chang Y, Moore PS, Said JW, Knowles DM (1995) Kaposi's sarcoma-associated herpesvirus-like DNA sequences in AIDS-related body-cavity-based lymphomas. *N Engl J Med* **332**: 1186–1191.

Cesarman E, Nador RG, Bai F, Bohenzky RA, Russo JJ, Moore PS, Chang Y, Knowles DM (1996) Kaposi's sarcoma-associated herpesvirus contains G protein-coupled receptor and cyclin D homologs which are expressed in Kaposi's sarcoma and malignant lymphoma. *J Virol* **70**: 8218–8223.

Cesarman E, Mesri EA, Gershengorn MC (2000) Viral G protein-coupled receptor and Kaposi's sarcoma: a model of paracrine neoplasia? *J Exp Med* **191**: 417–422.

Chang PJ, Shedd D, Gradoville L, Cho MS, Chen LW, Chang J, Miller G (2002) Open reading frame 50 protein of Kaposi's sarcoma-associated herpesvirus directly activates the viral PAN and K12 genes by binding to related response elements. *J Virol* **76**: 3168–3178.

Chang Y, Cesarman E, Pessin MS, Lee F, Culpepper J, Knowles DM, Moore PS (1994) Identification of herpesvirus-like DNA sequences in AIDS-associated Kaposi's sarcoma. *Science* **266**: 1865–1869.

Chang Y, Moore PS, Talbot SJ, Boshoff CH, Zarkowska T, Godden-Kent D, Paterson H, Weiss RA, Mittnacht S (1996) Cyclin encoded by KS herpesvirus. *Nature* **382**: 410.

Chatterjee M, Osborne J, Bestetti G, Chang Y, Moore PS (2002) Viral IL-6-induced cell proliferation and immune evasion of interferon activity. *Science* **298**: 1432–1435.

Chaudhary PM, Jasmin A, Eby MT, Hood L (1999) Modulation of the NF-kappa B pathway by virally encoded death effector domains-containing proteins. *Oncogene* **18**: 5738–5746.

Chauhan D, Bharti A, Raje N, Gustafson E, Pinkus GS, Pinkus JL, Teoh G, Hideshima T, Treon SP, Fingeroth JD, Anderson KC (1999) Detection of Kaposi's sarcoma herpesvirus DNA sequences in multiple myeloma bone marrow stromal cells. *Blood* **93**: 1482–1486.

Chen YB, Rahemtullah A, Hochberg E (2007) Primary effusion lymphoma. *Oncologist* **12**: 569–576.

Chiou CJ, Poole LJ, Kim PS, Ciufo DM, Cannon JS, ap Rhys CM, Alcendor DJ, Zong JC, Ambinder RF, Hayward GS (2002) Patterns of gene expression and a transactivation function exhibited by the vGCR (ORF74) chemokine receptor protein of Kaposi's sarcoma-associated herpesvirus. *J Virol* **76**: 3421–3439.

Choi J, Liu RM, Kundu RK, Sangiorgi F, Wu W, Maxson R, Forman, HJ (2000a) Molecular mechanism of decreased glutathione content in human immunodeficiency virus type 1 Tat-transgenic mice. *J Biol Chem* **275**: 3693–3698.

Choi JK, Lee BS, Shim SN, Li M, Jung JU (2000b) Identification of the novel K15 gene at the rightmost end of the Kaposi's sarcoma-associated herpesvirus genome. *J Virol* **74**: 436–446.

Cool CD, Rai PR, Yeager ME, Hernandez-Saavedra D, Serls AE, Bull TM, Geraci MW, Brown KK, Routes JM, Tuder RM, Voelkel NF (2003) Expression of human herpesvirus 8 in primary pulmonary hypertension. *N Engl J Med* **349**: 1113–1122.

Cotter MA 2nd, Robertson ES (1999) The latency-associated nuclear antigen tethers the Kaposi's sarcoma-associated herpesvirus genome to host chromosomes in body cavity-based lymphoma cells. *Virology* **264**: 254–264.

Damania B, Jeong JH, Bowser BS, DeWire SM, Staudt MR, Dittmer DP (2004) Comparison of the Rta/Orf50 transactivator proteins of gamma-2-herpesviruses. *J Virol* **78**: 5491–5499.

Damania B (2004) Oncogenic gamma-herpesviruses: comparison of viral proteins involved in tumorigenesis. *Nat Rev Microbiol* **2**: 656–668.

de Fraipont F, Nicholson AC, Feige JJ, Van Meir EG (2001) Thrombospondins and tumor angiogenesis. *Trends Mol Med* 7: 401–407.

Di Alberti L, Piattelli A, Artese L, Favia G, Patel S, Saunders N, Porter SR, Scully CM, Ngui SL, Teo CG (1997) Human herpesvirus 8 variants in sarcoid tissues. *Lancet* **350**: 1655–1661.

Di Bartolo DL, Cannon M, Liu YF, Renne R, Chadburn A, Boshoff C, Cesarman E (2008) KSHV LANA inhibits TGF-beta signaling through epigenetic silencing of the TGF-beta type II receptor. *Blood* **111**: 4731–4740.

Dittmer D, Lagunoff M, Renne R, Staskus K, Haase A, Ganem D (1998) A cluster of latently expressed genes in Kaposi's sarcoma-associated herpesvirus. *J Virol* **72**: 8309–8315.

Dou S, Zeng X, Cortes P, Erdjument-Bromage H, Tempst P, Honjo T, Vales LD (1994) The recombination signal sequence-binding protein RBP-2N functions as a transcriptional repressor. *Mol Cell Biol* **14**: 3310–3319.

Dourmishev LA, Dourmishev AL, Palmeri D, Schwartz RA, Lukac DM (2003) Molecular genetics of Kaposi's sarcoma-associated herpesvirus (human herpesvirus-8) epidemiology and pathogenesis. *Microbiol Mol Biol Rev* **67**: 175–212.

Dupin N, Grandadam M, Calvez V, Gorin I, Aubin JT, Havard S, Lamy F, Leibowitch M, Huraux JM, Escande JP *et al.* (1995) Herpesvirus-like DNA sequences in patients with Mediterranean Kaposi's sarcoma. *Lancet* **345**: 761–762.

Dupin N, Fisher C, Kellam P, Ariad S, Tulliez M, Franck N, van Marck E, Salmon D, Gorin I, Escande JP, Weiss RA, Alitalo K, Boshoff C (1999) Distribution of human herpesvirus-8 latently infected cells in Kaposi's sarcoma, multicentric Castleman's disease, and primary effusion lymphoma. *Proc Natl Acad Sci USA* **96**: 4546–4551.

Esteban M, García MA, Domingo-Gil E, Arroyo J, Nombela C, Rivas C (2003) The latency protein LANA2 from Kaposi's sarcoma-associated herpesvirus inhibits apoptosis induced by dsRNA-activated protein kinase but not RNase L activation. *J Gen Virol* **84**: 1463–1470.

Field N, Low W, Daniels M, Howell S, Daviet L, Boshoff C, Collins M (2003) KSHV vFLIP binds to IKK-gamma to activate IKK. *J Cell Sci* **15**: 3721–3728.

Friborg J Jr, Kong W, Hottiger MO, Nabel GJ (1999) p53 inhibition by the LANA protein of KSHV protects against cell death. *Nature* **402**: 889–894.

Fruehling S, Longnecker R (1997) The immunoreceptor tyrosine-based activation motif of Epstein-Barr virus LMP2A is essential for blocking BCR-mediated signal transduction. *Virology* **235**: 241–251.

Frizzera G, Massarelli G, Banks PM, Rosai J (1983) A systemic lymphoproliferative disorder with morphologic features of Castleman's disease. *Am J Surg Pathol* 7: 211–231.

Fujimuro M, Liu J, Zhu J, Yokosawa H, Hayward SD (2005) Regulation of the interaction between glycogen synthase kinase 3 and the Kaposi's sarcoma-associated herpesvirus latency-associated nuclear antigen. *J Virol* **79**: 10429–10441.

Ganem D (1998) Human herpesvirus 8 and its role in the genesis of Kaposi's sarcoma. *Curr Clin Top Infect Dis* **18**: 237–251.

Garber AC, Shu MA, Hu J, Renne R (2001) DNA binding and modulation of gene expression by the latency-associated nuclear antigen of Kaposi's sarcoma-associated herpesvirus. *J Virol* **75**: 7882–7892.

Geras-Raaka E, Varma A, Clark-Lewis I, Gershengorn MC (1998) Kaposi's sarcoma-associated herpesvirus (KSHV) chemokine vMIP-II and human SDF-1alpha inhibit signaling by KSHV G protein-coupled receptor. *Biochem Biophys Res Commun* **253**: 725–727.

Giancotti FG, Ruoslahti E (1999) Integrin signaling. *Science* **285**: 1028–1032.

Glenn M, Rainbow L, Auradé F, Davison A, Schulz TF (1999) Identification of a spliced gene from Kaposi's sarcoma-associated herpesvirus encoding a protein with similarities to latent membrane proteins 1 and 2A of Epstein-Barr virus. *J Virol* **73**: 6953–6963.

Godfrey A, Anderson J, Papanastasiou A, Takeuchi Y, Boshoff C (2005) Inhibiting primary effusion lymphoma by lentiviral vectors encoding short hairpin RNA. *Blood* **105**: 2510–2518.

Goudsmit J, Renwick N, Dukers NH, Coutinho RA, Heisterkamp S, Bakker M, Schulz TF, Cornelissen M, Weverling GJ (2000) Human herpesvirus 8 infections in the Amsterdam Cohort Studies (1984–1997): analysis of seroconversions to ORF65 and ORF73. *Proc Natl Acad Sci USA* **97**: 4838–4843.

Gradoville L, Gerlach J, Grogan E, Shedd D, Nikiforow S, Metroka C, Miller G (2000) Kaposi's sarcoma-associated herpesvirus open reading frame 50/Rta protein activates the entire viral lytic cycle in the HH-B2 primary effusion lymphoma cell line. *J Virol* **74**: 6207–6212.

Grandis JR, Drenning SD, Zeng Q, Watkins SC, Melhem MF, Endo S, Johnson DE, Huang L, He Y, Kim JD (2000) Constitutive activation of Stat3 signaling abrogates apoptosis in squamous cell carcinogenesis *in vivo*. *Proc Natl Acad Sci USA* **97**: 4227–4232.

Grisotto MG, Garin A, Martin AP, Jensen KK, Chan P, Sealfon SC, Lira SA (2006) The human herpesvirus 8 chemokine receptor vGPCR triggers autonomous proliferation of endothelial cells. *J Clin Invest* **116**: 1264–1273.

Grundhoff A, Ganem D (2003) The latency-associated nuclear antigen of Kaposi's sarcoma-associated herpesvirus permits replication of terminal repeat-containing plasmids. *J Virol* **77**: 2779–2783.

Guasparri I, Keller SA, Cesarman E (2004) KSHV vFLIP is essential for the survival of infected lymphoma cells. *J Exp Med* **199**: 993–1003.

Guasparri I, Wu H, Cesarman E (2006) The KSHV oncoprotein vFLIP contains a TRAF-interacting motif and requires TRAF2 and TRAF3 for signalling. *EMBO Rep* 7: 114–119.

Guo HG, Browning P, Nicholas J, Hayward GS, Tschachler E, Jiang YW, Sadowska M, Raffeld M, Colombini S, Gallo RC, Reitz MS Jr (1997) Characterization of a chemokine receptor-related gene in human herpesvirus 8 and its expression in Kaposi's sarcoma. *Virology* **228**: 371–378.

Gwack Y, Byun H, Hwang S, Lim C, Choe J (2001) CREB-binding protein and histone deacetylase regulate the transcriptional activity of Kaposi's sarcoma-associated herpesvirus open reading frame 50. *J Virol* **75**: 1909–1917.

Gwack Y, Nakamura H, Lee SH, Souvlis J, Yustein JT, Gygi S, Kung HJ, Jung JU (2003) Poly(ADP-ribose) polymerase 1 and Ste20-like kinase hKFC act as transcriptional repressors for gamma-2 herpesvirus lytic replication. *Mol Cell Biol* **23**: 8282–8294.

He Y, Pear WS (2003) Notch signalling in B cells. *Semin Cell Dev Biol* **14**: 135–142.

Henke-Gendo C, Schulz TF, Hoeper MM (2004) HHV-8 in pulmonary hypertension. *N Engl J Med* **350**: 194–195.

Henry M, Uthman A, Geusau A, Rieger A, Furci L, Lazzarin A, Lusso P, Tschachler E (1999) Infection of circulating $CD34^+$ cells by HHV-8 in patients with Kaposi's sarcoma. *J Invest Dermatol* **113**: 613–616.

Hideshima T, Chauhan D, Teoh G, Raje N, Treon SP, Tai YT, Shima Y, Anderson KC (2000) Characterization of signaling cascades triggered by human interleukin-6 versus Kaposi's sarcoma-associated herpes virus-encoded viral interleukin 6. *Clin Cancer Res* **6**: 1180–1189.

Hiscott J, Pitha P, Genin P, Nguyen H, Heylbroeck C, Mamane Y, Algarte M, Lin R (1999) Triggering the interferon response: the role of IRF-3 transcription factor. *J Interferon Cytokine Res* **19**: 1–13.

Ho HH, Du D, Gershengorn MC (1999) The N terminus of Kaposi's sarcoma-associated herpesvirus G protein-coupled receptor is necessary for high affinity chemokine binding but not for constitutive activity. *J Biol Chem* **274**: 31327–31332.

Honda K, Taniguchi T (2006) IRFs: master regulators of signalling by Toll-like receptors and cytosolic pattern-recognition receptors. *Nat Rev Immunol* **6**: 644–658.

Hyun TS, Subramanian C, Cotter MA 2nd, Thomas RA, Robertson ES (2001) Latency-associated nuclear antigen encoded by Kaposi's sarcoma-associated herpesvirus interacts with Tat and activates the long terminal repeat of human immunodeficiency virus type 1 in human cells. *J Virol* **75**: 8761–8771.

Inohara N, Koseki T, Hu Y, Chen S, Núñez G (1997) CLARP, a death effector domain-containing protein interacts with caspase-8 and regulates apoptosis. *Proc Natl Acad Sci USA* **94**: 10717–10722.

Inoue N, Winter J, Lal RB, Offermann MK, Koyano S (2003) Characterization of entry mechanisms of human herpesvirus 8 by using an Rta-dependent reporter cell line. *J Virol* 77: 8147–8152.

Irmler M, Thome M, Hahne M, Schneider P, Hofmann K, Steiner V, Bodmer JL, Schröter M, Burns K, Mattmann C, Rimoldi D, French LE, Tschopp J (1997) Inhibition of death receptor signals by cellular FLIP. *Nature* **388**: 190–195.

Izumiya Y, Lin SF, Ellison T, Chen LY, Izumiya C, Luciw P, Kung HJ (2003) Kaposi's sarcoma-associated herpesvirus K-bZIP is a coregulator of K-Rta: physical association and promoter-dependent transcriptional repression. *J Virol* 77: 1441–1451.

Jenner RG, Albà MM, Boshoff C, Kellam P (2001) Kaposi's sarcoma-associated herpesvirus latent and lytic gene expression as revealed by DNA arrays. *J Virol* **75**: 891–902.

Jones KD, Aoki Y, Chang Y, Moore PS, Yarchoan R, Tosato G (1999) Involvement of interleukin-10 (IL-10) and viral IL-6 in the spontaneous growth of Kaposi's sarcoma herpesvirus-associated infected primary effusion lymphoma cells. *Blood* **94**: 2871–2879.

Joo CH, Shin YC, Gack M, Wu L, Levy D, Jung JU (2007) Inhibition of interferon regulatory factor 7 (IRF7)-mediated interferon signal transduction by the Kaposi's sarcoma-associated herpesvirus viral IRF homolog vIRF3. *J Virol* **81**: 8282–8292.

Kaleeba JA, Berger EA (2006a) Kaposi's sarcoma-associated herpesvirus fusion-entry receptor: cystine transporter xCT. *Science* **311**: 1921–1924.

Kaleeba JA, Berger EA (2006b) Broad target cell selectivity of Kaposi's sarcoma-associated herpesvirus glycoprotein-mediated cell fusion and virion entry. *Virology* **354**: 7–14.

Kaposi M (1872) Idiopathisches multiples pigmentsarkom der haut arch dermatol syph **4**: 265–273.

Katano H, Sato Y, Sata T (2001) Expression of p53 and human herpesvirus-8 (HHV-8)-encoded latency-associated nuclear antigen with inhibition of apoptosis in HHV-8-associated malignancies. *Cancer* **92**: 3076–3084.

Keller SA, Schattner EJ, Cesarman E (2000) Inhibition of NF-kappa B induces apoptosis of KSHV-infected primary effusion lymphoma cells. *Blood* **96**: 2537–2542.

Kirshner JR, Staskus K, Haase A, Lagunoff M, Ganem D (1999) Expression of the open reading frame 74 (G-protein-coupled receptor) gene of Kaposi's sarcoma (KS)-associated herpesvirus: implications for KS pathogenesis. *J Virol* **73**: 6006–6014.

Krishnan HH, Naranatt PP, Smith MS, Zeng L, Bloomer C, Chandran B (2004) Concurrent expression of latent and a limited number of lytic genes with immune modulation and antiapoptotic function by Kaposi's sarcoma-associated herpesvirus early during infection of primary endothelial and fibroblast cells and subsequent decline of lytic gene expression. *J Virol* **78**: 3601–3620.

Krishnan HH, Sharma-Walia N, Streblow DN, Naranatt PP, Chandran B (2006) Focal adhesion kinase is critical for entry of Kaposi's sarcoma-associated herpesvirus into target cells. *J Virol* **80**: 1167–1180.

Kumar MS, Lu J, Mercer KL, Golub TR, Jacks T (2007) Impaired microRNA processing enhances cellular transformation and tumorigenesis. *Nat Genet* **39**: 673–677.

Lagunoff M, Ganem D (1997) The structure and coding organization of the genomic termini of Kaposi's sarcoma-associated herpesvirus. *Virology* **236**: 147–154.

Lagunoff M, Majeti R, Weiss A, Ganem D (1999) Deregulated signal transduction by the K1 gene product of Kaposi's sarcoma-associated herpesvirus. *Proc Natl Acad Sci USA* **96**: 5704–5709.

Laman H, Coverley D, Krude T, Laskey R, Jones N (2001) Viral cyclin-cyclin-dependent kinase 6 complexes initiate nuclear DNA replication. *Mol Cell Biol* **21**: 624–635.

Lan K, Kuppers DA, Verma SC, Robertson ES (2004) Kaposi's sarcoma-associated herpesvirus-encoded latency-associated nuclear antigen inhibits lytic replication by targeting Rta: a potential mechanism for virus-mediated control of latency. *J Virol* **78**: 6585–6594.

Lan K, Kuppers DA, Verma SC, Sharma N, Murakami M, Robertson ES (2005) Induction of Kaposi's sarcoma-associated herpesvirus latency-associated nuclear antigen by the lytic transactivator RTA: a novel mechanism for establishment of latency. *J Virol* **79**: 7453–7465.

Lawler J (2002) Thrombospondin-1 as an endogenous inhibitor of angiogenesis and tumor growth. *J Cell Mol Med* **6**: 1–12.

Lee BS, Alvarez X, Ishido S, Lackner AA, Jung JU (2000) Inhibition of intracellular transport of B cell antigen receptor complexes by Kaposi's sarcoma-associated herpesvirus K1. *J Exp Med* **192**: 11–21.

Lee BS, Connole M, Tang Z, Harris NL, Jung JU (2003) Structural analysis of the Kaposi's sarcoma-associated herpesvirus K1 protein. *J Virol* **77**: 8072–8086.

Lee BS, Lee SH, Feng P, Chang H, Cho NH, Jung JU (2005) Characterization of the Kaposi's sarcoma-associated herpesvirus K1 signalosome. *J Virol* **79**: 12173–12184.

Lee H, Veazey R, Williams K, Li M, Guo J, Neipel F, Fleckenstein B, Lackner A, Desrosiers RC, Jung JU (1998a) Deregulation of cell growth by the K1 gene of Kaposi's sarcoma-associated herpesvirus. *Nat Med* **4**: 435–440.

Lee H, Guo J, Li M, Choi JK, DeMaria M, Rosenzweig M, Jung JU (1998b) Identification of an immunoreceptor tyrosine-based activation motif of K1 transforming protein of Kaposi's sarcoma-associated herpesvirus. *Mol Cell Biol* **18**: 5219–5228.

Levy DE, Marié I, Smith E, Prakash A (2002) Enhancement and diversification of IFN induction by IRF-7-mediated positive feedback. *J Interferon Cytokine Res* **22**: 87–93.

Li M, Lee H, Yoon DW, Albrecht JC, Fleckenstein B, Neipel F, Jung JU (1997) Kaposi's sarcoma-associated herpesvirus encodes a functional cyclin. *J Virol* **71**: 1984–1991.

Li SS, Forslöw A, Sundqvist KG (2005) Autocrine regulation of T cell motility by calreticulin-thrombospondin-1 interaction. *J Immunol* **174**: 654–661.

Liang Y, Chang J, Lynch SJ, Lukac DM, Ganem D (2002) The lytic switch protein of KSHV activates gene expression via functional interaction with RBP-Jkappa (CSL), the target of the Notch signaling pathway. *Genes Dev* **16**: 1977–1989.

Liang Y, Ganem D (2003) Lytic but not latent infection by Kaposi's sarcoma-associated herpesvirus requires host CSL protein, the mediator of notch signaling. *Proc Natl Acad Sci USA* **100**: 8490–8495.

Liao W, Tang Y, Kuo YL, Liu BY, Xu CJ, Giam CZ (2003) Kaposi's sarcoma-associated herpesvirus/human herpesvirus 8 transcriptional activator Rta is an oligomeric DNA-binding protein that interacts with tandem arrays of phased A/T-trinucleotide motifs. *J Virol* **77**: 9399–9411.

Lim C, Sohn H, Gwack Y, Choe J (2000) Latency-associated nuclear antigen of Kaposi's sarcoma-associated herpesvirus (human herpesvirus-8) binds ATF4/CREB2 and inhibits its transcriptional activation activity. *J Gen Virol* **81**: 2645–2652.

Lim CS, Seet BT, Ingham RJ, Gish G, Matskova L, Winberg G, Ernberg I, Pawson T (2007) The K15 protein of Kaposi's sarcoma-associated herpesvirus recruits the endocytic regulator intersectin 2 through a selective SH3 domain interaction. *Biochemistry* **46**: 9874–9885.

Lin SF, Robinson DR, Miller G, Kung HJ (1999) Kaposi's sarcoma-associated herpesvirus encodes a bZIP protein with homology to BZLF1 of Epstein-Barr virus. *J Virol* **73**: 1909–1917.

Liu C, Okruzhnov Y, Li H, Nicholas J (2001) Human herpesvirus 8 (HHV-8)-encoded cytokines induce expression of and autocrine signaling by vascular endothelial growth factor (VEGF) in HHV-8-infected primary-effusion lymphoma cell lines and mediate VEGF-independent antiapoptotic effects. *J Virol* **75**: 10933–10940.

Liu L, Eby MT, Rathore N, Sinha SK, Kumar A, Chaudhary PM (2002) The human herpes virus 8-encoded viral FLICE inhibitory protein physically associates with and persistently activates the Ikappa B kinase complex. *J Biol Chem* **277**: 13745–13751.

Low W, Harries M, Ye H, Du MQ, Boshoff C, Collins M (2001) Internal ribosome entry site regulates translation of Kaposi's sarcoma-associated herpesvirus FLICE inhibitory protein. *J Virol* **75**: 2938–2945.

Lu M, Suen J, Frias C, Pfeiffer R, Tsai MH, Chuang E, Zeichner SL (2004) Dissection of the Kaposi's sarcoma-associated herpesvirus gene expression program by using the viral DNA replication inhibitor cidofovir. *J Virol* **78**: 13637–13652.

Lubyova B, Pitha PM (2000) Characterization of a novel human herpesvirus 8-encoded protein, vIRF-3, that shows homology to viral and cellular interferon regulatory factors. *J Virol* **74**: 8194–8201.

Lukac DM, Renne R, Kirshner JR, Ganem D (1998) Reactivation of Kaposi's sarcoma-associated herpesvirus infection from latency by expression of the ORF 50 transactivator, a homolog of the EBV R protein. *Virology* **252**: 304–312.

Lukac DM, Kirshner JR, Ganem D (1999) Transcriptional activation by the product of open reading frame 50 of Kaposi's sarcoma-associated herpesvirus is required for lytic viral reactivation in B cells. *J Virol* **73**: 9348–9361.

Lukac DM, Garibyan L, Kirshner JR, Palmeri D, Ganem D (2001) DNA binding by Kaposi's sarcoma-associated herpesvirus lytic switch protein is necessary for transcriptional activation of two viral delayed early promoters. *J Virol* **75**: 6786–6799.

Ma L, Teruya-Feldstein J, Weinberg RA (2007) Tumour invasion and metastasis initiated by microRNA-10b in breast cancer. *Nature* **449**: 682–688.

Maeda H, Niimi T, Sato S, Kawaguchi H, Sugiura Y, Mori S, Ueda R (2000) Human herpesvirus 8 is not associated with sarcoidosis in Japanese patients. *Chest* **118**: 923–927.

Martin DF, Kuppermann BD, Wolitz RA, Palestine AG, Li H, Robinson CA (1999) Oral ganciclovir for patients with cytomegalovirus retinitis treated with a ganciclovir implant. Roche Ganciclovir Study Group. *N Engl J Med* **340**: 1063–1070.

Matta H, Chaudhary PM (2004) Activation of alternative NF-kappa B pathway by human herpes virus 8-encoded Fas-associated death domain-like IL-1 beta-converting enzyme inhibitory protein (vFLIP). *Proc Natl Acad Sci USA* **101**: 9399–9404.

Matta H, Mazzacurati L, Schamus S, Yang T, Sun Q, Chaudhary PM (2007) Kaposi's sarcoma-associated herpesvirus (KSHV) oncoprotein K13 bypasses TRAFs and directly interacts with the IkappaB kinase complex to selectively activate NF-kappa B without JNK activation. *J Biol Chem* **282**: 24858–24865.

Mbulaiteye SM, Biggar RJ, Goedert JJ, Engels EA (2002) Pleural and peritoneal lymphoma among people with AIDS in the United States. *J Acquir Immune Defic Syndr* **29**: 418–421.

Mbulaiteye SM, Biggar RJ, Goedert JJ, Engels EA (2003) Immune deficiency and risk for malignancy among persons with AIDS. *J Acquir Immune Defic Syndr* **32**: 527–533.

McCormick C, Ganem D (2005) The kaposin B protein of KSHV activates the p38/MK2 pathway and stabilizes cytokine mRNAs. *Science* **307**: 739–741.

McGeoch DJ, Gatherer D, Dolan A (2005) On phylogenetic relationships among major lineages of the *Gammaherpesvirinae*. *J Gen Virol* **86**: 307–316.

Miles SA, Rezai AR, Salazar-González JF, Vander Meyden M, Stevens RH, Logan DM, Mitsuyasu RT, Taga T, Hirano T, Kishimoto T *et al.* (1990) AIDS Kaposi sarcoma-derived cells produce and respond to interleukin 6. *Proc Natl Acad Sci USA* **87**: 4068–4072.

Molden J, Chang Y, You Y, Moore PS, Goldsmith MA (1997) A Kaposi's sarcoma-associated herpesvirus-encoded cytokine homolog (vIL-6) activates signaling through the shared gp130 receptor subunit. *J Biol Chem* **272**: 19625–19631.

Montaner S, Sodhi A, Molinolo A, Bugge TH, Sawai ET, He Y, Li Y, Ray PE, Gutkind JS (2003) Endothelial infection with KSHV genes *in vivo* reveals that vGPCR initiates Kaposi's sarcomagenesis and can promote the tumorigenic potential of viral latent genes. *Cancer Cell* **3**: 23–36.

Montaner S (2007) Akt/TSC/mTOR activation by the KSHV G protein-coupled receptor: emerging insights into the molecular oncogenesis and treatment of Kaposi's sarcoma. *Cell Cycle* **6**: 438–443.

Moore PS, Boshoff C, Weiss RA, Chang Y (1996) Molecular mimicry of human cytokine and cytokine response pathway genes by KSHV. *Science* **274**: 1739–1744.

Moore PS, Chang Y (2003) Kaposi's sarcoma-associated herpesvirus immunoevasion and tumorigenesis: two sides of the same coin? *Annu Rev Microbiol* **57**: 609–639.

Müllberg J, Geib T, Jostock T, Hoischen SH, Vollmer P, Voltz N, Heinz D, Galle PR, Klouche M, Rose-John S (2000) IL-6 receptor independent stimulation of human gp130 by viral IL-6. *J Immunol* **164**: 4672–4677.

Muralidhar S, Pumfery AM, Hassani M, Sadaie MR, Kishishita M, Brady JN, Doniger J, Medveczky P, Rosenthal LJ (1998) Identification of kaposin (open reading frame K12) as a human herpesvirus 8 (Kaposi's sarcoma-associated herpesvirus) transforming gene. *J Virol* **72**: 4980–4988.

Nador RG, Cesarman E, Chadburn A, Dawson DB, Ansari MQ, Sald J, Knowles DM (1996) Primary effusion lymphoma: a distinct clinicopathologic entity associated with the Kaposi's sarcoma-associated herpes virus. *Blood* **88**: 645–656.

Nakamura H, Lu M, Gwack Y, Souvlis J, Zeichner SL, Jung JU (2003) Global changes in Kaposi's sarcoma-associated virus gene expression patterns following expression of a tetracycline-inducible Rta transactivator. *J Virol* **77**: 4205–4220.

Naranatt PP, Krishnan HH, Smith MS, Chandran B (2005) Kaposi's sarcoma-associated herpesvirus modulates microtubule dynamics via RhoA-GTP-diaphanous 2 signaling and utilizes the dynein motors to deliver its DNA to the nucleus. *J Virol* **79**: 1191–1206.

Narizhneva NV, Razorenova OV, Podrez EA, Chen J, Chandrasekharan UM, DiCorleto PE, Plow EF, Topol EJ, Byzova TV (2005)

Thrombospondin-1 up-regulates expression of cell adhesion molecules and promotes monocyte binding to endothelium. *FASEB J* **19**: 1158–1160.

Neipel F, Albrecht JC, Fleckenstein B (1997) Cell-homologous genes in the Kaposi's sarcoma-associated rhadinovirus human herpesvirus 8: determinants of its pathogenicity? *J Virol* **71**: 4187–4192.

Nicholas J, Ruvolo VR, Burns WH, Sandford G, Wan X, Ciufo D, Hendrickson SB, Guo HG, Hayward GS, Reitz MS (1997) Kaposi's sarcoma-associated human herpesvirus-8 encodes homologues of macrophage inflammatory protein-1 and interleukin-6. *Nat Med* **3**: 287–292.

Nicholas J (2007) Human herpesvirus 8-encoded proteins with potential roles in virus-associated neoplasia. *Front Biosci* **12**: 265–281.

Olsen SJ, Tarte K, Sherman W, Hale EE, Weisse MT, Orazi A, Klein B, Chang Y (1998) Evidence against KSHV infection in the pathogenesis of multiple myeloma. *Virus Res* **57**: 197–202.

Osborne J, Moore PS, Chang Y (1999) KSHV-encoded viral IL-6 activates multiple human IL-6 signaling pathways. *Hum Immunol* **60**: 921–927.

Papugani A, Coleman T, Jones C, Zhang L (2008) The interaction between KSHV RTA and cellular RBP-Jkappa and their subsequent DNA binding are not sufficient for activation of RBP-Jkappa. *Virus Res* **131**: 1–7.

Parravicini C, Corbellino M, Paulli M, Magrini U, Lazzarino M, Moore PS, Chang Y (1997) Expression of a virus-derived cytokine, KSHV vIL-6, in HIV-seronegative Castleman's disease. *Am J Pathol* **151**: 1517–1522.

Parravicini C, Chandran B, Corbellino M, Berti E, Paulli M, Moore PS, Chang Y (2000) Differential viral protein expression in Kaposi's sarcoma-associated herpesvirus-infected diseases: Kaposi's sarcoma, primary effusion lymphoma, and multicentric Castleman's disease. *Am J Pathol* **156**: 743–749.

Pellett PE, Roizman B (2007) The family Herpsesviridae: A brief introduction. In: Knipe D, Howley P (eds.), *Fields Virology*, 2479–2499. Philadelphia: Lippincott Williams & Wilkins.

Perna AM, Viviano E, Iannito E, Marceno R, Romano N (1998) No association between human herpesvirus type 8 infection and multiple myeloma. *J Natl Cancer Inst* **90**: 1013–1014.

Pertel PE (2002) Human herpesvirus 8 glycoprotein B (gB), gH, and gL can mediate cell fusion. *J Virol* **76**: 4390–4400.

Pfeffer S, Sewer A, Lagos-Quintana M, Sheridan R, Sander C, Grässer FA, van Dyk LF, Ho CK, Shuman S, Chien M, Russo JJ, Ju J, Randall G, Lindenbach BD, Rice CM, Simon V, Ho DD, Zavolan M, Tuschl T

(2005) Identification of microRNAs of the herpesvirus family. *Nat Methods* **2**: 269–276.

Polson AG, Wang D, DeRisi J, Ganem D (2002) Modulation of host gene expression by the constitutively active G protein-coupled receptor of Kaposi's sarcoma-associated herpesvirus. *Cancer Res* **62**: 4525–4530.

Poole LJ, Zong JC, Ciufo DM, Alcendor DJ, Cannon JS, Ambinder R, Orenstein JM, Reitz MS, Hayward GS (1999) Comparison of genetic variability at multiple loci across the genomes of the major subtypes of Kaposi's sarcoma-associated herpesvirus reveals evidence for recombination and for two distinct types of open reading frame K15 alleles at the right-hand end. *J Virol* **73**: 6646–6660.

Qiang W, Cahill JM, Liu J, Kuang X, Liu N, Scofield VL, Voorhees JR, Reid AJ, Yan M, Lynn WS, Wong PK (2004) Activation of transcription factor Nrf-2 and its downstream targets in response to moloney murine leukemia virus ts1-induced thiol depletion and oxidative stress in astrocytes. *J Virol* **78**: 11926–11938.

Radkov SA, Kellam P, Boshoff C (2000) The latent nuclear antigen of Kaposi sarcoma-associated herpesvirus targets the retinoblastoma-E2F pathway and with the oncogene Hras transforms primary rat cells. *Nat Med* **6**: 1121–1127.

Radtke F, Raj K (2003) The role of Notch in tumorigenesis: oncogene or tumour suppressor? *Nat Rev Cancer* **3**: 756–767.

Rappocciolo G, Jenkins FJ, Hensler HR, Piazza P, Jais M, Borowski L, Watkins SC, Rinaldo CR Jr (2006) DC-SIGN is a receptor for human herpesvirus 8 on dendritic cells and macrophages. *J Immunol* **176**: 1741–1749.

Renne R, Zhong W, Herndier B, McGrath M, Abbey N, Kedes D, Ganem D (1996) Lytic growth of Kaposi's sarcoma-associated herpesvirus (human herpesvirus 8) in culture. *Nat Med* **2**: 342–346.

Renne R, Barry C, Dittmer D, Compitello N, Brown PO, Ganem D (2001) Modulation of cellular and viral gene expression by the latency-associated nuclear antigen of Kaposi's sarcoma-associated herpesvirus. *J Virol* **75**: 458–468.

Rettig M, Ma H, Vescio R, Pold M, Schiller G, Belson D, Savage A, Nishikubo C, Wu C, Fraser J, Said J, Berenson J (1997) Kaposi's sarcoma-associated herpesvirus infection of bone marrow dendritic cells from myeloma patients. *Science* **276**: 1851–1854.

Rivas C, Thlick AE, Parravicini C, Moore PS, Chang Y (2001) Kaposi's sarcoma-associated herpesvirus LANA2 is a B-cell-specific latent viral protein that inhibits p53. *J Virol* **75**: 429–438.

Rosenkilde MM, Kledal TN, Bräuner-Osborne H, Schwartz TW (1999) Agonists and inverse agonists for the herpesvirus 8-encoded constitutively active seven-transmembrane oncogene product, ORF-74. *J Biol Chem* **274**: 956–961.

Rozen R, Sathish N, Li Y, Yuan Y (2008) Virion-wide protein interactions of Kaposi's sarcoma-associated herpesvirus. *J Virol* **82**: 4742–4750.

Russo JJ, Bohenzky RA, Chien MC, Chen J, Yan M, Maddalena D, Parry JP, Peruzzi D, Edelman IS, Chang Y, Moore PS (1996) Nucleotide sequence of the Kaposi sarcoma-associated herpesvirus (HHV8). *Proc Natl Acad Sci USA* **93**: 14862–14867.

Sadler R, Wu L, Forghani B, Renne R, Zhong W, Herndier B, Ganem D (1999) A complex translational program generates multiple novel proteins from the latently expressed kaposin (K12) locus of Kaposi's sarcoma-associated herpesvirus. *J Virol* **73**: 5722–5730.

Sakakibara S, Ueda K, Chen J, Okuno T, Yamanishi K (2001) Octamer-binding sequence is a key element for the autoregulation of Kaposi's sarcoma-associated herpesvirus ORF50/Lyta gene expression. *J Virol* **75**: 6894–6900.

Saldanha G, Ghura V, Potter L, Fletcher A (2004) Nuclear beta-catenin in basal cell carcinoma correlates with increased proliferation. *Br J Dermatol* **151**: 157–164.

Samaniego F, Pati S, Karp JE, Prakash O, Bose D (2001) Human herpesvirus 8 K1-associated nuclear factor-kappa B-dependent promoter activity: role in Kaposi's sarcoma inflammation? *J Natl Cancer Inst Monogr* **28**: 15–23.

Samols MA, Hu J, Skalsky RL, Renne R (2005) Cloning and identification of a microRNA cluster within the latency-associated region of Kaposi's sarcoma-associated herpesvirus. *J Virol* **79**: 9301–9305.

Samols MA, Skalsky RL, Maldonado AM, Riva A, Lopez MC, Baker HV, Renne R (2007) Identification of cellular genes targeted by KSHV-encoded microRNAs. *PLoS Pathog* **3**: e65.

Sánchez I, Dynlacht BD (2005) New insights into cyclins, CDKs, and cell cycle control. *Semin Cell Dev Biol* **16**: 311–321.

Sarid R, Wiezorek JS, Moore PS, Chang Y (1999) Characterization and cell cycle regulation of the major Kaposi's sarcoma-associated herpesvirus (human herpesvirus 8) latent genes and their promoter. *J Virol* **73**: 1438–1446.

Sasaki H, Sato H, Kuriyama-Matsumura K, Sato K, Maebara K, Wang H, Tamba M, Itoh K, Yamamoto M, Bannai S (2002) Electrophile response element-mediated induction of the cystine/glutamate exchange transporter gene expression. *J Biol Chem* **277**: 44765–44771.

Schulz TF, Sheldon J, Greensill J (2002) Kaposi's sarcoma associated herpesvirus (KSHV) or human herpesvirus 8 (HHV8). *Virus Res* **82**: 115–126.

Schwam DR, Luciano RL, Mahajan SS, Wong L, Wilson AC (2000) Carboxy terminus of human herpesvirus 8 latency-associated nuclear antigen mediates dimerization, transcriptional repression, and targeting to nuclear bodies. *J Virol* **74**: 8532–8540.

Schwarz M, Murphy PM (2001) Kaposi's sarcoma-associated herpesvirus G protein-coupled receptor constitutively activates NF-kappa B and induces proinflammatory cytokine and chemokine production via a C-terminal signaling determinant. *J Immunol* **167**: 505–513.

Seo T, Park J, Lim C, Choe J (2004) Inhibition of nuclear factor kappa B activity by viral interferon regulatory factor 3 of Kaposi's sarcoma-associated herpesvirus. *Oncogene* **23**: 6146–6155.

Sharp TV, Wang HW, Koumi A, Hollyman D, Endo Y, Ye H, Du MQ, Boshoff C (2002) K15 protein of Kaposi's sarcoma-associated herpesvirus is latently expressed and binds to HAX-1, a protein with antiapoptotic function. *J Virol* **76**: 802–816.

Shelby BD, LaMarca HL, McFerrin HE, Nelson AB, Lasky JA, Sun G, Myatt L, Offermann MK, Morris CA, Sullivan DE (2007) Kaposi's sarcoma associated herpesvirus G-protein coupled receptor activation of cyclooxygenase-2 in vascular endothelial cells. *Virol J* **4**: 87.

Sodhi A, Montaner S, Gutkind JS (2004) Does dysregulated expression of a deregulated viral GPCR trigger Kaposi's sarcomagenesis? *FASEB J* **18**: 422–427.

Song MJ, Li X, Brown HJ, Sun R (2002) Characterization of interactions between RTA and the promoter of polyadenylated nuclear RNA in Kaposi's sarcoma-associated herpesvirus/human herpesvirus 8. *J Virol* **76**: 5000–5013.

Soulier J, Grollet L, Oksenhendler E, Cacoub P, Cazals-Hatem D, Babinet P, D'Agay M-F, Clauvel J-P, Raphael M, Degos L, Sigaux F (1995) Kaposi's sarcoma-associated herpesvirus-like DNA sequences in multicentric Castleman's disease. *Blood* **86**: 1276–1280.

Spear PG, Longnecker R (2003) Herpesvirus entry: an update. *J Virol* **77**: 10179–10185.

Staskus KA, Zhong W, Gebhard K, Herndier B, Wang H, Renne R, Beneke J, Pudney J, Anderson DJ, Ganem D, Haase AT (1997) Kaposi's sarcoma-associated herpesvirus gene expression in endothelial (spindle) tumor cells. *J Virol* **71**: 715–719.

Staskus KA, Sun R, Miller G, Racz P, Jaslowski A, Metroka C, Brett-Smith H, Haase AT (1999) Cellular tropism and viral interleukin-6 expression distinguish human herpesvirus 8 involvement in Kaposi's sarcoma, primary effusion lymphoma, and multicentric Castleman's disease. *J Virol* **73**: 4181–4187.

Staudt MR, Kanan Y, Jeong JH, Papin JF, Hines-Boykin R, Dittmer DP (2004) The tumor microenvironment controls primary effusion lymphoma growth *in vivo*. *Cancer Res* **64**: 4790–4799.

Sun Q, Matta H, Chaudhary PM (2003) The human herpes virus 8-encoded viral FLICE inhibitory protein protects against growth factor withdrawal-induced apoptosis via NF-kappa B activation. *Blood* **101**: 1956–1961.

Sun Q, Matta H, Lu G, Chaudhary PM (2006) Induction of IL-8 expression by human herpesvirus 8 encoded vFLIP K13 via NF-kappaB activation. *Oncogene* **25**: 2717–2726.

Sun R, Lin SF, Gradoville L, Yuan Y, Zhu F, Miller G (1998) A viral gene that activates lytic cycle expression of Kaposi's sarcoma-associated herpesvirus. *Proc Natl Acad Sci USA* **95**: 10866–10871.

Swanton C, Mann DJ, Fleckenstein B, Neipel F, Peters G, Jones N (1997) Herpes viral cyclin/Cdk6 complexes evade inhibition by CDK inhibitor proteins. *Nature* **390**: 184–187.

Talbot SJ, Weiss RA, Kellam P, Boshoff C (1999) Transcriptional analysis of human herpesvirus-8 open reading frames 71, 72, 73, K14, and 74 in a primary effusion lymphoma cell line. *Virology* **257**: 84–94.

Taraboletti G, Benelli R, Borsotti P, Rusnati M, Presta M, Giavazzi R, Ruco L, Albini A (1999) Thrombospondin-1 inhibits Kaposi's sarcoma (KS) cell and HIV-1 Tat-induced angiogenesis and is poorly expressed in KS lesions. *J Pathol* **188**: 76–81.

Taylor JF, Templeton AC, Vogel CL, Ziegler JL, Kyalwazi SK (1971) Kaposi's sarcoma in Uganda: a clinico-pathological study. *Int J Cancer* **8**: 122–135.

Thome M, Schneider P, Hofmann K, Fickenscher H, Meinl E, Neipel F, Mattmann C, Burns K, Bodmer JL, Schröter M, Scaffidi C, Krammer PH, Peter ME, Tschopp J (1997) Viral FLICE-inhibitory proteins (FLIPs) prevent apoptosis induced by death receptors. *Nature* **386**: 517–521.

Tomlinson C, Damania B (2004) The K1 protein of Kaposi's sarcoma-associated herpesvirus activates the Akt signaling pathway. *J Virol* **78**: 1918–1927.

Trus BL, Heymann JB, Nealon K, Cheng N, Newcomb WW, Brown JC, Kedes DH, Steven AC (2001) Capsid structure of Kaposi's sarcoma-associated herpesvirus, a gammaherpesvirus, compared to those of an alphaherpesvirus, herpes simplex virus type 1, and a betaherpesvirus, cytomegalovirus. *J Virol* **75**: 2879–2890.

Verschuren EW, Klefstrom J, Evan GI, Jones N (2002) The oncogenic potential of Kaposi's sarcoma-associated herpesvirus cyclin is exposed by p53 loss *in vitro* and *in vivo*. *Cancer Cell* **2**: 229–241.

Voorhoeve PM, le Sage C, Schrier M, Gillis AJ, Stoop H, Nagel R, Liu YP, van Duijse J, Drost J, Griekspoor A, Zlotorynski E, Yabuta N, De Vita G, Nojima H, Looijenga LH, Agami R (2006) A genetic screen implicates miRNA-372 and miRNA-373 as oncogenes in testicular germ cell tumors. *Cell* **124**: 1169–1181.

Wang FZ, Akula SM, Pramod NP, Zeng L, Chandran B (2001) Human herpesvirus 8 envelope glycoprotein K8.1A interaction with the target cells involves heparan sulfate. *J Virol* **75**: 7517–7527.

Wang FZ, Akula SM, Sharma-Walia N, Zeng L, Chandran B (2003) Human herpesvirus 8 envelope glycoprotein B mediates cell adhesion via its RGD sequence. *J Virol* 77: 3131–3147.

Wang HW, Trotter MW, Lagos D, Bourboulia D, Henderson S, Mäkinen T, Elliman S, Flanagan AM, Alitalo K, Boshoff C (2004) Kaposi sarcoma herpesvirus-induced cellular reprogramming contributes to the lymphatic endothelial gene expression in Kaposi sarcoma. *Nat Genet* **36**: 687–693.

Wang J, Zhang J, Zhang L, Harrington W Jr, West JT, Wood C (2005) Modulation of human herpesvirus 8/Kaposi's sarcoma-associated herpesvirus replication and transcription activator transactivation by interferon regulatory factor 7. *J Virol* **79**: 2420–2431.

Wang L, Wakisaka N, Tomlinson CC, DeWire SM, Krall S, Pagano JS, Damania B (2004) The Kaposi's sarcoma-associated herpesvirus (KSHV/HHV-8) K1 protein induces expression of angiogenic and invasion factors. *Cancer Res* **64**: 2774–2781.

Wang L, Dittmer DP, Tomlinson CC, Fakhari FD, Damania B (2006) Immortalization of primary endothelial cells by the K1 protein of Kaposi's sarcoma-associated herpesvirus. *Cancer Res* **66**: 3658–3666.

Wang S, Liu S, Wu M, Geng Y, Wood C (2001) Kaposi's sarcoma-associated herpesvirus/human herpesvirus-8 ORF50 gene product contains a potent C-terminal activation domain which activates gene expression via a specific target sequence. *Arch Virol* **146**: 1415–1426.

Wang SE, Wu FY, Chen H, Shamay M, Zheng Q, Hayward GS (2004) Early activation of the Kaposi's sarcoma-associated herpesvirus RTA, RAP, and

MTA promoters by the tetradecanoyl phorbol acetate-induced AP1 pathway. *J Virol* **78**: 4248–4267.

Weng AP, Ferrando AA, Lee W, Morris JP, Silverman LB, Sanchez-Irizarry C, Blacklow SC, Look AT, Aster JC (2004) Activating mutations of NOTCH1 in human T cell acute lymphoblastic leukemia. *Science* **306**: 269–271.

Winzen R, Kracht M, Ritter B, Wilhelm A, Chen CY, Shyu AB, Müller M, Gaestel M, Resch K, Holtmann H (1999) The p38 MAP kinase pathway signals for cytokine-induced mRNA stabilization via MAP kinase-activated protein kinase 2 and an AU-rich region-targeted mechanism. *EMBO J* **18**: 496949–80.

Wong EL, Damania B (2005) Linking KSHV to human cancer. *Curr Oncol Rep* 7: 349–356.

Wong EL, Damania B (2006) Transcriptional regulation of the Kaposi's sarcoma-associated herpesvirus K15 gene. *J Virol* **80**: 1385–1392.

Wu L, Lo P, Yu X, Stoops JK, Forghani B., Zhou ZH (2000) Three-dimensional structure of the human herpesvirus 8 capsid. *J Virol* **74**: 9646–9654.

Wu W, Vieira J, Fiore N, Banerjee P, Sieburg M, Rochford R, Harrington W Jr, Feuer G (2006) KSHV/HHV-8 infection of human hematopoietic progenitor ($CD34^+$) cells: persistence of infection during hematopoiesis *in vitro* and *in vivo*. *Blood* **108**: 141–151.

Yang TY, Chen SC, Leach MW, Manfra D, Homey B, Wiekowski M, Sullivan L, Jenh CH, Narula SK, Chensue SW., Lira SA (2000) Transgenic expression of the chemokine receptor encoded by human herpesvirus 8 induces an angioproliferative disease resembling Kaposi's sarcoma. *J Exp Med* **191**: 445–454.

Yang Z, Wood C (2007) The transcriptional repressor K-RBP modulates RTA-mediated transactivation and lytic replication of Kaposi's sarcoma-associated herpesvirus. *J Virol* **81**: 6294–6306.

Yang Z, Yan Z, Wood C (2008) Kaposi's sarcoma-associated herpesvirus transactivator RTA promotes degradation of the repressors to regulate viral lytic replication. *J Virol* **82**: 3590–3603.

Ye FC, Zhou FC, Xie JP, Kang T, Greene W, Kuhne K, Lei XF, Li QH, Gao SJ (2008) Kaposi's sarcoma-associated herpesvirus latent gene vFLIP inhibits viral lytic replication through NF-kappaB-mediated suppression of the AP-1 pathway: a novel mechanism of virus control of latency. *J Virol* **82**: 4235–4249.

Yoshizaki K, Matsuda T, Nishimoto N, Kuritani T, Taeho L, Aozasa K, Nakahata T, Kawai H, Tagoh H, Komori T, Kishimoto S, Hirano T, Kishimoto T (1989) Pathogenic significance of interleukin-6 (IL-6/BSF-2) in Castleman's disease. *Blood* **74**: 1360–1367.
Yu Y, Wang SE, Hayward GS (2005) The KSHV immediate-early transcription factor RTA encodes ubiquitin E3 ligase activity that targets IRF7 for proteosome-mediated degradation. *Immunity* **22**: 59–70.
Zheng ZM (2003) Split genes and their expression in Kaposi's sarcoma-associated herpesvirus. *Rev Med Virol* **13**: 173–184.
Zhong W, Wang H, Herndier B, Ganem D (1996) Restricted expression of Kaposi sarcoma-associated herpesvirus (human herpesvirus 8) genes in Kaposi sarcoma. *Proc Natl Acad Sci USA* **93**: 6641–6646.
Zhu FX, Chong JM, Wu L, Yuan Y (2005) Virion proteins of Kaposi's sarcoma-associated herpesvirus. *J Virol* **79**: 800–811.

Chapter 7

Human T-Cell Leukemia Virus 1 and Cellular Transformation

Ya-Hui Chi* and Kuan-Teh Jeang*

Abstract: Human T-cell leukemia virus 1 (HTLV-1), a retrovirus that infects approximately 20 million people worldwide, is the first retrovirus demonstrated to be causal for a human cancer [adult T-cell leukemia (ATL)]. After a prolonged asymptomatic period of 20–40 years, 1–5% of HTLV-1-infected individuals develop ATL. Although HTLV-1's leukemogenic mechanism for ATL is not fully understood, its viral transactivator protein, Tax, is the key component for cellular transformation. In addition to activating viral transcription to facilitate viral replication, Tax disturbs several regulatory mechanisms that are critical for cell growth and proliferation. However, leukemic ATL cells frequently lack Tax expression, and this seems to be due to genetic and epigenetic changes in the integrated HTLV-1 provirus. Such observations suggest that Tax is needed for the initiation of the transformation but not for the maintenance of the transformed phenotype. Here we discuss, in brief, the roles played by the Tax oncoprotein in cellular transformation that leads to ATL.

1. The Discovery of HTLV-1

In the late 1970s, Kiyoshi Takatsuki and his colleagues reported a clear geographic clustering of a unique leukemia in western Japan

*Molecular Virology Section, Laboratory of Molecular Microbiology, National Institute of Allergy and Infectious Diseases, National Institutes of Health, Bethesda, Maryland.

named the adult T-cell leukemia (ATL). This leukemia has an unusual morphology with multi-lobulated nuclei. The HTLV-1 is a retrovirus, which was later (1980s) isolated from ATL cells through the independent efforts of American and Japanese scientists, and this retrovirus was established as the causal agent for ATL (Gallo, 2005; Yoshida, 2005). HTLV-1, a member of the *Deltaretrovirus* family, is the first human retrovirus directly associated with a malignancy.

1.1. Structure of HTLV-1 Genome

The HTLV-1 virion is approximately 100 nm in diameter, and is surrounded by a proteolipid envelope bilayer embedded with viral transmembrane and surface proteins. The inner envelope sheaths the matrix layer, the nucleocapsid, the reverse transcriptase, and the integrase (Verdonck *et al.*, 2007). The genome of HTLV-1 is a positive, single-stranded RNA, and two copies of genomic RNA are present within each virion. After infection, the retroviral RNA is first converted by reverse transcription to double-stranded DNA, which is then inserted randomly into the host genome. This inserted DNA form of a retrovirus is referred to as a provirus.

The HTLV-1 proviral genome encodes the viral group-specific antigen (gag), protease (pro)/polymerase (pol), and envelope (env) proteins (Fig. 1). The HTLV-1 genome is flanked at either ends by long terminal repeats (LTRs) composed of U3, R, and U5 regions (Fig. 1). The viral promoter in the U3 region of the 5′-LTR plays a role in determining gene expression. HTLV-1 has an additional pX sequence between the 3′-end of the env gene and the 3′-LTR. This region includes seven alternative open reading frames which can encode several regulatory proteins (Fig. 1).

Amongst the seven pX-encoded proteins, Tax is the viral transactivator that can increase viral gene transcription through its interaction with cellular factors and 5′-LTR of the proviral genome. Rex, a second accessory protein, acts post-transcriptionally to enhance the export of unspliced and partially spliced viral RNAs from the nucleus to the cytoplasm.

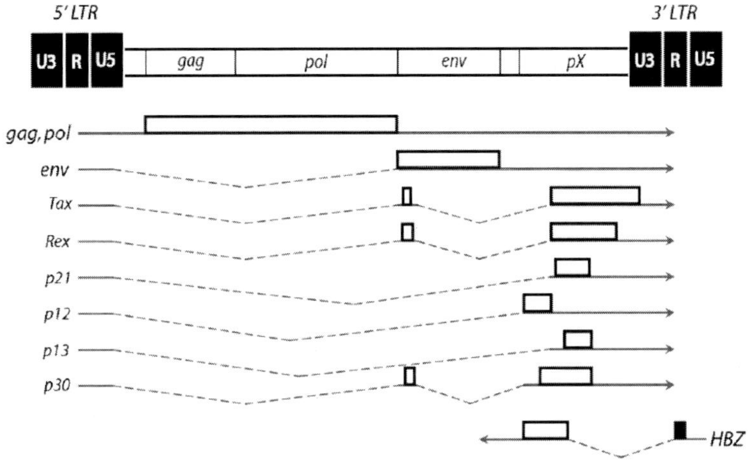

Fig. 1. Structure of the HTLV-1 proviral genome. The various spliced viral RNA species and the encoded proteins are shown. In addition to the structural genes *gag*, *pol*, and *env*, the pX region of the provirus encodes the Tax, Rex, p21, p12, p13, and p30 accessory proteins. The HTLV-1 genome also encodes a basic leucine zipper factor (HBZ) which is expressed from the antisense strand.

Additionally, the pX region encodes accessory proteins including p21, p12, p13, p30, and the recently characterized HTLV-1 basic ZIP factor (HBZ, Fig. 1). The p12 protein, which is present in endoplasmic reticulum and the Golgi (Ding *et al.*, 2001), has been shown to interact with calreticulin and calnexin and it has been proposed to influence the proliferation and differentiation of T lymphocytes. The p30 accessory protein binds Tax and Rex mRNAs and retains both transcripts in the nucleus (Nicot *et al.*, 2004), thereby preventing their translation in the cytoplasm. By suppressing Tax protein synthesis, p30 attenuates HTLV-1 transcription and possibly regulates a switch between productive vs. latent viral infection *in vivo*. HBZ is a newly identified viral protein, which is encoded by the minus strand of the provirus (Fig. 1). Current evidence suggests that the HBZ protein suppresses Tax-mediated transactivation of viral transcription via the 5′-LTR and HBZ RNA promotes ATL cellular proliferation (Satou *et al.*, 2006; Lemasson *et al.*, 2007). The functions of the other pX region proteins remain unclear (Nicot *et al.*, 2005).

1.2. HTLV-1-associated Diseases

Worldwide, HTLV-1 infections are clustered in many endemic areas including south western Japan, Iran, the Caribbean islands, and parts of South Africa (Proietti *et al.*, 2005). HTLV-1 has been associated with several diseases including ATL, HTLV-associated myelopathy/tropical spastic paraparesis (HAM/TSP), uveitis, and infective dermatitis. The virus has also been linked to cases of polymyositis, synovitis, thyroiditis, and bronchioalveolar pneumonitis, although definitive epidemiologic proof of HTLV-1 association for some of these pathologies is lacking.

ATL is a lethal T-cell malignancy characterized by hypercalcemia, hepatomegaly, splenomegaly, lymphadenopathy, skin involvement, and the presence of abnormal lymphocytes (Takatsuki, 2005). ATL has four subtypes: acute, lymphoma-type, chronic, and smoldering. The first two types show aggressive clinical courses while the latter two types progress more indolently. The survival time of the patients ranges between 7 and 24 months, depending on the clinical form of the disease. Although a recently developed approach using a combination of antiretroviral drugs (e.g. AZT) and interferon-α shows some promise, there is currently no curative chemotherapy for ATL.

HAM/TSP typically develops in up to 4% of HTLV-1-infected persons, and more frequently in women than in men. Patients are afflicted with a debilitating process characterized by a slow-onset spastic paraparesis associated with sphincter disturbance and variable degrees of proprioceptive and sensory dysfunction. HAM/TSP is constituted pathologically by parenchymal infiltration of mononuclear cells into the gray and white matter of the thoracic spinal cord, resulting in severe white matter degeneration and fibrosis. This syndrome is also currently poorly responsive to treatment.

1.3. HTLV-1 Infectivity and Latency

Cell-free infection by HTLV-1 is highly inefficient; most viral infection occurs via cell–cell contact. HTLV-1 is transmitted primarily in three ways: mother-to-infant (mainly through breast feeding), sexual contact, and blood transfusion. *In vivo*, HTLV-1 is mostly detected in CD4$^+$ helper T lymphocytes in both asymptomatic and symptomatic carriers, thus suggesting that the CD4$^+$ cell compartment constitutes a preferred component of HTLV-1 tropism. Nonetheless, during the lifetime of an infected individual, other hematopoietic cells (non-CD4$^+$ T-cell subsets, B lymphocytes, monocytes and macrophages, dendritic cells, and megakaryocytes) as well as glial cells (astrocytes and microglial cells) can also be part of HTLV-1's tropism (Manel *et al.*, 2005).

HTLV-1 causes ATL in a small percentage (1–5%) of infected individuals after a long latency of up to 20–40 years. During the latent period, the proviral load in the peripheral blood lymphocytes and the viral gene expression in the infected cells are very low. The mechanism(s) conferring latency is still unclear. A recent report suggests that suppression of Tax expression by genetic changes in the provirus genome or by deletion/hypermethylation of 5′-LTR may contribute to this latency (Taniguchi *et al.*, 2005).

Unlike asymptomatic carriers with low HTLV-1 expression, HAM/TSP patients have significantly higher proviral loads, suggesting that active HTLV-1 viral replication plays a key role in the development of this disease. A recent study has shown that a high level of Tax expression and low CD8$^+$ antiviral efficiency are correlated with high proviral load and HAM/TSP development (Asquith *et al.*, 2005).

2. Pleiotropic Functions of the HTLV-1 Oncoprotein Tax

HTLV-1 encodes a transforming protein, Tax. Tax is a 40-kDa viral phosphoprotein that is a transcriptional activator of viral gene expression.

The Tax-responsive elements (TRE) in the 5′-LTR of the HTLV-1 provirus are composed of three imperfectly conserved 21 bp repeats which are also cAMP-responsive elements (CRE). Tax activates LTR-directed transcription through CRE-binding protein (CREB) in conjunction with CBP, p300, and PCAF (Beimling & Moelling, 1992; Yin *et al.*, 1995; Jiang *et al.*, 1999).

Tax also activates and represses cellular genes. A couple of examples include activation of proliferating cell nuclear antigen (PCNA) expression and repression of human β-polymerase (huβ-pol) (Jeang *et al.*, 1990). More will be discussed below.

2.1. Tax Transgenic Mouse Models

Currently, the ability of Tax to transform experimentally human cells has not been established, although Tax can transform many rodent cells. There is good evidence that Tax can singularly induce tumor formation in several transgenic mouse models. For example, Tax transgenic mice under the regulation of the human granzyme B promoter (GrmB, expressed in activated T- and natural killer [NK] cells) develop lymphoproliferative diseases (leukemia, lymphomas, and splenomegaly) partially resembling ATL. However, the GrmB-Tax transgenic mice predominantly develop a large granular leukemia/lymphoma (LGL) rather than the $CD4^+$ lymphoma/leukemia most commonly seen in ATL (Grossman *et al.*, 1995).

Although mice from the early Tax transgenic mouse models develop tumors, most of the tumor types failed to recapitulate the T-cell leukemic presentation of ATL. It was only until a recent report by Hasegawa and his colleagues (Hasegawa *et al.*, 2006) that the development of ATL/lymphoma (ATLL)-like T-cell lymphoma/leukemia in mice was shown. In Hasegawa's study, Tax expression was restricted to thymocytes and T lymphocytes through the use of a tissue-specific Lck promoter. After a prolonged latency period, these transgenic mice developed diffuse large-cell lymphomas/leukemia. In addition, the mice were functionally immunocompromised and developed opportunistic infections. Flow cytometry showed that the cells were $CD4^-$ and $CD8^-$, but not $CD44^+$, $CD25^+$, and cytoplasmic $CD3^+$. This phenotype is indicative of a thymus-derived pre-T-cell phenotype, and disease development was associated with the constitutive activation of NF-κB. Although this mouse model most closely reflected human disease, the T lymphoma cells in this work were of immature T cells, whereas human ATLs are generally of mature T lymphocytes. More recently, in a second Tax transgenic mouse model that used Lck promoter, the major leukemic cells that developed were $CD4^+$ or $CD8^+$ mature T cells (Ohsugi *et al.*, 2007). Taken together the two studies provide models that can be used to advance our understanding of how HTLV-1 may transform both immature and mature T cells.

2.2. Tax and DNA Structural Damage

Cancers commonly have structurally damaged DNA. Like other cancers, ATL cells have frequent clastogenic DNA damage. There are three major biochemical pathways employed to repair DNA damage: the mismatch repair (MMR), the nucleotide excision repair (NER), and the base excision repair (BER) pathways (Charames & Bapat, 2003). Defects in intracellular mechanisms of DNA damage repair have been inferred to play critical roles in genomic instability. Two sets of current evidence support that the HTLV-1 Tax protein abrogates DNA repair functions. First, Tax can repress NER by activating PCNA expression (Lemoine *et al.*, 2000). PCNA is a eukaryotic DNA pol processivity factor that is involved in both DNA replication and repair. PCNA recruits crucial players to the DNA replication fork. The presence of PCNA increases the processivity of DNA pols from tens to thousands of nucleotides (Moldovan *et al.*, 2007). Thus, overactivated PCNA reduces the amount of time available for the repair of DNA errors. PCNA has been used as a marker for cellular proliferation in a variety of tumors and is expressed at a higher level in virally transformed cells than in their uninfected counterparts. Second, Tax downregulates the expression of huβ-pol, a cellular DNA pol involved in BER.

2.3. Tax and Cell Survival

DNA-damaged cells usually succumb to apoptosis. However, transformed cells, while maintaining damaged genomes, must survive and continue to expand. HTLV-1-infected cells appear to acquire survival mechanism(s) to combat an otherwise expected proclivity for apoptosis. Findings suggest that the Tax oncoprotein can engage two cellular survival factors, NF-κB and Akt (Ruben *et al.*, 1988; Ballard *et al.*, 1988; Liu *et al.*, 2001; Peloponese Jr & Jeang, 2006).

NF-κB regulates diverse biological processes, including the growth and survival of both lymphoid and nonlymphoid cells (Jost & Ruland, 2007). The NF-κB family includes the p50 (NF-κB1), p52 (NF-κB2), p65 (RelA), RelB, and c-Rel factors that share a common Rel homology domain (RHD) (Horie, 2007). In non-activated state, NF-κB dimers are retained in the cytoplasm by inhibitory proteins comprising the IκB family, which includes the I-κBα, I-κBβ, I-κBγ, I-κBε, p105, and p100 proteins. These proteins bind to the RHD of the NF-κB factors and mask their nuclear localization signal (NLS). Upon activation by extracellular stimuli such as interleukin-1 (IL-1), tumor necrosis factor-α (TNF-α) or bacterial lipopolysaccharide (LPS), I-κB becomes serine phosphorylated by I-κB kinases (IKKs). This action triggers a polyubiquination event that leads to degradation of I-κB by proteolysis. The degradation of I-κB causes the release of cytoplasmic NF-κB, which migrates into the nucleus to activate the transcription of NF-κB-responsive genes.

NF-κB factors are constitutively activated in HTLV-1-infected cells. It has been observed that Tax activates both the canonical and non-canonical NF-κB pathways by targeting two different IKK complexes. First, Tax associates with the canonical IKK$\alpha\beta\gamma$ complex via IKKγ/NEMO, and triggers the nuclear migration of NF-κB p65 (Sun & Yamaoka, 2005). Second, Tax can stimulate NF-κB through an IKKα-dependant pathway. Here, binding of Tax to IKKγ and p100 in an IKKα–IKKγ–p100 complex leads to the processing of NF-κB p100 precursor protein to its active p52 product form. Activation of NF-κB produces transcription of "survival" genes that counters the propensity of virus-infected cells to commit apoptosis.

Tax can also activate the Akt pathway. Akt, also known as protein kinase B (PKB), is a serine/threonine kinase that mediates PI3K-initiated signaling. Akt is able to prevent apoptosis in some cells through phosphorylation and inhibition of pro-apoptotic mediators such as Bad and caspase-9 (Datta *et al.*, 1999). Activated Akt is also thought to trigger transcriptional factors, such as AP-1, in many human cancers. Tax promotes Akt phosphorylation by binding PI3K directly.

2.4. Tax and Cell Cycle Progression

The cell cycle is regulated by cyclins and cyclin-dependent kinases (Cdks). Progression of the cell cycle is tightly controlled at various stages by different cyclin–Cdk complexes. For instance, cyclins D and E mediate passage through the G1 phase and the G1/S transition, and the A cyclins accumulate and function during the S phase, whereas the B cyclins are active during mitosis.

Cyclin D–Cdk4 and cyclin D–Cdk6 complexes are also active in G1. Tax-expressing cells display an accelerated progression through G1, which is in part contributed by elevated expression of cyclin D2 in some cells. Elevated cyclin D2 expression occurs through interleukin-2 (IL-2) receptor signaling and via direct Tax activation of the cyclin D2 promoter (Santiago *et al.*, 1999). The former is consistent with findings of increased IL-2 secretion from HTLV-1-infected T-lymphocytes. Tax can also directly bind cyclin D3, cyclin D2, and Cdk4 and can stabilize cyclin D–Cdk4 complexes (Marriott & Semmes, 2005). Further reports reveal that Tax expression activates transcription of Cdk2 and Cdk4, and represses transcription of Cdk inhibitors p18INK4c and p19INK4d (Suzuki *et al.*, 1999; Kehn *et al.*, 2004). Through the binding of Cdks Tax can inactivate the retinoblastoma protein (pRB) (Neuveut *et al.*, 1998). The phosphorylation and/or degradation of pRB release the E2F1 transcription factor; this release of E2F1 can accelerate the cell cycle and promote premature exit from G1 into S phase.

The p53 tumor suppressor proteins monitor for DNA damage prior to the cell entering the DNA synthesis S phase. Activation of p53 delays the cell cycle progression between G1 and S (the G1/S checkpoint) and allows time for DNA repair. Impaired p53 function creates an accumulation of damaged DNA; and this finding has been invoked as a significant contributor to the genesis of human cancers. Although mutation of the p53 tumor suppressor gene is found in only 30% of ATLs, actual p53 function has been proposed to be inactivated by the viral Tax protein. Tax inactivation of p53 has been correlated with signaling through NF-κB (Pise-Masison *et al.*, 2000a,b) or through CREB/CBP (Ariumi *et al.*, 2000) or through additional yet characterized means (Miyazato *et al.*, 2005).

2.5. Tax and Mitosis

ATL cells have multi-lobulated nuclei and are called "flower cells." These cells are aneuploid with numerical chromosomal abnormalities. How the virus causes aneuploidy is not fully understood. There are, however, some suggested mechanisms. Of note, cultured human cells that express Tax are frequently multi-nucleated (Majone *et al.*, 1993; Jin *et al.*, 1998), suggesting that Tax perturbs mitosis and disturbs euploidy.

One way that Tax affects aneuploidy is through a disturbance of centrosome numbers. Centrosomes serve as the microtubule-organizing centers (MTOC) that form the bipolar mitotic spindle poles, which anchor the apparatus for the correct segregation of replicated chromosomes in mitosis. Prior to mitosis, centrosome duplicates precisely once during the S phase, concurrent with DNA replication. Cells with supernumerary (>2) centrosomes may form tri- or multi-polar spindle poles that result in improper chromosome segregation and aneuploidy. Ching and his colleagues (Ching *et al.*, 2006) and Peloponese and his colleagues (Peloponese *et al.*, 2005) showed that Tax can disturb centrosome numbers through two different mechanisms (Fig. 2). First, Tax creates centrosome over-duplication by targeting a cellular coiled-coil protein Tax1BP2, which normally blocks centriole replication. Second, Tax binds Ran-binding protein-1 (RANBP1), which is located at spindle poles and causes centrosome fragmentation in the M phase (Peloponese Jr *et al.*, 2005). These

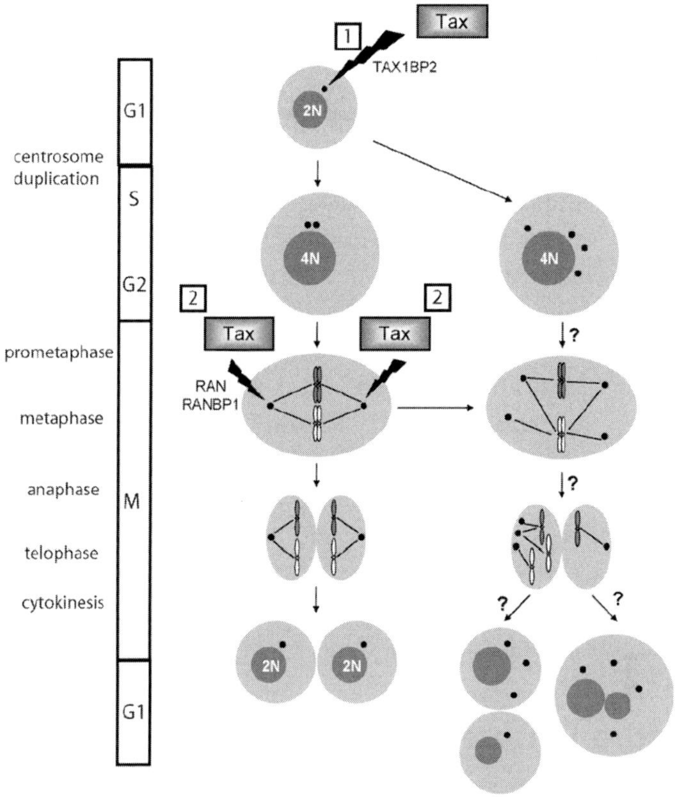

Fig. 2. Possible pathways to the induction of supernumerary centrosomes by Tax. Tax may disturb centrosome maturation by interacting with TAX1BP2 which is associated with centrosome duplication in G1/S phase or by binding RAN and RANBP1, two factors that are required for microtubule nucleation and spindle formation in mitosis.

mechanisms help to explain the long-standing observations of aneuploidy and frequent presentations of multipolar spindles in ATL cells (Kamihira *et al.*, 1994).

Aneuploid cells should normally be arrested by the spindle assembly checkpoint (SAC). The SAC guards against chromosome mis-segregation in mitosis. In cells with perturbed SAC, aberrant mitoses progress unchecked through the cell cycle to produce progenies with aneuploid genomes (Chi & Jeang, 2007). For HTLV-1, Jin and his colleagues first reported that Mad1, a component of the SAC, is targeted by Tax.

Through direct protein–protein binding, Tax is thought to abrogate the SAC checkpoint function of Mad1 in M phase. Recently, additional evidence has emerged that the mitotic pathology inflicted by Tax may also be associated with unscheduled and premature activation of the anaphase promoting complex/cyclosome (APC/C), an E3-ubiquitin ligase in SAC regulation that is required for the onset of anaphase and the exit of mitosis. The expression of APC/C substrate, securin/Pds1p (precocious dissociation of sister chromatids), was found to be significantly reduced in Tax-expressing HeLa, MT4, and *Saccharomyces cerevisiae* cells. Through direct interaction with APC/C–Cdc20 and Cdc27–APC3 complexes, Tax is thought to promote premature activation of APC/C and exit mitosis ahead of schedule (Liu *et al.*, 2005). However, other findings suggest that the APC/C may not be prematurely activated by Tax (Sheleg *et al.*, 2007). The role of APC/C in HTLV-1 transformation requires further experimental clarification.

3. Future Perspectives

It has been three decades since the discovery of HTLV-1 as the causal agent for ATL (Takatsuki, 2005; Gallo, 2005; Yoshida, 2005). Despite the enormous progress that has been made in understanding the mechanisms for cellular transformation, prognosis for ATL patients and even those treated intensively with chemotherapy, remains poor. Currently, the mean survival time of aggressive ATL after diagnosis is less than one year, with chemotherapy improving life span marginally (Yamada *et al.*, 2001). The main obstacles to a successful outcome include: (1) resistance of ATL cells to anticancer drugs and (2) immunodeficiency in ATL patients with its complication in opportunistic infections. To date, it is unclear how one could make advances in ATL therapy; however, what seems helpful is to have a better understanding of how ATL cells are transformed and what the necessary cellular changes that guide the survival and proliferation of these leukemic cells. In these respects, the continued molecular investigations of the biology of HTLV-1 infections have made great strides over the past 30 years such research promises to uncover additional important discoveries in the coming years.

Acknowledgment

Research in KT Jeang's laboratory is supported by intramural funds from NIAID, NIH.

References

Ariumi Y, Kaida A, Lin JY, Hirota M, Masui O, Yamaoka S, Taya Y, Shimotohno K (2000) HTLV-1 tax oncoprotein represses the p53-mediated trans-activation function through coactivator CBP sequestration. *Oncogene* **19**: 1491–1499.

Asquith B, Mosley AJ, Heaps A, Tanaka Y, Taylor GP, McLean AR, Bangham CR (2005) Quantification of the virus-host interaction in human T lymphotropic virus I infection. *Retrovirology* **2**: 75.

Ballard DW, Bohnlein E, Lowenthal JW, Wano Y, Franza BR, Greene WC (1988) HTLV-I tax induces cellular proteins that activate the kappa B element in the IL-2 receptor alpha gene. *Science* **241**: 1652–1655.

Beimling P, Moelling K (1992) Direct interaction of CREB protein with 21 bp Tax-response elements of HTLV-ILTR. *Oncogene* **7**: 257–262.

Charames GS, Bapat B (2003) Genomic instability and cancer. *Curr Mol Med* **3**: 589–596.

Chi YH, Jeang KT (2007) Aneuploidy and cancer. *J Cell Biochem* **102**: 531–538.

Ching YP, Chan SF, Jeang KT, Jin DY (2006) The retroviral oncoprotein Tax targets the coiled-coil centrosomal protein TAX1BP2 to induce centrosome overduplication. *Nat Cell Biol* **8**: 717–724.

Datta SR, Brunet A, Greenberg ME (1999) Cellular survival: a play in three Akts. *Genes Dev* **13**: 2905–2927.

Ding W, Albrecht B, Luo R, Zhang W, Stanley JR, Newbound GC, Lairmore MD (2001) Endoplasmic reticulum and cis-Golgi localization of human T-lymphotropic virus type 1 p12(I): association with calreticulin and calnexin. *J Virol* **75**: 7672–7682.

Gallo RC (2005) The discovery of the first human retrovirus: HTLV-1 and HTLV-2. *Retrovirology* **2**: 17.

Grossman WJ, Kimata JT, Wong FH, Zutter M, Ley TJ, Ratner L (1995) Development of leukemia in mice transgenic for the tax gene of human T-cell leukemia virus type I. *Proc Natl Acad Sci USA* **92**: 1057–1061.

Hasegawa H, Sawa H, Lewis MJ, Orba Y, Sheehy N, Yamamoto Y, Ichinohe T, Tsunetsugu-Yokota Y, Katano H, Takahashi H, Matsuda J, Sata T, Kurata T, Nagashima K, Hall WW (2006) Thymus-derived leukemia-lymphoma in mice transgenic for the Tax gene of human T-lymphotropic virus type I. *Nat Med* **12**: 466–472.

Horie R (2007) NF-kappaB in pathogenesis and treatment of adult T-cell leukemia/lymphoma. *Int Rev Immunol* **26**: 269–281.

Jeang KT, Widen SG, Semmes OJ, Wilson SH (1990) HTLV-I trans-activator protein, tax, is a trans-repressor of the human beta-polymerase gene. *Science* **247**: 1082–1084.

Jiang H, Lu H, Schiltz RL, Pise-Masison CA, Ogryzko VV, Nakatani Y, Brady JN (1999) PCAF interacts with tax and stimulates tax transactivation in a histone acetyltransferase-independent manner. *Mol Cell Biol* **19**: 8136–8145.

Jin DY, Spencer F, Jeang KT (1998) Human T-cell leukemia virus type 1 oncoprotein Tax targets the human mitotic checkpoint protein MAD1. *Cell* **93**: 81–91.

Jost PJ, Ruland J (2007) Aberrant NF-kappaB signaling in lymphoma: mechanisms, consequences, and therapeutic implications. *Blood* **109**: 2700–2707.

Kamihira S, Atogami S, Sohda H, Momita S, Toryia K, Ikeda S, Yamada Y, Tomonaga M (1994) DNA aneuploidy of adult T-cell leukemia cells. *Leuk Res* **18**: 79–84.

Kehn K, Deng L, de la FC, Strouss K, Wu K, Maddukuri A, Baylor S, Rufner R, Pumfery A, Bottazzi ME, Kashanchi F (2004) The role of cyclin D2 and p21/waf1 in human T-cell leukemia virus type 1 infected cells. *Retrovirology* **1**: 6.

Lemasson I, Lewis MR, Polakowski N, Hivin P, Cavanagh MH, Thebault S, Barbeau B, Nyborg JK, Mesnard JM (2007) Human T-cell leukemia virus type 1 (HTLV-1) bZIP protein interacts with the cellular transcription factor CREB to inhibit HTLV-1 transcription. *J Virol* **81**: 1543–1553.

Lemoine FJ, Kao SY, Marriott SJ (2000) Suppression of DNA repair by HTLV type 1 Tax correlates with Tax trans-activation of proliferating cell nuclear antigen gene expression. *AIDS Res Hum Retroviruses* **16**: 1623–1627.

Liu B, Hong S, Tang Z, Yu H, Giam CZ (2005) HTLV-I Tax directly binds the Cdc20-associated anaphase-promoting complex and activates it ahead of schedule. *Proc Natl Acad Sci USA* **102**: 63–68.

Liu Y, Wang Y, Yamakuchi M, Masuda S, Tokioka T, Yamaoka S, Maruyama I, Kitajima I (2001) Phosphoinositide-3 kinase-PKB/Akt pathway activation is involved in fibroblast Rat-1 transformation by human T-cell leukemia virus type I tax. *Oncogene* **20**: 2514–2526.

Majone F, Semmes OJ, Jeang KT (1993) Induction of micronuclei by HTLV-I Tax: a cellular assay for function. *Virology* **193**: 456–459.

Manel N, Battini JL, Taylor N, Sitbon M (2005) HTLV-1 tropism and envelope receptor. *Oncogene* **24**: 6016–6025.

Marriott SJ, Semmes OJ (2005) Impact of HTLV-I Tax on cell cycle progression and the cellular DNA damage repair response. *Oncogene* **24**: 5986–5995.

Miyazato A, Sheleg S, Iha H, Li Y, Jeang KT (2005) Evidence for NF-kappaB- and CBP-independent repression of p53's transcriptional activity by human T-cell leukemia virus type 1 Tax in mouse embryo and primary human fibroblasts. *J Virol* **79**: 9346–9350.

Moldovan GL, Pfander B, Jentsch S (2007) PCNA, the maestro of the replication fork. *Cell* **129**: 665–679.

Neuveut C, Low KG, Maldarelli F, Schmitt I, Majone F, Grassmann R, Jeang KT (1998) Human T-cell leukemia virus type 1 Tax and cell cycle progression: role of cyclin D-cdk and p110Rb. *Mol Cell Biol* **18**(6): 3620–3632.

Nicot C, Dundr M, Johnson JM, Fullen JR, Alonzo N, Fukumoto R, Princler GL, Derse D, Misteli T, Franchini G (2004) HTLV-1-encoded p30II is a post-transcriptional negative regulator of viral replication. *Nat Med* **10**: 197–201.

Nicot C, Harrod RL, Ciminale V, Franchini G (2005) Human T-cell leukemia/lymphoma virus type 1 nonstructural genes and their functions. *Oncogene* **24**: 6026–6034.

Ohsugi T, Kumasaka T, Okada S, Urano T (2007) The Tax protein of HTLV-1 promotes oncogenesis in not only immature T cells but also mature T cells. *Nat Med* **13**: 527–528.

Peloponese Jr, JM, Haller K, Miyazato A, Jeang KT (2005) Abnormal centrosome amplification in cells through the targeting of Ran-binding protein-1 by the human T-cell leukemia virus type-1 Tax oncoprotein. *Proc Natl Acad Sci USA* **102**: 18974–18979.

Peloponese Jr JM, Jeang KT (2006) Role for Akt/protein kinase B and activator protein-1 in cellular proliferation induced by the human T-cell leukemia virus type 1 tax oncoprotein. *J Biol Chem* **281**: 8927–8938.

Pise-Masison CA, Mahieux R, Jiang H, Ashcroft M, Radonovich M, Duvall J, Guillerm C, Brady JN (2000a) Inactivation of p53 by human T-cell lymphotropic virus type 1 Tax requires activation of the NF-kappaB pathway and is dependent on p53 phosphorylation. *Mol Cell Biol* **20**: 3377–3386.

Pise-Masison CA, Mahieux R, Radonovich M, Jiang H, Duvall J, Guillerm C, Brady JN (2000b) Insights into the molecular mechanism of p53 inhibition by HTLV type 1 Tax. *AIDS Res Hum Retroviruses* **16**: 1669–1675.

Proietti FA, Carneiro-Proietti AB, Catalan-Soares BC, Murphy EL (2005) Global epidemiology of HTLV-I infection and associated diseases. *Oncogene* **24**: 6058–6068.

Ruben S, Poteat H, Tan TH, Kawakami K, Roeder R, Haseltine W, Rosen CA (1988) Cellular transcription factors and regulation of IL-2 receptor gene expression by HTLV-I tax gene product. *Science* **241**: 89–92.

Santiago F, Clark E, Chong S, Molina C, Mozafari F, Mahieux R, Fujii M, Azimi N, Kashanchi F (1999) Transcriptional up-regulation of the cyclin D2 gene and acquisition of new cyclin-dependent kinase partners in human T-cell leukemia virus type 1-infected cells. *J Virol* **73**: 9917–9927.

Satou Y, Yasunaga J, Yoshida M, Matsuoka M (2006) HTLV-I basic leucine zipper factor gene mRNA supports proliferation of adult T-cell leukemia cells. *Proc Natl Acad Sci USA* **103**: 720–725.

Sheleg SV, Peloponese JM, Chi YH, Li Y, Eckhaus M, Jeang KT (2007) Evidence for cooperative transforming activity of the human pituitary tumor transforming gene and human T-cell leukemia virus type 1 Tax. *J Virol* **81**: 7894–7901.

Sun SC, Yamaoka S (2005) Activation of NF-kappaB by HTLV-I and implications for cell transformation. *Oncogene* **24**: 5952–5964.

Suzuki T, Narita T, Uchida-Toita M, Yoshida M (1999) Down-regulation of the INK4 family of cyclin-dependent kinase inhibitors by tax protein of HTLV-1 through two distinct mechanisms. *Virology* **259**: 384–391.

Takatsuki K (2005) Discovery of adult T-cell leukemia. *Retrovirology* **2**: 16.

Taniguchi Y, Nosaka K, Yasunaga J, Maeda M, Mueller N, Okayama A, Matsuoka M (2005) Silencing of human T-cell leukemia virus type I gene transcription by epigenetic mechanisms. *Retrovirology* **2**: 64.

Verdonck K, Gonzalez E, Van DS, Vandamme AM, Vanham G, Gotuzzo E (2007) Human T-lymphotropic virus 1: recent knowledge about an ancient infection. *Lancet Infect Dis* **7**: 266–281.

Yamada Y, Tomonaga M, Fukuda H, Hanada S, Utsunomiya A, Tara M, Sano M, Ikeda S, Takatsuki K, Kozuru M, Araki K, Kawano F, Niimi M, Tobinai K, Hotta T, Shimoyama M (2001) A new G-CSF-supported combination chemotherapy, LSG15, for adult T-cell leukaemia-lymphoma: Japan Clinical Oncology Group Study 9303. *Br J Haematol* **113**: 375–382.

Yin MJ, Paulssen EJ, Seeler JS, Gaynor RB (1995) Protein domains involved in both *in vivo* and *in vitro* interactions between human T-cell leukemia virus type I tax and CREB. *J Virol* **69**: 3420–3432.

Yoshida M (2005) Discovery of HTLV-1, the first human retrovirus, its unique regulatory mechanisms, and insights into pathogenesis. *Oncogene* **24**: 5931–5937.

Index